American Medical Association
Physicians dedicated to the health of America

cpt® changes

An Insider's View

2003

AMA press

Michael Beebe, Director, CPT Editorial and Information Services
Catherine Duffy, Director, CPT Education and Information Services
Desiree Evans, Project Coordinator
Rejina Glenn, Project Coordinator
DeHandro Hayden, Coding Consultant
Elizabeth Lumakovska, Coding Consultant
Marie Mindeman, Director, CPT Editorial Research and Development
Karen O'Hara, Senior Coding Consultant
Mary O'Heron, Senior Coding Consultant
Dan Reyes, Director, CPT Product Development
Desiree Rozell, Senior Coding Consultant
Lianne Stancik, Coding Consultant
Ron Friedmann, Coding Associate
Ada Walker, Coding Associate
Joan Zacharias, Coding Consultant

CPT® 2003 Changes: An Insider's View

Copyright © 2002 American Medical Association
Printed in the United States of America. All rights reserved.

http://www.ama-assn.org

No part of this publication may be reproduced, stored in a retrieval system, transmitted in any form, or by any means, electronic, mechanical, photocopying, recording, or otherwise, without prior written permission of the publisher.

CPT is a registered trademark of the American Medical Association.

For information regarding the reprinting or licensing of CPT® 2003 Changes: An Insider's View, please contact:

CPT Intellectual Property Services
American Medical Association
515 N. State St.
Chicago, IL 60610
312 464-5022

This book is intended for information purposes only. It is not intended to constitute legal advice. If legal advice is desired or needed, a licensed attorney should be consulted.

ISBN: 1-57947-313-X
AC25:02-P-004:11/02

Additional copies of this book (Product Number OP512903) may be ordered by calling: 800 621-8335.

Table of Contents

Foreword vii

Acknowledgments viii

Using This Book ix
    The Symbols ix
    The Rationale ix
    Reading the Clinical Examples ix
    The Tabular Review of the Changes x
    CPT Book Text/Guidelines x
    Modifier '-63' x

Evaluation and Management 1
    Pediatric Critical Care Patient Transport 3
    Critical Care Services 5
    Neonatal and Pediatric Critical Care Services 6
    Intensive (Non-Critical) Low Birth Weight Services 12
    Prolonged Services 16

Anesthesia 17
    Neck 19
    Intrathoracic 20
    Spine and Spinal Cord 23
    Lower Abdomen 24
    Perineum 27
    Knee and Popliteal Area 28
    Lower Leg (Below Knee, Includes Ankle and Foot) 28
    Shoulder and Axilla 29
    Upper Arm and Elbow 29
    Forearm, Wrist, and Hand 29
    Obstetric 31
    Other Procedures 40

Surgery **45**

    General 47

    Integumentary System 47

    Musculoskeletal System 54

    Respiratory System 68

    Cardiovascular System 69

    Hemic and Lymphatic Systems 100

    Mediastinum and Diaphragm 107

    Digestive System 108

    Urinary System 128

    Male Genital System 136

    Female Genital System 138

    Nervous System 152

    Eye and Ocular Adnexa 177

    Auditory System 179

Radiology **181**

    Radiology Guidelines (Including Nuclear Medicine and Diagnostic Ultrasound) 183

    Administration of Contrast Materials 183

    Diagnostic Radiology (Diagnostic Imaging) 183

    Diagnostic Ultrasound 190

    Radiation Oncology 194

Pathology and Laboratory **195**

    Organ or Disease Oriented Panels 197

        Urinalysis 197

        Chemistry 197

        Hematology and Coagulation 199

    Immunology 202

    Transfusion Medicine 203

        Microbiology 203

        Cytopathology 205

Cytogenetic Studies 206

Other Procedures 206

Medicine 207

Vaccines, Toxoids 209

Therapeutic, Prophylactic or Diagnostic Injections 209

Biofeedback 209

    Special Otorhinolaryngologic Services 210

    Evaluative and Therapeutic Services 210

    Cardiovascular 217

    Non-Invasive Vascular Diagnostic Studies 222

    Pulmonary 223

    Allergy and Clinical Immunology Allergy Testing 223

    Neurology and Neuromuscular Procedures 224

Health and Behavior Assessment/Intervention 227

Chemotherapy Administration 228

Special Dermatological Procedures 229

Special Services, Procedures and Reports 232

Qualifying Circumstances for Anesthesia 232

Home Health Procedures/Services 232

Home Infusion Procedures/Services 234

Appendix —Modifiers 237

    Modifiers Approved for Ambulatory Surgery Center (ASC) Hospital Outpatient Use 242

Category III Codes 245

Tabular Review of the Changes 259

CPT 2003 Errata 291

Foreword

The American Medical Association is pleased to offer *CPT Changes 2003: An Insider's View*. Since this publication first came out in 2000 it has served as the definitive text on additions, revisions, and deletions to the CPT code set. In developing this book it was our intention to provide CPT users with a glimpse of the logic, rationale and proposed function of CPT changes that resulted from the decisions of the CPT Editorial Panel and the yearly update process. AMA staff members have the unique perspective of being both participants in the CPT editorial process, and users of the CPT code set. *CPT Changes* is intended to bridge understanding between clinical decisions made at the CPT Editorial Panel regarding appropriate service/procedure descriptions, with functional interpretations of coding guidelines and code combinations necessary for users of the CPT code set. A new edition of the book is published every year.

To assist CPT users in applying new and revised CPT codes, this book uses clinical examples that describe the typical patient who might receive the procedure and detailed descriptions of the procedure. Both of these are required as part of the CPT code change proposal process and are used by the CPT Editorial Panel in crafting language, guidelines, and parenthetical notes associated with the new or revised codes. In addition, the clinical examples and descriptions of the procedures are used in the AMA/Specialty Society RVS Update process for conducting surveys on physician work and in developing work relative value recommendations to the Centers for Medicare and Medicaid Services as part of the Medicare Physician Fee Schedule.

We are confident that the information contained in *CPT Changes* each year will prove to be a valuable resource to CPT users not only as they apply changes for any given year, but also as they continue their education in CPT coding during the course of several years. The American Medical Association makes every effort to be a voice of clarity and consistency in an otherwise confusing system of health care claims and payment and *CPT Changes 2003: An Insider's View* demonstrates our continued commitment to assist users of the CPT code set.

Acknowledgments

Thank you to these members of the AMA Press:

Anthony J. Frankos, Vice President, Business Products

Mary Lou White, Executive Director, Editorial

Jean Roberts, Director, Production and Manufacturing

Elise Schumacher, Senior Acquisitions Editor

Erin Kalitowski, Marketing Manager

Pat Lee, Technical Developmental Editor

Rosalyn Carlton, Senior Production Coordinator

Ronnie Summers, Senior Print Coordinator

Boon Ai Tan, Senior Production Coordinator

Using This Book

This book is designed to serve as a reference guide to understanding the changes contained in *Current Procedural Terminology (CPT®) 2003* and is not intended to replace the CPT book. We make every effort to ensure accuracy; however, if differences exist, you should always defer to the information contained in *CPT 2003*.

The Symbols

This book uses the same coding conventions that appear in the CPT nomenclature.

- ● Indicates that new procedure numbers were added to the CPT nomenclature
- ▲ Indicates that a code revision has resulted in a substantially altered procedure descriptor
- + Indicates CPT add-on codes
- ⊘ Indicates codes that are exempt from the use of modifier '-51,' but are not designated as CPT add-on procedures/services
- ►◄ Indicate revised guidelines, cross-references, and/or explanatory text

Whenever possible, we tried to include complete segments of text from the CPT book; however, in some cases, the text has been abbreviated.

The Rationale

After each change or series of changes is a rationale. The rationale is intended to provide a brief explanation as to why the change(s) occurred, but may not answer every question that may arise as a result of the change(s).

Reading the Clinical Examples

The clinical examples/procedural descriptions included in this text are presented to give practical situations for which the new and/or revised codes in *CPT 2003* would be appropriately reported. It is important to note that these examples do not suggest limiting the use of a code, but only represent the typical patient and service/procedure. They do not describe the universe of patients for whom the service/procedure would be appropriate. In addition, third-party payer reporting practices may differ.

The Tabular Review of the Changes

The table beginning on page 261 allows you to see all of the code changes at a glance. By reviewing the table you can easily determine the level to which your particular field of interest has been affected by the changes in *CPT 2003*.

CPT Book Text/Guidelines

Guideline and revised CPT book text appears indented. Any revised text, guidelines, and/or headings are indicated with the ►◄ symbols.

Modifier '–63'

Rationales have not been placed for any issues related to modifier '-63.'

Please refer to p. 244 for more information.

Evaluation and Management

The revisions to the Evaluation and Management Services section reflect the extensive revisions to the Neonatal Intensive Care section of the CPT code set, with the addition of a new subsection and new codes to report the critical care of children 24 months of age or less. To correlate, the Critical Care guidelines have been revised to instruct the appropriate reporting for these services. The neonatal intensive subsequent care codes have also been revised to more accurately describe the care of the post-neonatal care low birth weight infant. In addition, the Patient Transport services codes have been revised to indicate that these codes are appropriately reported only for physician services for those patients 24 months of age or less.

Evaluation and Management

▶Pediatric Critical Care◀ Patient Transport

The following codes 99289 and 99290 are used to report the physical attendance and direct face-to-face care by a physician during the interfacility transport of a critically ill or ▶critically◀ injured ▶pediatric◀ patient. For the purpose of reporting codes 99289 and 99290, face-to-face care begins when the physician assumes primary responsibility of the ▶pediatric◀ patient at the referring hospital/facility, and ends when the receiving hospital/facility accepts responsibility for the ▶pediatric◀ patient's care. Only the time the physician spends in direct face-to-face contact with the patient during the transport should be reported. ▶Pediatric◀ patient transport services involving less than 30 minutes of face-to-face physician care should not be reported using codes 99289, 99290. Procedure(s) or service(s) performed by other members of the transporting team may not be reported by the supervising physician.

▶The following services are included when performed during the pediatric patient transport by the physician providing critical care and may not be reported separately: routine monitoring evaluations (eg, heart rate, respiratory rate, blood pressure, and pulse oximetry), the interpretation of cardiac output measurements (93561, 93562), chest x-rays (71010, 71015, 71020), pulse oximetry (94760, 94761, 94762), blood gases and information data stored in computers (eg, ECGs, blood pressures, hematologic data) (99090), gastric intubation (43752, 91105), temporary transcutaneous pacing (92953), ventilatory management (94656, 94660, 94662) and vascular access procedures (36000, 36400, 36405, 36406, 36410, 36415, 36540, 36600). Any services performed which are not listed above should be reported separately.

Critical care is the direct delivery by a physician(s) of medical care for a critically ill or critically injured patient. A critical illness or injury acutely impairs one or more vital organ systems such that there is a high probability of imminent or life threatening deterioration in the patient's condition. Critical care involves high complexity decision making to assess, manipulate, and support vital system function(s) to treat single or multiple vital organ system failure and/or to prevent further life-threatening deterioration of the patient's condition. Examples of vital organ system failure include, but are not limited to: central nervous system failure; circulatory failure; shock; renal, hepatic, metabolic, and/or respiratory failure.

Providing medical care to a critically ill, injured, or post-operative patient qualifies as a critical care service only if both the illness or injury and the treatment being provided meet the above requirements.◀

The direction of emergency care to transporting staff ...

The emergency department services codes (99281-99285), initial hospital care codes (99221-99223), hourly critical care codes (99291, 99292), ...

Code 99289 is used to report the first 30-74 minutes of direct face-to-face time with the transport ▶pediatric◀ patient and should be reported only once on a given date. Code 99290 is used to report each additional 30 minutes provided on a given date. Face-to-face services less than 30 minutes should not be reported with these codes.

▲**99289** Critical care services delivered by a physician, face-to-face, during an interfacility transport of critically ill or critically injured pediatric patient, 24 months of age or less; first 30-74 minutes of hands on care during transport

+**99290** each additional 30 minutes (List separately in addition to code for primary service)

(Use 99290 in conjunction with 99289)

▶(Critical care of less than 30 minutes total duration should be reported with the appropriate E/M code)◀

Rationale

To avoid redundancy with CMS-established "G" codes for adult transport services for critically ill or critically injured patients, and to comply with reporting mechanisms, the patient transport codes 99289 and 99290 were revised to 1) limit application to pediatric patients; 2) meet the requirements of critical care; 3) provide clear beginning and ending times for the face-to-face service; and 4) bundle the same services in the codes that are bundled into the critical care codes (99291-99292).

The revised codes have the same services bundled into them as do the hourly critical care codes, including: interpretation of cardiac output measurements (93561, 93562); chest x-rays (71010, 71015, 71020); pulse oximetry (94760, 94761, 94762); blood gases and information data stored in computers (99090); gastric intubation (43752, 91105); temporary transcutaneous pacing (92953); ventilatory management (94656, 94660, 94662); and vascular access procedures (36000, 36400, 36405, 36406, 36410, 36415, 36540, 36600).

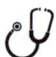
Clinical Example (99289)

A previously healthy patient is struck by a vehicle while crossing a busy street. The patient is not run over, but is thrown and impacts the road 15 feet from the point of the accident. The patient is taken by EMS to the nearest hospital, a non-trauma facility. During initial stabilization, the ED physician finds significant injuries to the head, chest, and abdomen requiring trauma specialty care that is unavailable at the facility. After consultation with the receiving trauma center, a specialized transport team consisting of a physician, nurse, respiratory therapist, and paramedic is dispatched to the local hospital.

At the local hospital, with the ED physician, the transport physician reviews the patient's history, clinical progress, lab tests, and radiographs, and assists in further stabilization of the patient, including endotracheal intubation (following rapid sequence induction), and the placement of central lines and a chest tube. The patient has unstable vital signs, but requires the trauma center's services. The patient is moved to the transport unit where he is placed on continuous heart, respiratory, blood pressure, pulse oximetry, and end-tidal CO_2 monitors. All IVs and medications are on electronic monitoring pumps. The patient is placed on a transport ventilator. The physician remains at the patient's side in continuous attendance providing direct care and directing the activities of the team. The transport unit has limited space and resources. Bedside blood tests are used to adjust respiratory and medical treatment. The vehicle is in constant motion and patient observation and intervention are challenging.

Upon arrival at the trauma center, there has been no further deterioration in the patient's condition. Care is transferred to the trauma service after review of the patient's records from the transferring facility and events that occurred and care that was provided during the transport.

Critical Care Services

Critical care is the direct delivery …

Providing medical care to a critically ill …

Critical care services provided to infants ►31 days up through 24 months of age◄ are reported with ►pediatric critical care codes 99293 and 99294. The pediatric critical care codes are reported as long as the infant/young child qualifies for critical care services during the hospital stay.◄ Critical care services provided to neonates (30 days of age or less) are reported with the neonatal critical care codes 99295 ►and◄ 99296. The neonatal critical care codes are reported as long as the neonate qualifies for critical care services ►through the 30th postnatal day◄. The reporting of ►the pediatric and◄ neonatal critical care services is not based on time ►or◄ the type of unit (eg, pediatric or neonatal critical care unit) ►and it is not dependent upon◄ the type of provider delivering the care. For additional instructions on reporting these services, see the Neonatal ►and Pediatric Critical Care◄ section and codes ►99293-99296.◄

Services for a patient …

Critical care and other E/M services …

The following services are included …

Codes 99291-99292 should be reported for the physician's attendance during the transport of critically ill or ►critically◄ injured patients ►over 24 months of age◄ to or from a facility or hospital. ►For◄ physician transport services of critically ill or ►critically◄ injured ►pediatric◄ patients ►24 months of age or less◄ see 99289, 99290.

The critical care codes 99291 and 99292 are used to report …

Time spent with the individual patient should be …

Time spent in activities that occur …

Code 99291 is used to report the first …

Code 99292 is used to report each ...

The following examples illustrate ...

 Rationale

The Critical Care notes were editorially revised to clarify an inconsistency in the language, in which the term "critically" was inadvertently omitted from the guidelines. The addition of this term indicates the appropriate reporting for both critically ill and critically injured patients.

Further revisions to the Critical Care Services subsection reflect the changes to the NICU-PICU code series. This includes the expansion of the Critical Care services subsection with the addition of two new codes 99293 and 99294 to report Pediatric Critical Care Services. These revisions also reflect clarification of the terminology related to the age of the non-pediatric patient, the deletion of code 99297, and the addition of the Low Birth Weight Services subsection, in which code 99298 was incorporated into this series of codes and separated out from the Neonatal Intensive Care codes.

Neonatal ▶and Pediatric Critical Care Services◀

The following codes ▶(99293-99296)◀ are used to report services provided by a physician directing the care of a critically ill ▶neonate/infant. The same definitions for critical care services apply for the adult, child, and neonate.◀

The ▶initial day◀ neonatal critical care code ▶(99295) can◀ be used in addition to codes 99360, 99436, or 99440 as appropriate, when the physician is present for the delivery and newborn resuscitation is required. ▶Other procedures performed as a necessary part of the resuscitation (eg, endotracheal intubation) are also reported separately.◀

▶Codes 99295, 99296 are used to report services provided by a physician directing the care of a critically ill neonate through the first 30 days of life. They represent care starting with the date of admission (99295) and subsequent day(s) (99296) and may be reported only once per day, per patient. Once the neonate is no longer considered to be critically ill, the Intensive Low Birth Weight Services codes for those with present body weight of less than 2500 grams (99298, 99299) or the codes for Subsequent Hospital Care (99231-99233) for those with present body weight over 2500 grams should be utilized.◀

▶Codes 99293-99294 are used to report services provided by a physician directing the care of a critically ill infant or young child from 31 days of postnatal age up through 24 months of age. They represent care starting with the date of admission (99293) and subsequent day(s) (99294) and may be reported by a single physician only once per day, per patient in a given setting. The critically ill or critically injured child older than two years when admitted to an intensive care unit would be reported with hourly critical care service codes (99291, 99292). Once an infant is no longer considered to be critically ill but continues to require intensive care, the Intensive Low Birth Weight Services codes (99298, 99299) should be used to report services for infants with present body weight of less than 2500 grams. When the present body weight of those infants exceeds 2500 grams, the Subsequent Hospital Care (99231-99233) codes should be utilized.◄

Care rendered ►under 99293-99296◄ includes management, monitoring and treatment of the patient including ►respiratory, pharmacologic control of the circulatory system,◄ enteral and parenteral nutrition, metabolic and hematologic maintenance, parent ►/family◄ counseling, case management services, and personal direct supervision of the health care team in the performance of cognitive and procedural activities.

►The pediatric and neonatal critical care codes include those procedures◄ listed above for ►the◄ hourly ►critical care◄ codes ►(99291, 99292). In addition,◄ the following procedures are also included in the bundled (global) ►pediatric and◄ neonatal ►critical care service◄ codes ►(99293-99296):◄ umbilical venous (36510) and umbilical arterial ►(36660)◄ catheters, central (36488, 36490) or peripheral vessel catheterization (36000), other arterial catheters (36140, 36620), oral or nasogastric tube placement ►(43752)◄, endotracheal intubation (31500), lumbar puncture (62270), suprapubic bladder aspiration (51000), bladder catheterization (53670), initiation and management of mechanical ventilation (94656, 94657) or continuous positive airway pressure (CPAP) (94660), surfactant administration, intravascular fluid administration ►(90780, 90781)◄, transfusion of blood components (36430, 36440), vascular punctures (36420, 36600), invasive or non-invasive electronic monitoring of vital signs, bedside pulmonary function testing ►(94375)◄, and/or monitoring or interpretation of blood gases or oxygen saturation (94760-94762). Any services performed which are not listed above should be reported separately.

For additional instructions, see descriptions listed for 99293-►99296◄.

►Pediatric Critical Care◄

●99293 **Initial pediatric critical care,** 31 days up through 24 months of age, per day, for the evaluation and management of a critically ill infant or young child

●99294 **Subsequent pediatric critical care,** 31 days up through 24 months of age, per day, for the evaluation and management of a critically ill infant or young child

►Neonatal Critical Care◄

▲99295 **Initial neonatal critical care,** per day, for the evaluation and management of a critically ill neonate, 30 days of age or less

This code is reserved for the date of admission for neonates who are critically ill. Critically ill neonates require cardiac and/or respiratory support (including ventilator or nasal CPAP when indicated), continuous or frequent vital sign monitoring, laboratory and blood gas interpretations, follow-up physician re-evaluations, and constant observation by the health care team under direct physician supervision. Immediate preoperative evaluation and stabilization of neonates with life threatening surgical or cardiac conditions are included under this code. ▶Neonates with life threatening surgical or cardiac conditions are included under this code.◀

▶Care for neonates who require an intensive care setting but who are not critically ill is reported using the initial hospital care codes (99221-99223).◀

▲ 99296   **Subsequent neonatal critical care,** per day, for the evaluation and management of a critically ill neonate, 30 days of age or less

A critically ill neonate will require cardiac and/or respiratory support (including ventilator or nasal CPAP when indicated), continuous or frequent vital sign monitoring, laboratory and blood gas interpretations, follow-up physician re-evaluations throughout a 24-hour period, and constant observation by the health care team under direct physician supervision.

▶(99297 has been deleted. To report, use 99296)◀

 Rationale

The guidelines for the Critical Care Services and Neonatal Intensive Care subsections of the E/M section of the CPT code set were revised with added text to reflect the revisions to the NICU-PICU code series and the addition of Pediatric Intensive Care Service codes. Two new codes, 99293 and 99294, were established to report initial and subsequent pediatric intensive care for critically ill infants or young pediatric patients 31 days of postnatal age up through 24 months of age. Codes 99295 and 99296 were revised to clarify the description of initial and subsequent NICU care of the recovering, low birth weight infant and the critically ill neonate. Code 99297 was deleted to accommodate these revisions.

The establishment of codes 99293 and 99294 for pediatric critical care services created a new subsection for the Evaluation and Management-Critical Care Services section of the CPT code set, to define critical care services for the patient over 30 days of age through 24 months of age. The creation of these codes reflects the additional work related to the age of these young patients due to small size, previous therapy, and limited mechanisms of physiological compensation. In addition to the establishment of these codes, a new heading and introductory notes were added to define the Pediatric Intensive Care Services, with revision of the title of the subsection from "Neonatal Intensive Care" to "Neonatal and Pediatric Critical Care Services."

The Pediatric Critical Care Services codes are intended to report the work required in the care of pediatric patients 24 months of age or less. These patients typically suffer from a chronic (often genetic) condition or disease, or late pulmonary or neurologic sequelae of premature birth, requiring readmission to a critical care unit for a life-threatening illness. The most common physiologic abnormality in infants and children less than two years of age is primarily respiratory failure or respiratory distress with impending failure. However, many other critically ill pediatric patients such as post-operative, trauma, head injury, transplant, etc, will have the respiratory or cardiorespiratory system involved. Along with respiratory compromise or failure, these patients typically present with multi-organ system dysfunction or failure. This pediatric age group is physiologically different from adult patients covered under the Critical Care Services codes 99291-99292.

Code 99293 is intended to report the admission of the patient 24 months of age or less to an intensive care unit, usually a PICU. The initial care services include rapid assessment of the patient's condition; therapy initiation; evaluation of the patient's extent of the current illness; discussion of the current illness with the primary care physician and/or the specialist; family interview; review of old and new laboratory data and radiographs (chest x-rays, CT scans, etc); and decision concerning whether the patient's chronic condition will be compromised or will compromise further the new onset critical illness.

The patients described in the Pediatric Critical Care codes are infants beyond the neonatal period and up through 24 months of age who meet the accepted definition of critically ill or injured with single or multiple organ failure where the physician's presence is required frequently and intermittently over a 24-hour period. The services included in codes 99293 and 99294 include repetitive evaluation of the patient, therapy adjustment, and supervision of the health care team by the physician. Since these evaluations occur in both brief and long encounters throughout the day and cannot reasonably be "counted" or documented at each patient contact (often representing a dozen or more per day), the Pediatric Critical Care codes are reported only one time per day, as indicated in the code descriptor.

There are various treatments that are necessary to stabilize and prevent further decompensation of these multiply compromised children. These treatments are inherent in the Pediatric Critical Care codes and include endotracheal intubation to secure the airway, vascular access to provide vasoactive infusions, correction of acid-base balance, and provision of other medications. Also inherent in these procedures is the establishment of vascular access, including but not limited to, peripheral, arterial as well as central venous lines for these patients with chronic disease. These patients are typically infants who have previously spent several months in the Neonatal ICU. Venous access through the central circulation often requires placement of a femoral, internal jugular, or subclavian catheter. These sites pose additional risk to the patient and require additional skill and training on the part of the physician since umbilical vessels cannot be accessed beyond the immediate neonatal period.

Also inherent in the Pediatric Critical Care codes is the performance of some of the more repetitive procedures, often in series, including intubation, interpretation of blood gas results, family interviews, records review, communication with prior or primary care physicians, and review of initial laboratory data. Multi-system organ management requires frequent and multiple laboratory testing and evaluation during the initial hours following admission, with subsequent changes made in ventilator settings, IV fluid rates and composition, initiation and manipulation of vasoactive or inotropic drugs, antibiotics, and other therapeutic maneuvers. Optimal patient management will require frequent visits and ongoing supervision of the health care team by the physician in order to perform complex, integrated decision making and applications.

Codes 99295 and 99296 were revised and 99297 deleted to clarify the description of initial and subsequent NICU care of the critically ill neonate and to remove ambiguity from the interpretation of physician services. Prior to 2003, the definitions of the terms "stable" and "unstable" that distinguished these two codes were unclear. Therefore, code 99297 was deleted and 99296 revised to develop a single subsequent day NICU code for critically ill neonates to allow more accurate reporting for this service.

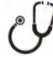

Clinical Example (99293)

A 6-month-old female, former 28-week gestational age premature infant, now with chronic lung disease (bronchopulmonary dysplasia) following her neonatal course is admitted to the PICU from home with respiratory distress and impending respiratory failure. She had been stable on a low flow of nasal oxygen until 2 days prior to admission when she developed a fever, cough, and increased oxygen requirement. She gradually developed tachypnea, wheezing, and retractions despite increased bronchodilator therapy at home (in addition to her daily diuretics, supplemental oxygen, and maintenance bronchodilator therapy for her CLD).

In the ER she was found to have an oxygen saturation of 83% on 1 L of nasal cannula O_2. An ABG revealed acute and chronic hypercarbia and hypoxia. A CXR revealed bilateral diffuse pneumonia, as well as hyperinflation. She was transferred to the PICU for evaluation and management by the pediatric intensivist. Despite aggressive therapy to treat her pulmonary disease, she progressed to respiratory failure requiring intubation and mechanical ventilation. Central venous and arterial access was obtained by the pediatric intensivist after numerous attempts at peripheral arterial and venous catheterization were unsuccessful due to scarring from line placement during her NICU stay. Arterial blood pressure and central venous pressure monitoring revealed hypotension and intravascular volume depletion. Blood, urine, and respiratory cultures were obtained and broad-spectrum antibiotic coverage was instituted for presumed sepsis. The patient's hypotension responded to treatment with fluid boluses and low doses of pressors. Her respiratory failure worsened and she developed acute respiratory distress syndrome (ARDS), circulatory failure, and fluid and electrolyte disturbances that required high frequency oscillatory ventilation and increased inotropic support for 7 days. She was eventually converted back to conventional ventilation and weaned to extubation. The pediatric intensivist spent many hours throughout the child's admission coordinating the activities of other subspecialists, nursing staff, respiratory therapists, nutritionists, and social workers, as well as providing daily communications to the family and the patient's primary care physician.

Description of Procedure (99293)

A complete examination of the head, eyes, nose, mouth, chest, lungs, heart, abdomen, genitals, rectum, joints, spine, extremities, and a neurologic appraisal of movement, reflexes, cranial nerves, and degree of arousal and activity are performed. All attached monitors and tubes are checked for secure placement and proper function.

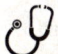
Clinical Example (99294)

A 1½-year-old male, who was in his usual state of health, now presented with acute respiratory distress to the emergency department. The patient's ongoing medications included home nebulized bronchodilator therapy and low dose steroids for significant reactive airway disease. After evaluation and failure to clear with bronchodilator therapy in the ED he was admitted to the Pediatric ICU with increasing respiratory distress and impending respiratory failure. Over the next few hours he demonstrated increasing oxygen requirements, tachypnea, cough, and a mild rash. He was placed on bronchodilator therapy; constant cardiopulmonary, blood pressure, and oxygen saturation monitoring; IV infusions; antibiotics; chest radiographs; blood gases; and intravenous steroids. He was placed on a 100% nonrebreather mask and multiple laboratory examinations for bacterial and viral studies were performed. His response to therapy was variable over the first 12 hours and he then gradually deteriorated.

The patient's deteriorating clinical state was discussed extensively with the family, including the need to intubate the patient for ventilatory support. He required endotracheal intubation and mechanical ventilation for respiratory failure. His chest x-ray at that time showed a diffuse, interstitial pattern consistent with progressive diffuse alveolar disease. The patient was placed on IV continuous sedation of fentanyl and midazolam to assist with ventilator/patient asynchrony. The patient's family and primary care physician were contacted daily for daily updates and therapeutic planning. The patient continued to show a deteriorating state of oxygenation and ventilation over the first 48 hours, and increasing lung congestion consistent with non-cardiogenic pulmonary edema. Initially this was treated with diuretic therapy and increasing the mechanical ventilatory support with positive expiratory pressure. The patient had associated glucose and electrolyte abnormalities, which were treated with additional diuretic therapy and changes in intravenous solutions. Nutritional support was provided in the form of hyperalimentation.

Over the next 72 hours he continued to require increased FIO_2 to 80% and increasing ventilatory support resulting in high airway pressures, necessitating placement on high frequency oscillatory ventilation. Due to the child's unstable condition he required 1:1 nursing care. An arterial line and central venous pressure monitoring line were placed to closely monitor the patient's hemodynamics and his intravascular fluid status. During the course of high frequency oscillation, progressive anemia from blood obtained for laboratory tests and from hemodilution was treated with packed red blood cell transfusions. Over the course of the first week of high frequency oscillation, the patient developed improvement of his chest radiograph and a decrease in oxygen requirements to less than 50%. By the end of the second week his respiratory status had improved and he was transferred to conventional mechanical ventilation with moderate settings on pressure regulated volume control. The family was given daily updates and discussion about his progress. His primary physician received daily calls with clinical changes discussed. At this time the patient was weaned down to minimum ventilator and oxygen levels. By the end of the third week the patient had been successfully weaned down to CPAP and subsequently extubated to a nasal cannula. His clinical condition was no longer considered critical, but he continued to require close observation and evaluation.

Description of Procedure
A complete examination of the head, eyes, nose, mouth, chest, lungs, heart, abdomen, genitals, rectum, joints, spine, extremities, and a neurologic appraisal of movement, reflexes, cranial nerves, and degree of arousal and activity are performed. All attached monitors and tubes are checked for secure placement and proper function.

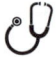

Clinical Example (99295)
Under the care of the attending physician, either personally or by direct supervision, a 28-week gestational 900-gram male infant is admitted. The infant is examined and determined to have respiratory distress syndrome. The infant is intubated and placed on a ventilator. Umbilical artery and vein catheters are placed. Blood culture is obtained and antibiotics started. The infant is placed on continuous cardiovascular, respiratory, and blood pressure monitoring. The mother's record is reviewed and she is interviewed for her history. A family history is obtained from the father. Arterial blood gases, x-ray, and laboratory results are reviewed. The surfactant is administered. The parents are counseled as to diagnosis and prognosis, and appropriate informed consent is obtained. Throughout the first 24 hours, the infant is examined repeatedly and arterial blood gases, x-rays, and laboratory values are evaluated repeatedly. The infant is given volume expansion and started on dopamine. An additional dose of surfactant is given. The medical records including history, physical assessment, plan orders, and progress notes are prepared. The parents are informed and counseled as to the infant's condition, progress, and prognosis.

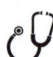

Clinical Example (99296)
This infant is now 3 days old and is under the care and direct supervision of the attending physician. The infant remains intubated and on intermittent mandatory ventilation. The infant has both umbilical artery and view catheters in place and is on continuous cardiac, respiratory, and blood pressure monitoring. Blood pressure is being supported with dopamine. Hyperalimentation has been started. After evaluation, indomethacin has been started for a patent ductus arteriosus. Evaluation for intraventricular hemorrhage with ultrasound has been completed. A packed red blood cell transfusion is given. The infant is examined repeatedly and laboratory, x-rays, and arterial blood gases are repeatedly evaluated. The parents are informed and counseled as to the infant's condition and prognosis. Medical records are maintained including orders and progress notes. Fluids and ventilator changes are made frequently as required.

▶Intensive (Non-Critical) Low Birth Weight Services◀

▶Codes 99298-99299 are used to report services subsequent to the day of admission provided by a physician directing the continuing intensive care of the low birth weight (LBW) or very low birth weight (VLBW) infant who no longer meets the definition of critically ill. They represent subsequent day(s) of care and may be reported only once per day, per patient. Low birth weight services are reported for those neonates less than 2500 grams who do not meet the definition of critical care but continue to require intensive observation and frequent services and interventions only available in an intensive care setting. The level and frequency of services required for the LBW and the VLBW infant exceed those available in less intensive hospital areas or medical floors. Codes 99298-99299 are global 24-hour codes with the same services bundled as outlined under codes 99293-99296.◄

►For additional instructions, see descriptions listed for 99298-99299.◄

▲99298 **Subsequent intensive care,** per day, for the evaluation and management of the recovering very low birth weight infant (present body weight less than 1500 grams)

►Infants with present body weight less than 1500 grams◄ who are no longer critically ill continue to require intensive cardiac and respiratory monitoring, continuous and/or frequent vital sign monitoring, heat maintenance, enteral and/or parenteral nutritional adjustments, laboratory and oxygen monitoring, and constant observation by the health care team under direct physician supervision.

●99299 **Subsequent intensive care,** per day, for the evaluation and management of the recovering low birth weight infant (present body weight of 1500-2500 grams)

Infants with present body weight of 1500-2500 grams who are no longer critically ill continue to require intensive cardiac and respiratory monitoring, continuous and/or frequent vital sign monitoring, heat maintenance, enteral and/or parenteral nutritional adjustments, laboratory and oxygen monitoring, and constant observation by the health care team under direct physician supervision.

Rationale

Code 99298 was revised, and code 99299 was established to define the provision of intensive care services related to the neonatal body weight of the infant. In support of this, a new heading and notes were added to define care for the low birth weight infant.

The revision of code 99298 and the creation of a new subsection are intended to support the definition of a new category of patients for neonates whose present body weight is less than 1500 grams and who still require intensive care. The revision is also intended to clarify the previous definition of this code for the provision of neonatal intensive care services encompassing medical, cardiac, and surgical conditions and diseases for neonates with a present body weight of less than 1500 grams. Prior to this, the language in the guidelines and descriptors for Neonatal Intensive Care prevented providers from using the code in appropriate cases, such as when a neonate's weight dropped to below 1500 grams, but still required intensive care. The terms "critically ill though stable" or "critically ill and unstable" rendered the previous codes 99296 and 99297 inadequate to report these services.

The services that are inherent in code 99298 include management, monitoring, and treatment of the patient including enteral and parenteral nutritional maintenance; metabolic and hematologic maintenance; pharmacologic control of the circulatory system; parent counseling; case management services; and personal direct supervision of the health care team in the performance of cognitive and procedural activities. Additionally, as described in the Pediatric and Neonatal Critical Care services codes, 99298 includes the following procedures: umbilical venous (36510) and umbilical arterial (36660) catheters, central (36488, 36490) or peripheral vessel catheterization (36000), other arterial catheters (36140, 36620), oral or nasogastric tube placement (43752), endotracheal intubation (31500), lumbar puncture (62270), suprapubic bladder aspiration (51000), bladder catheterization (53670), initiation and management of mechanical ventilation (94656, 94657) or continuous positive airway pressure (CPAP) (94660), surfactant administration, intravascular fluid administration (90780, 90781), transfusion of blood components (36430, 36440), vascular punctures (36420, 36600), invasive or non-invasive electronic monitoring of vital signs, bedside pulmonary function testing (94375), and/or monitoring or interpretation of blood gases or oxygen saturation (94760-94762).

Code 99299 was established to report services provided for infants previously classified into critical care or subsequent routine hospital care groupings. These low birth weight infants (1500-2500 grams) are recovering from the most critical phase of their illness and are still unstable and have increased mortality and morbidity. Though not meeting commonly held definitions of "critically ill," they are still not healthy "feeding and growing" infants. This code is intended to bridge the "critically ill" and subsequent hospital care coding gap in low birth weight infants (1500-2500 grams). Advances in technology, nutrition, and infectious disease therapy will require treatment of many of these infants between 1500 and 2500 grams in the neonatal intensive care unit, where they must continue to receive intensive care before transition to regular hospital care and finally to home. These patients will generally still require oxygen supplementation and/or administration of respiratory stimulant drugs to treat frequent and recurrent apnea, some level of total parenteral nutrition (TPN) support while enteral nutrition is being introduced and increased, and monitoring or treatment for one or more of the complications of their prematurity.

The care for newborns who have achieved a level of observation, monitoring, and clinical care that is safely and effectively delivered on a routine medical-surgical floor (regardless of the hospital's decision of where to provide the care) is reported with subsequent hospital codes (99231-99233).

The decision to place a newborn or infant in an intensive care or critical care unit does not qualify automatically for reporting this code. The following examples illustrate situations that would and would not qualify for reporting critical care:

- Neonates recovering from a critical phase of their illness who are requiring only nutritional supplementation, thermal support, multiple medications, or observation for possible apnea spells would not qualify for a critically ill code. In contrast, a neonate with a hypoplastic left heart syndrome not receiving mechanical ventilation, but requiring nitrogen, dopamine, and prostaglandin to prevent death or immediate morbidity from hypotension or ductal closure would be considered critically ill.

- Mechanical ventilation, which is expected in the majority of neonates or infants considered critically ill, is not a prerequisite for the use of these codes. A neonate whose cardiovascular and neurologic systems are stable but who requires low flow oxygen by cannula or hood would not qualify for critical care codes. Neonates and young infants requiring low flow oxygen are routinely managed on standard hospital medical-surgical floors.

- The preoperative child with upper intestinal obstruction who demonstrates cardiovascular and neurological stability would not be considered critically ill.

- Neonates admitted to an intensive care unit for observation for the possibility of infection (ie, septic workup) and routine antibiotic therapy are not considered critically ill. The pre-catheter or pre-operative neonate who demonstrates cardiovascular and neurologic stability, whose admission is for the evaluation of a possible cardiac lesion, would not be considered critically ill. This same child who is admitted on prostaglandin, pressors, and oxygen/nitrogen therapy would be considered critically ill.

- The postoperative neonate who has not yet established normal urine output, who is at risk for postanesthesia respiratory arrest, who has not regained normal bowel function, and whose blood pressure is variable would qualify as critically ill in either a stable or an unstable category.

Clinical Example (99298)

An 1100-gram, 30-week preterm infant is now three weeks of age and weighs 1200 grams. The child was ventilated from birth and received two doses of surfactant. By 7 days of age, the neonate was extubated and is now on a nasal cannula of one-fourth liter of oxygen. His umbilical venous and arterial catheters were removed at 10 days of age. A percutaneous central venous line was then placed for total parenteral nutrition. Feedings were begun at 10 days of age and he is now receiving 75% of his total calorie requirement by the enteral route. He has been moved from a radiant warmer to an isolette for continued heat maintenance. Antibiotic maintenance was started for the first 7 days. All cultures were subsequently negative. His initial ultrasound examination on day 3 detected a grade one subependymal bleed; a repeat study on day 7 showed progression into the ventricles with dilation on the right side. His most recent chest radiograph is compatible with mild chronic lung disease. He has completed a single short course of steroids. His first eye examination demonstrated Grade I ROP. The infant continues with recurrent episodes of apnea and was placed on caffeine therapy. His family lives 60 miles from the NICU and visits 2 to 3 times weekly. A review of the child's flow sheet, discussion with the nursing staff, a complete physical examination, review of laboratory and medical imaging data, and conversations with the family occur daily. The referring physician is updated by telephone twice a week.

Description of Procedure (99298)

A complete examination of the head, eyes, nose, mouth, chest, lungs, heart, abdomen, genitals, rectum, joints, spine, extremities, and a neurologic appraisal of movement, reflexes, cranial nerves, and degree or arousal and reactivity are performed. All attached monitors and tubes are checked for secure placement and proper function.

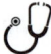
Clinical Example (99299)
A neonate, now weighing 2080 grams, is 9 days of age. He was born at 35 weeks gestation and weighed 2000 grams. His mother presented to the hospital with a temperature of 103.5F. Membranes had been ruptured for 6 hours. The fetal monitoring strip was non-reassuring with a tachycardia and persistent variable declarations. Mother received one dose of penicillin and delivery via cesarean section was performed. Cervical culture was positive for Group B streptococcus. The infant was flaccid at birth. Apgar scores were 2, 4, and 7 at 1, 5, and 10 minutes, respectively. The infant was intubated and needed 5 days of conventional ventilation. Chest x-ray was consistent with pneumonia and the baby was started on a 10-day course of antibiotics. He was weaned to nasal continuous positive airway pressure (CPAP) on day 6 and nasal cannula oxygen on day 7. Hyperalimentation was begun on day 3 and gavage feedings on day 7. He currently is on nasal cannula oxygen (30%-½ liter) and 50% TPN through a (PICC) line. There is no apnea but there are 2 to 3 brief desaturation episodes per day which are self-resolving. X-ray is improved but still not normal. He remains in an isolette on cardiorespiratory and oxygen saturation monitoring.

Description of Procedure
A complete examination of the head, eyes, nose, mouth, chest, lungs, heart, abdomen, genitals, rectum, joints, spine, extremities, and a neurologic appraisal of movement, reflexes, cranial nerves, and degree of arousal and activity are performed. All attached monitors and tubes are checked for secure placement and proper function.

Prolonged Services

Physician Standby Services

99360 **Physician standby service,** requiring prolonged physician attendance, each 30 minutes (eg, operative standby, standby for frozen section, for cesarean/high risk delivery, for monitoring EEG)

▶(For hospital mandated on call services, see 99026, 99027)◀

Rationale
Two new codes 99026 and 99027 were established in the Medicine subsection of the CPT code set to report physician hospital mandated on-call services. In support of this action, a cross-reference was added following 99360 to instruct users that hospital mandated on-call services are reported with codes 99026 and 99027.

Anesthesia

In continuation of the updates to the Anesthesia section, most significant are the revision of eight musculoskeletal arthroscopic procedure codes to delineate the diagnostic procedures from therapeutic procedures to create a consistent structure with the existing surgical procedure codes. Other major revisions include the addition of two new codes to report the administration of anesthetic for nerve block procedures, and restructuring of the Obstetric subsection codes to create non-indent (parent) codes for this section.

Anesthesia

Neck

▲ 00320 Anesthesia for all procedures on esophagus, thyroid, larynx, trachea and lymphatic system of neck; not otherwise specified, age 1 year or older

● 00326 Anesthesia for all procedures on the larynx and trachea in children less than 1 year of age

▶(Do not report 00326 in conjunction with code 99100)◀

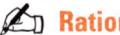 **Rationale**

Code 00320 previously encompassed all cases in which anesthesia was provided for procedures on the esophagus, thyroid, larynx, trachea, and lymphatic system of the neck. Within this group were included laryngoscopy and tracheostomy in infants less than 1 year of age. The work, method, and risk of anesthesia for these services are far greater for these patients than any other procedure or patient previously identified by this code. Therefore, code 00326 has been created to reflect the additional effort necessary for anesthesia provided in support of procedures performed on the larynx and trachea in children less than 1 year of age. In addition, code 00320 has been revised to reflect provision of these services for patients age 1 year or older.

The anesthetic technique (general/regional/MAC) utilized in the clinical examples is for illustrative purposes only. It is not a consideration in selecting an anesthesia code.

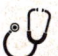 **Clinical Example** (00326)

The patient is a 4-month-old noted to have noisy breathing worsening on excitement. The patient was born at 35 weeks gestational age. The patient was discharged home on day four after bilirubin levels were noted to be decreasing. Stridor was noted to be present on inspiration when crying and has become worse in the past 2 weeks. There is no significant family history for congenital diseases or adverse anesthesia reactions. The patient is on iron fortified formula and takes no medications. There are no known allergies. The patient weighs 5 kg. Vital signs are appropriate for age. The baby is noted to be of normal color and has a mild suprasternal notch tug on quiet inspiration. When crying there is inspiratory stridor associated with significant chest retractions. No change in color is noted. The airway is noted to be of normal appearance. The breath sounds are clear bilaterally. The heart is auscultated finding normal rate and rhythm. No murmur is heard. No other obvious congenital abnormalities are noted. Significant laboratory test results include a hematocrit of 32%.

Description of Procedure (00326)

A general anesthesia with induction by mask is agreed to by the parents. An intramuscular injection of atropine is administered. The baby is transported to the operating room where monitors are placed. A forced air mattress is in place as are heating lamps. Anesthesia is gradually induced by volatile agent through a mask.

Intravenous access is secured. The anesthetic is slowly deepened with careful attention to blood pressure, heart rate, and oxygenation. When the baby is sufficiently anesthetized, laryngoscopy is performed and topical local anesthesia is sprayed in the trachea and on the larynx. The airway is again secured by mask, and vital signs are checked. Caffeine 10 mg/kg is intravenously administered. The baby is turned to the bronchoscopist with careful attention to the patency of the airway. The mask is removed and the bronchoscopist performs laryngoscopy and placement of a rigid bronchoscope into the trachea. The anesthesia circuit is attached to the bronchoscope and adequate ventilation is determined by carbon dioxide monitoring, chest excursion with positive pressure ventilation, and, if necessary, auscultation of breath sounds. Pulse oximetry and end tidal carbon dioxide are continuously and closely monitored throughout the procedure. The bronchoscopy continues and nearing the end of the procedure the anesthetic gases are decreased and eventually turned off. An endotracheal tube is placed by the anesthesiologist after bronchoscopy if airway patency is in question. Emergence from anesthesia ensues. When the infant demonstrates sufficient strength and awareness by opening the eyes, the endotracheal tube is removed and the patient observed for air movement with inspiration. Pulse oximetry and end tidal carbon dioxide are verified. When the patient is stable, transport to recovery with monitors and supplemental oxygen takes place. The patient is monitored for a prolonged period in the recovery room prior to transfer to the inpatient unit. The infant is placed on continuous pulse oximetry and respiratory monitors. When the baby has been stable for a period of 6 hours, with no evidence of apnea, discharge to home occurs.

Intrathoracic

00520 Anesthesia for closed chest procedures; (including bronchoscopy) not otherwise specified

00528 mediastinoscopy and diagnostic thoracoscopy

▶(For tracheobronchial reconstruction, use 00539)◀

●**00539** Anesthesia for tracheobronchial reconstruction

00540 Anesthesia for thoracotomy procedures involving lungs, pleura, diaphragm, and mediastinum (including surgical thoracoscopy); not otherwise specified

●**00541** utilizing one lung ventilation

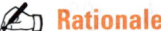 **Rationale**

These codes reflect change in clinical practice for anesthetic management of patients undergoing thoracic surgical procedures necessitating isolation of one lung. Previous codes did not reflect the additional physician work and complexity of clinical management when isolation of one lung is required to provide the surgeon with optimal clinical conditions for the procedure. Therefore, the revisions and additions were necessary to reflect this effort. In addition, code

00539 reflects a change in clinical practice for anesthetic management of patients undergoing thoracic surgery that involves tracheobronchial reconstruction.

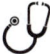
Clinical Example (00539)

A 47-year-old woman is scheduled to undergo tracheal resection and reconstruction for tracheal stenosis. The patient sustained chest and abdominal trauma from a motor vehicle accident 5 years ago. As a result of the injuries, she had a prolonged hospitalization complicated by ARDS, sepsis, and renal failure. The patient required mechanical ventilatory support for 6 weeks. During that hospitalization the patient underwent tracheotomy to facilitate long-term mechanical ventilation and bronchopulmonary hygiene. Since removal of the tracheotomy tube, the patient has had clinical evidence of severe tracheal stenosis and several episodes of severe stridor.

Description of Procedure (00539)

Pre-anesthesia: The patient requiring tracheobronchial reconstruction has known abnormalities of the airways, necessitating a more thorough preoperative evaluation and more careful planning for airway management at the time of surgery. The evaluation includes review of neck and chest radiographs, cine-radiographs and CT or MRI scans to assess the caliber of the airway and the degree of tracheomalacia. This assessment is essential to determine the most appropriate approach to tracheal intubation and airway management during the procedure. Because of the known tracheal abnormalities, the patient is also at increased risk for infection and aspiration, necessitating preoperative preparation with medications to reduce the likelihood of respiratory failure.

Intra-operative: In order to provide the surgical conditions necessary to complete the tracheal reconstruction, the surgeon and anesthesiologist must carefully coordinate the intraoperative management of the patient's airway, ventilation, and gas exchange. Since both the surgeon and anesthesiologist are sharing the airway during tracheobronchial reconstruction, the anesthesiologist and surgeon must coordinate the manipulation of the trachea and artificial airway to allow the surgical procedure to be completed without loss of airway integrity or life-threatening compromise in ventilation and oxygenation. The anesthesiologist must carefully coordinate mechanical ventilation, hand ventilation, and airway suctioning to ensure that the airway remains clear of blood and secretions that would be aspirated into the lungs. The endotracheal tube position must be frequently adjusted to provide surgical conditions that facilitate the repair of the trachea and ensure ventilation and oxygenation of the patient. Because of the blood and secretions in the surgical field, the anesthesiologist must provide regular suctioning of the airway and repositioning of the endotracheal tube. After completion of the surgical repair, the anesthesiologist must ensure that the airway is properly positioned to protect the airway from aspiration, ensure gas exchange, and prevent pressure necrosis on surgical suture lines.

Postanesthesia: The patient who undergoes tracheal resection requires meticulous management after the surgical procedure to ensure that the suture line remains intact and that there is no compromise in tracheal blood flow. The initial goal is to remove the endotracheal tube as soon as possible, after the procedure, while also ensuring that the patient has a clear airway. After the tracheal resection, mucociliary clearance is impaired, necessitating intensive respiratory care and careful suctioning of pulmonary secretions to optimize bronchopulmonary hygiene without disrupting the tracheal anastomosis. Pain relief is carefully titrated to achieve patient comfort.

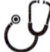

Clinical Example (00541)

A 64-year-old male is scheduled for a thoracoscopic left upper lobectomy for carcinoma of the lung. The patient has a long smoking history. He has coronary artery disease with previous myocardial infarction, although his ventricular function is good. He has had no recent chest pain. The surgeon is concerned about possible post-obstructive infection in the left upper lobe. To facilitate the surgical procedure, the surgeon has requested isolation of the lung. A double lumen endotracheal tube will be placed and the positioning of the tube confirmed by fiberoptic bronchoscopy.

Description of Procedure

Intra-operative: To isolate one lung from another and provide one lung ventilation, a placement of double lumen endotracheal tube or, less commonly, placement of a bronchial blocker is required. The placement of a double lumen endotracheal tube required intubation of the trachea with a special endotracheal tube that has a tracheal and bronchial lumen. The tube is initially placed through the vocal cords and subsequently passed into the mainstem bronchus. To guide proper tube positioning, a fiberoptic bronchoscope is placed through the special double lumen endotracheal tube into the mainstem bronchus. Once the airways are properly identified, the double lumen endotracheal tube is placed in the mainstem bronchus, its positioning confirmed by bronchoscopy. Once the tube is in proper position, the tracheal and bronchial cuffs of the tube are inflated and ventilation is provided to each lung independently to confirm proper positioning. After confirming proper positioning of the tube with the patient in the supine position, the patient is turned to the position required for the surgical procedure, most often the lateral decubitus position. Once positioned for the surgery, the patient undergoes repeat bronchoscopy to confirm proper position of the endotracheal tube.

Postanesthesia: After completion of the surgical procedure, the patient who has undergone a procedure that isolated one lung from another is at greater risk for atelectasis, lung consolidation, and impaired gas exchange. Prior to tracheal extubation, the non-ventilated lung must be re-expanded without compromising pulmonary vascular resistance or lung perfusion. Many of the patients require postoperative mechanical ventilatory support, necessitating tracheal reintubation with a single lumen endotracheal tube to prevent trauma to the mainstem bronchi and minimize the risk of tracheobronchial malacia or stenosis.

Spine and Spinal Cord

●**00640** Anesthesia for manipulation of the spine or for closed procedures on the cervical, thoracic or lumbar spine

 Rationale

Code 00640 has been added to *CPT 2003* to identify anesthesia performed for closed manipulation procedures of the spine provided separate from the actual manipulation procedure (as identified by code 22505). This code is intended to be used by the individual who provides the separately administered anesthesia. Previously, there was not an applicable anesthesia code in the CPT code set to use when the anesthesia services were provided by a physician. Therefore, this anesthesia code was created to allow the physician who administers separately provided anesthesia to identify his/her services when manipulation of the spine is performed by another physician (22505).

 Clinical Example (00640)

The typical patient is one in whom office manipulations have failed to relieve the pain syndrome. The patient may not be able to work and resists further office therapy because of the pain involved. Further manipulation via manipulation under anesthesia should be determined after a conservative approach to manual therapy.

Description of Procedure (00640)

The patient is evaluated preoperatively by an anesthesiologist to determine the presence of coexisting medical illness, drug therapy, allergies, previous surgical history, and applicable family history. For example, if the patient is known to be taking cardiac medication or antihypertensives, instructions would be given to him or her regarding the medications. Also, cardiovascular and other end organ damage due to chronic hypertension would be sought after and emphasized during the examination. The airway is evaluated as a critical part of the physical examination. Physical examination would also include the cardiopulmonary exam.

At this point the patient is advised of the type of anesthesia that will be used for the procedure and the risks, benefits, and alternatives are given. Instructions for the day of surgery are given to the patient, including the appropriate period of time for fasting prior to the surgery.

On the day of the procedure, after obtaining informed consent, the patient is again evaluated by the anesthesia provider who will start a peripheral intravenous line and begin an infusion of lactated ringers. The anesthesia provider will have assured that all equipment and drugs necessary for resuscitation are available and working. The patient is placed on the OR table and monitoring devices are applied (ECG, NIBP, pulse oximetry) and baseline values are obtained. Intravenous anesthetics, with or without benzodiazepines and/or narcotics, are most commonly used. Supplemental oxygen is given and the airway is maintained throughout. This is especially important during manipulations of the cervical spine. Additional intravenous medication is given as required. Blood pressure is monitored every 3 to 5 minutes, more frequently if indicated. As the procedure nears completion, anesthetic agents are withdrawn to prepare the patient for wakefulness. Hemodynamic stability, adequacy of ventilation, and level of consciousness are examined. If these parameters are acceptable, the patient is transferred to the postanesthesia care unit. A complete record is maintained by the anesthesia provider.

In the postanesthesia care unit, the patient is managed according to ASA guidelines. Any side effects of anesthesia, most commonly nausea and vomiting, are assessed and treated if necessary. Prior to discharge, level of consciousness, respiratory function, ability to ambulate, and availability of an escort are assessed, and discharge instructions are issued and documented in the patient's record.

Lower Abdomen

00830 Anesthesia for hernia repairs in lower abdomen; not otherwise specified

00832   ventral and incisional hernias

▶(For hernia repairs in the infant 1 year of age or younger, see 00834, 00836)◀

●**00834** Anesthesia for hernia repairs in lower abdomen not otherwise specified, under 1 year of age

▶(Do not report 00834 in conjunction with code 99100)◀

●**00836** Anesthesia for hernia repair in the lower abdomen not otherwise specified, infants less than 37 weeks gestational age at birth and less than 50 weeks gestational age at time of surgery

▶(Do not report 00836 in conjunction with code 99100)◀

00860 Anesthesia for extraperitoneal procedures in lower abdomen, including urinary tract; not otherwise specified

▶(00869 has been renumbered. To report, use 00921)◀

 Rationale

Over the past several years the pediatric general surgeons have recognized the increased work and risk necessary to care for younger and smaller children by developing CPT codes that are stratified by age for children undergoing inguinal hernia repair. Increased work and risk also exist in anesthetizing these children for these procedures. These codes were created to recognize the anesthetic complexity involved. This also correlates with current surgical CPT codes.

Existing literature demonstrates an increased risk of caring for children less than 1 year of age. Therefore, the new code does not identically match the existing surgical inguinal hernia repair (49495) of less than 6 months age.

Lastly, code 00869 Anesthesia for extraperitoneal procedures in lower abdomen, including urinary tract; vasectomy, unilateral/bilateral, was renumbered as new code 00921.

Clinical Example (00834)
The patient is an 11-month-old male who was noted to have a groin mass by the mother. The pediatrician diagnosed an inguinal hernia and referred the patient to a pediatric surgeon. The patient now presents for bilateral inguinal hernia repair. The patient's birth history was normal. The only history of significance is recent middle ear infection, managed successfully with a course of antibiotics. Family history did not reveal significant diseases or difficulty with anesthesia. The patient is on no medications and has no allergies. Physical examination with emphasis on the airway, lungs, heart, and nervous system is performed. After discussing anesthetic options with the parents, an inhalational general anesthesia is planned.

Description of Procedure (00834)
The patient is transferred to the operating room and ECG, pulse oximeter, and blood pressure monitors are applied. Anesthesia is induced with a volatile agent by mask. Intravenous access is obtained in the lower extremity. Muscle relaxation is administered and monitored by a twitch monitor. The airway is secured with an orally placed endotracheal tube. Proper tracheal tube placement is determined by carbon dioxide monitoring and auscultation of breath sounds bilaterally. A temperature monitor is placed. The patient is placed in the left lateral decubitus position and the sacrum is palpated for sacral cornua and a sterile preparation is performed. Using a 22-gauge styletted blunt needle, the epidural space is entered by the caudal route. After ascertaining safe needle placement, 1 mL/kg of local anesthetic is injected. The patient is then returned to the supine position. Breath sounds are again auscultated. Continuous monitoring and charting ensue with adjustments to the anesthesia as necessary. A forced warm air heater is placed around the patient. Intravenous fluids are administered accounting for hourly maintenance and deficit from denial of oral intake preoperatively. At the end of the surgical procedure the anesthetic gases are discontinued and the muscle relaxation is pharmacologically reversed. When the patient is making strong purposeful movement the trachea is extubated. The patient is observed prior to transfer to the postanesthesia care unit for stability of vital signs and satisfactory pulse oximetry results. In the postoperative period the patient is observed in the postanesthesia care unit (PACU) for a minumum of 30 minutes or until the patient satisfies discharge criteria. Additional analgesia is provided as needed. The patient is then transferred to the ambulatory care unit and observed for at least another 30 minutes until deemed ready to be discharged home.

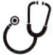 **Clinical Example (00836)**
The patient is a 4-week-old male born at 28 weeks gestational age. The patient was endotracheally intubated in the delivery room with Apgar scores of 2 and 5. The patient's trachea was extubated at 1 week of age after the administration of surfactant and indomethacin. A grade 2 intraventricular hemorrhage was diagnosed in week 2. At present there are no significant sequelae from the previous problems. The patient is presently gaining weight with oral nutritional supplementation. Discharge planning is taking place, but hindered by the presence of a large right inguinal hernia. Currently the patient receives calcium

supplementation. There are no allergies. The patient's weight is currently 2 kg. The heart rate is 140 beats per minute, respiratory rate of 45 breaths per minute and a systolic blood pressure of 50 mm Hg. Laboratory data includes normal electrolytes and a hematocrit of 30%. Aside from the patient's extremely small size and the presence of a large right inguinal hernia, the airway appears appropriate and patent, the lung fields are clear, and the heart is auscultated revealing normal rate and rhythm with no appreciable murmur. Also noted are multiple ecchymotic areas from previous venous access attempts. There is no venous access at present nor are any veins easily visible. The parents are not present or available for discussion regarding anesthetic plans. Surgical consent was obtained by phone a day earlier. General anesthesia is planned with induction by intravenous technique. A caudal block is planned for intraoperative and postoperative pain relief (separately reportable).

Description of Procedure (00836)

The patient is transferred from the neonatal intensive care unit and monitored to the operating room. The operating room has been preheated to 80°F. The patient is transferred to the operating table and the monitors are placed for ECG, pulse oximetry, and blood pressure. A warming mattress and heat lamps are used to keep the patient normothermic. A 22-gauge intravenous catheter is placed in the saphenous vein blindly. Anesthesia is induced slowly with intravenous agents constantly monitoring the vital signs. A muscle relaxant is administered. A volatile anesthetic agent is slowly titrated to effect with careful attention to blood pressure. The baby's trachea is intubated with a 2.5-mm endotracheal tube. After determining appropriate placement by the presence of carbon dioxide and auscultation of bilateral breath sounds, the endotracheal tube is secured. The baby is turned to the left lateral decubitus position and the sacrum is prepared by sterile technique. A caudal block is performed with a 22-gauge stylleted blunt needle placed in the epidural space at the level of the sacrum. After ascertaining correct needle placement, 2 mL of local anesthetic is slowly injected. The baby is returned to the supine position and bilateral breath sounds are auscultated. The inspired oxygen concentration is decreased as possible by monitoring pulse oximetry to 25% oxygen or less. Surgery is performed with continuous monitoring of vital signs, recording all pertinent data on the anesthesia chart. To prevent postoperative apnea that is possible in this age group, 10 mg/kg of caffeine is administered by intravenous route. At the end of the surgical procedure, the anesthetic agents are discontinued and the muscle relaxant is reversed. Upon demonstration of adequate emergence from anesthesia as noted by purposeful movement and adequate reversal of muscle relaxation demonstrated by spontaneous flexion of the hips off the bed, the endotracheal tube is removed. The patient is observed for stability of vital signs. The patient is transferred to the isolette and monitored. An emergency resuscitation kit is prepared specific to the baby's weight and includes airway equipment and resuscitative medications. The baby is transported back to the neonatal intensive care unit with continuous pulse oximetry and EKG monitor. Vital signs are again taken and a full report is given to the nurse and the primary care physician. Analgesic needs are assessed and medication given as necessary to achieve patient comfort.

Perineum

00920 Anesthesia for procedures on male genitalia (including open urethral procedures); not otherwise specified

●**00921** vasectomy, unilateral/bilateral

 Rationale

Code 00921 was added to identify anesthesia provided for unilateral or bilateral vasectomy on the male genitalia. This anesthesia care was previously reported with code 00869. Code 00869 has been renumbered and relocated to the perineum section.

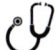 **Clinical Example** (00921)

A 42-year-old married male with three children, ages 11, 8, and 3, desires permanent sterilization. He and his wife prefer not to use mechanical means of contraception. They have chosen vasectomy for him, preferring to avoid general anesthesia for her, which is necessary for a tubal ligation. He is in excellent health, exercising 45 minutes or so 5 days a week.

Description of Procedure (00921)

The anesthesiologist saw the patient in the holding area of the outpatient surgery center. The holding room nurse had inserted a 20-gauge intravenous (IV) line in the dorsum of his left hand. The patient's past medical and anesthetic history were quickly reviewed: his last oral intake was 10 hours previously, and his airway was rated a Mallampati Class I. The anesthetic management discussed with the patient included intravenous sedation.

The patient was taken to the operating room, placed on the table in the supine position, and had the usual monitoring devices attached (ECG, non-invasive blood pressure, and pulse oximetry). Supplemental oxygen was given via a face mask, to which had been attached an end-tidal CO_2 sampling tube.

The patient was sedated. His scrotum was prepped, and systemic anesthesia was administered. When the patient stopped responding to verbal stimulation, the surgeon injected a local anesthetic into each side of the patient's upper scrotum, after having identified the spermatic cord.

During the procedure, the patient was given additional anesthesia. After the bilateral incisions had been closed, and the patient was easily arousable, the monitors were removed, and the patient moved himself to the recovery stretcher. His mental status was sufficient to allow him to be taken to the second-stage recovery area.

Knee and Popliteal Area

▶Surgical endoscopy/arthroscopy always includes a diagnostic endoscopy/arthroscopy.◀

▲ **01382** Anesthesia for diagnostic arthroscopic procedures of knee joint

▲ **01400** Anesthesia for open or surgical arthroscopic procedures on knee joint; not otherwise specified

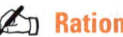
Rationale
Codes 01382 and 01400 were editorially revised to reflect the current practice of medicine, as arthroscopy is now provided not only as a diagnostic tool but as an interventional tool as well. Previously, code 01382 reflected all arthroscopic procedures provided for the knee and popliteal area. This code was changed to reflect provision of anesthesia for diagnostic procedures alone. In addition, code 01400 was revised to reflect anesthesia provided for both open and surgical arthroscopic procedures, as anesthesia for surgical arthroscopy requires effort beyond that identified as part of anesthesia provided for diagnostic arthroscopy. Therefore, these codes were revised to reflect the difference in effort for providing each type of anesthesia service.

In addition, similar to the guideline provided in the Surgery section of the CPT coding manual, a guideline was added to the Knee and Popliteal Area Anesthesia section to identify that surgical endoscopy always includes diagnostic endoscopy/arthroscopy.

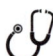
Clinical Example (01400)
A typical patient is a young adult athlete, male or female, who has sustained an injury to the knee and now has a painful and unstable knee, which precludes participation in his/her sport. An MRI reveals a torn anterior cruciate ligament and arthroscopic-assisted surgical repair of the torn anterior cruciate ligament is scheduled.

Description of Procedure
The general anesthetic is begun after assessing the baseline vital functions. An inhalation anesthetic is used with a laryngeal mask airway (LMA). The procedure, which includes an open harvest of the patellar tendon graft and the arthroscopic preparation of the joint and placement of the graft, proceeds without problem. Vital signs are monitored continuously during the procedure. At the end of the procedure, and after the placement of a brace on the operated knee, the patient is awakened and taken to the post-anesthesia care unit (PACU).

Lower Leg (Below Knee, Includes Ankle and Foot)

▶Surgical endoscopy/arthroscopy always includes a diagnostic endoscopy/arthroscopy.◀

▲ **01464** Anesthesia for arthroscopic procedures of ankle and/or foot

Rationale

An editorial revision was made to code 01464 to include anesthesia provided for arthroscopic procedures of the foot as well as the ankle.

Shoulder and Axilla

▶Surgical endoscopy/arthroscopy always includes a diagnostic endoscopy/arthroscopy.◀

▲01622   Anesthesia for diagnostic arthroscopic procedures of shoulder joint

▲01630   Anesthesia for open or surgical arthroscopic procedures on humeral head and neck, sternoclavicular joint, acromioclavicular joint, and shoulder joint; not otherwise specified

 Rationale

Codes 01622 and 01630 were editorially revised to reflect improvements in surgical care of the shoulder as a result of arthroscopic techniques. Arthroscopy was initially a diagnostic procedure only. Surgical techniques now quite often include an open component and an arthroscopic component. This revision was made to acknowledge this fact, resulting in codes that are more representative of current practice.

Upper Arm and Elbow

▶Surgical endoscopy/arthroscopy always includes a diagnostic endoscopy/arthroscopy.◀

▲01732   Anesthesia for diagnostic arthroscopic procedures of elbow joint

▲01740   Anesthesia for open or surgical arthroscopic procedures of the elbow; not otherwise specified

 Rationale

Codes 01732 and 01740 were editorially revised to reflect improvements in surgical care of the elbow as a result of arthroscopic techniques. Arthroscopy was initially a diagnostic procedure only. Surgical techniques now quite often include an open component and an arthroscopic component. This revision was made to acknowledge this fact and to provide codes that are more representative of current practice.

Forearm, Wrist, and Hand

●01829   Anesthesia for diagnostic arthroscopic procedures on the wrist

▲01830   Anesthesia for open or surgical arthroscopic/endoscopic procedures on distal radius, distal ulna, wrist, or hand joints; not otherwise specified

01832   total wrist replacement

Rationale
Code 01830 was revised and code 01829 was added to describe provision of anesthesia for arthroscopic procedures of the wrist. The descriptor for code 01830 was revised to reflect provision of anesthesia for either open or surgical arthroscopic procedures of the radius, ulna, wrist, or hand. Code 01829 was created to identify diagnostic arthroscopic procedures of the wrist.

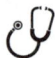 ### Clinical Example (01829)
A 25-year-old baseball pitcher has developed marked pain and significant swelling in his right wrist. There is no history of significant trauma. Cold packs, anti-inflammatory medications, and immobilization have not relieved his wrist pain. Radiographs do not reveal an obvious fracture. He is otherwise healthy. He is scheduled for a diagnostic arthroscopy of his right wrist.

Description of Procedure (01829)
In the operating room the patient is safely transferred to the operating table. Pulse oximetry, blood pressure, and ECG monitors are placed. Oxygen by mask is given to achieve 100% saturation for several minutes, then general anesthesia is induced using intravenous fentanyl and propofol. A #4 laryngeal mask airway (LMA) is carefully inserted through the mouth into the hypopharynx. The presence of end tidal CO_2 is documented, a good fit is established and the tube is taped in place. Inhalation anesthesia agents are added to the oxygen. Eyes are padded and protective tape is applied to maintain closure. Peripheral nerves and pressure points are padded and protected. The patient is further secured to the operating table with surgical tape and straps. Warm blankets are placed to achieve normothermia. Anesthesia is maintained with inhalation anesthesia agents. Intravenous fluids are given to maintain hydration and to treat hypotension. Depth of anesthesia is maintained by continuous assessment of blood pressure, pulse rate, and respiratory effort. Additional narcotics and inhalation agents are provided as needed. Toward the end of the procedure, the inhalation agents are gradually withdrawn and narcotics are slowly added, titrating the dose to maintain the patient's respiration. At the end of the surgical procedure, adequacy of spontaneous ventilation, tidal volume, and emergence from anesthesia is determined and if these are adequate, the LMA is removed. A mask providing O_2 is placed on the patient's face, and if ventilation and oxygenation are satisfactory, the patient is then moved to a stretcher and transferred to the post-anesthesia care unit.

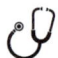 ### Clinical Example (01830)
A 15-year-old female develops a compound fracture of her right distal radius and ulna in a fall. Closed reduction is not feasible due to the extent of the fractures and an open reduction with internal fixation is planned. She is on no medications and is otherwise healthy. Last meal was 8 hours ago.

Description of Procedure (01830)

In the operating room the patient is safely transferred to the operating table. Pulse oximetry, blood pressure, and ECG monitors are placed. Oxygen by mask is given to achieve 100% saturation for several minutes, then general anesthesia is induced. After carbon dioxide is detected in the exhaled gas, and after breath sounds are detected bilaterally, the endotracheal tube is secured to the face with tape. Inhalation anesthesia agents are added to the oxygen. Eyes are padded and protective tape is applied to maintain closure. Anesthesia is maintained with inhalation anesthesia agents. Peripheral nerves and pressure points are padded and protected. The patient is further secured to the operating table. A forced air-warming blanket is applied to maintain normothermia. Intravenous fluids are given to maintain hydration and treat hypotension. Depth of anesthesia is maintained by assessing blood pressure, pulse rate, respiratory effort, and neuromuscular blockade. Additional narcotics, neuromuscular blocking drugs, and inhalation agents are provided as needed. Following completion of the surgical procedure, the inhalation agents are withdrawn and residual neuromuscular blockade is reversed using anticholinesterase and anticholinergic drugs. Additionally, narcotics are slowly titrated to maintain adequate respiratory rate and achieve analgesia. At the end of the surgical procedure, adequacy of spontaneous ventilation, tidal volume, and emergence from anesthesia are determined and, if adequate, the patient is suctioned and the endotracheal tube is removed. A green mask and O_2 are placed on the patient's face and, if ventilation and oxygenation are satisfactory, the patient is then moved to a stretcher and transferred to the postanesthesia care unit.

Obstetric

01960 Anesthesia for vaginal delivery only

▲**01961** Anesthesia for cesarean delivery only

▲**01962** Anesthesia for urgent hysterectomy following delivery

▲**01963** Anesthesia for cesarean hysterectomy without any labor analgesia/anesthesia care

▲**01964** Anesthesia for abortion procedures

+▲**01968** Anesthesia for cesarean delivery following neuraxial labor analgesia/anesthesia (List separately in addition to code for primary procedure performed)

(Use 01968 in conjunction with code 01967)

+▲**01969** Anesthesia for cesarean hysterectomy following neuraxial labor analgesia/anesthesia (List separately in addition to code for primary procedure performed)

(Use 01969 in conjunction with code 01967)

Rationale

The phrase "Anesthesia for" was added to codes 01968 and 01969 as an editorial change to identify provision of anesthesia services. The same phrase was added to codes 01960-01964 for consistency.

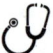
Clinical Example (01960)

A 27-year-old gravida 3 para 2 female at 36 weeks gestation arrives in labor and delivery in active labor and fully dilated. Vaginal exam shows that she is complete with breech presentation. The obstetrician believes that it is too late for an epidural anesthetic. The patient cannot be delivered vaginally with local analgesia and general anesthesia is required for delivery.

Description of Procedure (01960)

The patient is given 100% oxygen via the anesthesia mask/circuit. General anesthesia is induced intravenously with rocuronium followed by thiopental sodium Pentothal and succinylcholine, while cricoid pressure is being applied. After the patient was anesthetized and adequate neuromuscular blockade was achieved, the trachea is intubated with a 7-mm cuffed endotracheal tube. Proper placement of the tube is assured by condensation in the tube, chest movement, auscultation of the lungs, and a satisfactory wave form and numerical value on the end-tidal CO_2 monitor. The tube was secured with tape and the eyes were taped closed. Via the endotracheal tube, the patient is given oxygen, nitrous oxide, and desflurane. The obstetrician, after infiltrating the perineum with a local anesthetic and performing an episiotomy, proceeds to deliver the breech presentation vaginally. During this, the anesthesiologist passes an 18-gauge oro-gastric tube to decompress the stomach.

After delivery of the baby, and prior to delivery of the placenta, additional thiopental and fentanyl are administered intravenously. After delivery of the placenta, oxytocin is added to the intravenous infusion. After the episiotomy is repaired, the patient is taken out of the lithotomy position and her uterus massaged. The nitrous oxide and desflurane are discontinued, and the patient began to emerge from anesthesia. When her level of consciousness and respiratory effort are judged to be adequate, the endotracheal tube is removed.

The patient is moved to a recovery stretcher, and taken to the Post-Anesthesia Care Unit (PACU). Report is given to the PACU nurse as the usual PACU monitors and an oxygen mask are being applied. After vital signs are taken, and the PACU nurse's questions are answered, the anesthesiologist leaves the PACU.

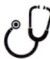
Clinical Example (01961)

A 25-year-old gravida 1 para 0 presents to the obstetrical suite with prolonged active labor and failure to progress. The patient did not want neuraxial analgesia for labor. A non-reassuring fetal heart rate tracing is noted. A cesarean section is planned.

Description of Procedure

After having received additional Ringer's lactate, the patient is taken to the delivery room and moved to the operating table. She is helped to sit on the table with her legs over the side, and the usual monitors (eg, ECG, non-invasive blood pressure, and a pulse oximeter) are applied. After having been positioned by the labor nurse, who is helping her maintain that position, her lower back is prepared with an iodine solution and alcohol. A solution of 1% Lidocaine is infiltrated into the skin and subcutaneous tissue and an 18-gauge introducer needle is inserted at the L-3-4 interspace. Through the introducer needle, a 24-gauge pencil-point spinal needle is inserted into the subarachnoid space; no paresthesia is noted by the patient, and the cerebrospinal fluid is clear. Fentanyl in "spinal bupivacaine" (0.75% bupivacaine in 8.25% dextrose) is injected intrathecally for surgical anesthesia. After 30 seconds, the patient is placed in the supine position, with her head elevated approximately 15 degrees, and a roll is placed under her right hip to provide left uterine displacement. An oxygen mask is placed on the patient, and she is given ephedrine intravenously, as prophylaxis against hypotension.

After the fetal heart tones are checked and a urinary catheter is inserted, the patient's abdomen is prepped and draped. The sensory level of the spinal anesthetic has been frequently checked during this time, and her blood pressure is being checked every 3 minutes. A satisfactory sensory level of the anesthetic was confirmed, and the patient's husband is brought into the room and placed at the head of the table. As had been discussed in the labor room, what the patient is likely to experience during the surgical procedure is explained to her and her husband. The patient's hand-grip strength is checked from time to time, as is the appearance and affect of her husband. Although she is aware of "something going on" in her abdomen, she denies any discomfort.

As the baby is being delivered through the uterine incision, she does comment on some pressure in her upper abdomen, which ends with the delivery of her baby. At the time of delivery, the father is given the opportunity to stand up and witness the delivery. After the delivery, the oxygen mask is removed from the patient, and the drapes are briefly lowered so that she can see her baby before it is given to the neonatologist in attendance. Oxytocin is added to the intravenous fluid bag, and an antibiotic is given intravenously.

The vital signs continue to be monitored during the remainder of the operation, and the patient is kept apprised of the progress of the procedure. After being evaluated by the neonatologist, the baby is brought to the patient for several minutes before being taken to the nursery. After the incision is closed and a dressing applied, the patient is moved to a recovery stretcher and taken to the Post-Anesthesia Care Unit (PACU).

Report is given to the PACU nurse, including the drugs given and the orders pertaining to postoperative pain management. After the vital signs are taken, and any questions by the patient and the PACU nurse are answered, the anesthesiologist returned to the Labor and Delivery Suite but remained available via pager to manage issues such as nausea and postsurgical pain.

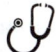

Clinical Example (01962)

The patient, a 37-year-old gravida 5 female, presents to the labor and delivery suite in active labor at 39 weeks gestation. Her obstetric history is remarkable for three uncomplicated vaginal deliveries that did not require labor analgesia services. Her fourth pregnancy was complicated by a cesarean section for breech presentation. This labor reveals a reassuring fetal heart rate tracing and rapid progression to the second stage of labor, without augmentation. The patient tolerated the discomfort of labor and delivery without any anesthetic intervention. After uneventful delivery of a healthy male neonate, adherent placenta (placenta accreta) complicates delivery of the placenta. Due to increasing hemorrhage and partial inversion of the uterus during attempted manual extraction of retained placenta, the obstetrician decides to perform an emergent laparotomy for control of hemorrhage. The obstetrician administers oxytocin intravenously and methylergonovine intramuscularly without apparent improvement.

Description of Procedure (01962)
The anesthesiologist instructs the nurse to apply and maintain cricoid pressure. After uncomplicated rapid-sequence intubation, the anesthesiologist confirms endotracheal tube placement via auscultation and presence of end-tidal carbon dioxide. Vital signs demonstrate continued hypotension and tachycardia; peripheral nerve stimulator indicates the need for additional muscle relaxation. The anesthesiologist also administers incremental doses of fentanyl and low-dose (less than 0.5 MAC) inhalational anesthesia to achieve analgesia and amnesia, adjusting the anesthetic depth to minimize hypotension. While the surgical team rapidly prepares the patient's abdomen and applies sterile drapes, the anesthesiologist places a 14-gauge, antecubital intravenous catheter, which she connects to a rapid infusion device (Level One).

The obstetrician makes the skin incision. Due to the continuing hemorrhage and associated hypotension, the anesthesiologist rapidly infuses hydroxyethyl starch. Arterial blood gas demonstrates metabolic acidosis and adequate oxygenation. Hemoglobin is 6 g/dL and platelet count is 80,000/cc^3. The anesthesiologist orders appropriate blood products and administers sodium bicarbonate intravenously. The surgeon quickly exposes the uterus, which demonstrates atony. Clamping the uterine arteries only minimally reduces the ongoing hemorrhage. A nurse delivers four units of crossmatched packed red blood cells to the operating room. The anesthesiologist begins a rapid infusion of the red cells after confirming with the nurse that the unit is in date and that the crossmatch is correct. Given the ongoing hemorrhage, the obstetrician decides to proceed with urgent hysterectomy. Despite continued rapid infusion of blood and crystalloid, the patient's hypotension only minimally improves. The obstetrician reports increasing bleeding from serosal surfaces, and the anesthesiologist notes bleeding around the intravenous catheter sites. The platelets arrive and the anesthesiologist administers the platelets after confirming the blood bank tag with the nurse. Oxygen saturation declines from 99% to 93% despite administration of 100% oxygen. Lung auscultation demonstrates diffuse rales. A nurse delivers the results of the coagulation panel, which demonstrate low fibrinogen, elevated D-dimers, prothrombin time of 25 seconds (INR 2.3), and activated thromboplastin time of 60 seconds. The anesthesiologist makes a diagnosis of disseminated intravascular coagulation and possible adult respiratory distress syndrome. The anesthesiologist orders additional platelets, cryoprecipitate, and fresh frozen plasma. To address the respiratory compromise, the anesthesiologist adds positive end-expiratory pressure (PEEP); however, the patient's hypotension worsens, and the PEEP is discontinued. To help support blood pressure, the anesthesiologist initiates an infusion of dopamine, which increases the blood pressure to 80-90/35-45 mm Hg. At the end of surgery, the anesthesiologist and the nurse transfer the patient to the ICU bed. The anesthesiologist connects the transport monitor and observes ECG, oxygen saturation and arterial blood pressure. Using an Ambu bag, the anesthesiologist ventilates the patient manually during transport to the ICU.

On arrival, the anesthesiologist orders initial ventilator settings, reviews hemodynamics, orders sedatives and analgesics for patient comfort, and provides a detailed report to the admitting nurse. In addition, the anesthesiologist orders admitting laboratory studies that include complete blood count and arterial blood gas, reviews the results of the coagulation profile obtained at the end of surgery, reviews the chest x-ray obtained after pulmonary artery catheter placement, and provides a detailed report to the intensivist, who will be assuming care of the patient. The anesthesiologist and the surgeon then visit with the patient's family to discuss the anesthetic and the surgery and the patient's condition and to answer the family's questions.

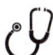

Clinical Example (01963)

A 30-year-old gravida 4 para 3 female presents to the delivery suite in active labor. A non-reassuring fetal heart rate is noted and an urgent cesarean section is planned with the patient under general anesthesia. After cesarean delivery of the infant, separation of the placenta is incomplete, and severe ongoing blood loss occurs. A cesarean hysterectomy is required.

Description of Procedure (01963)

The patient is taken to the operating room and placed on the table in the supine position, with a roll under her right hip. While the usual monitors (eg, ECG, non-invasive blood pressure and a pulse oximeter) are being applied, the patient is given oxygen via a mask and the anesthesia breathing circuit. The patient's abdomen is prepped and draped, and when the obstetrician and the surgical team are ready, general anesthesia is induced while cricoid pressure is being applied. After approximately 45 seconds, the trachea is intubated with a 7-mm oral endotracheal tube with some sight difficulty because of the patient's body habitus and airway architecture. Proper position is assured by seeing condensation in the tube, movement of the chest, auscultation of the lungs, and a satisfactory wave form and numerical value on the end-tidal CO_2 monitor. Oxygen, nitrous oxide, and desflurane are administered via the endotracheal tube.

The operative delivery is accomplished within approximately 5 minutes; the baby is given to the attending neonatologist. Additional thiopental, fentanyl, and rocuronium are administered intravenously, and oxytocin is added to the intravenous solution. An 18-gauge oro-gastric tube is inserted to decompress the stomach.

The obstetrician reports that the uterine tone is not satisfactory, and 4 mg of blood vessel constrictor is administered intramuscularly. More than the usual amount of bleeding is occurring and the obstetrician is concerned that in trying to separate the placenta, a tear in the lateral wall of the uterus has occurred. Except for a slight increase in the patient's pulse rate, the vital signs remain stable. Methergine is given intramuscularly, and the blood bank is called and 4 units of packed red blood cells (PRBC) are ordered. Another 18-gauge intravenous catheter is inserted in the patient's right forearm, and an esophageal stethoscope/temperature probe is inserted into her esophagus.

Over the next 10 minutes the bleeding continues and the exact origin cannot be identified. The obstetrician asks a colleague who is finishing a vaginal delivery to assist; they agree that in the face of not being able to control the bleeding, a hysterectomy is necessary. While the second obstetrician remains scrubbed, the patient's obstetrician steps outside to explain the situation to the patient's husband.

The anesthesiologist has called for two fluid warming devices and an upper body forced air-warming blanket; when they arrive, they are immediately employed.

The patient's blood pressure has dropped into the 80s and her pulse rate is 110-120. The blood loss at this time is estimated to be 2000 cc. The four units of PRBC arrive, and after being checked by the circulator and the anesthesiologist, two units are immediately hung. The blood bank is asked to stay four units of PRBC ahead.

The primary obstetrician has returned, and an emergency hysterectomy is initiated. Once the blood supply to the uterus has been identified and ligated, the bleeding is controlled; by this time the blood loss is thought to be approximately 2500 cc. Two additional units of PRBC are administered. The blood pressure has stabilized at 104-112 mm Hg systolic, and the pulse rate is in the low 90s. The anesthetic continues to be a combination of intravenous drugs and inhalation anesthesia.

The hysterectomy is completed, and a posterior lateral tear in the uterine wall is seen; this is identified as the site of the bleeding. The abdomen is explored to be sure that no surgical packs/sponges were retained, and the abdomen is closed.

The patient's temperature is 35.5°C, and her other vital signs are stable. Her urine, somewhat pink in color, is flowing at about 60 cc per hour. Following closure of the abdomen, the inhalation anesthesia is discontinued and the residual paralysis reversed. When the patient's mental status, respiratory effort, and head lift are judged adequate, the endotracheal tube is removed.

The patient is moved to a recovery stretcher and taken to the Post-Anesthesia Care Unit (PACU) while being administered oxygen via a face mask. The anesthesiologist gives report to the PACU nurse, including reviewing the blood products (four units of PRBC) and fluids she received, and told her of the four units of PRBC remaining in the blood bank. The patient's vital signs are taken and are acceptable. After discussing the plans for pain management, monitoring and fluid administration with the obstetrician, the anesthesiologist leaves word with the PACU nurse as to how he can be reached, and returns to the labor and delivery suite.

Clinical Example (01964)

A 22-year-old unmarried female discovers she is pregnant. For a variety of reasons, she does not wish to have a child at this point in her life. At approximately 8 weeks estimated gestational age, she consults her obstetrician about an elective termination of the pregnancy. Except for some seasonal reactive airway disease, she is in otherwise good health.

Description of Procedure (01964)

An 18-gauge intravenous (IV) catheter is inserted in her left forearm; she is given 2 mg of midazolam and 10 mg of metoclopramide and taken to the operating room (OR). After moving to the OR table, ECG, non-invasive blood pressure, and pulse oximetry monitors are attached. She breathes 100% oxygen by mask, and anesthesia is induced. Anesthetic is added to the inspired oxygen, and she is ventilated by hand. After approximately 60 seconds, a #4 laryngeal mask airway (LMA) is inserted. Proper positioning is assured by chest movement and a satisfactory wave form and numerical value on the end-tidal CO_2 monitor. The patient is gently ventilated by hand for an additional 4 to 5 minutes before spontaneous respirations resume.

The patient is put in the lithotomy position, and after a vaginal prep, the procedure commences. At the request of the surgeon, oxytocin is added to the solution that is infusing via the IV.

The procedure lasts 20 minutes. At the conclusion of the procedure, the patient was placed in the supine position. The inhalation anesthesia is discontinued when the surgeon announces that she had completed the procedure. The patient is still breathing spontaneously and the LMA is removed 1 or 2 minutes later.

The patient is moved to a recovery stretcher and taken to the Post-Anesthesia Care Unit (PACU). Report is given to the PACU nurse as the monitors are being applied. After assuring that the patient's condition is satisfactory, the anesthesiologist gives his pager number to the PACU nurse and leaves to see his next patient.

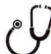

Clinical Example (01968)

A 30-year-old primiparous female with an estimated fetal age of 41 weeks is admitted for induction of labor following spontaneous rupture of membranes. At the request of both the obstetrician and the patient herself, the anesthesiologist has been consulted for additional pain management of labor. A lumbar epidural has been placed. The patient's labor, augmented by oxytocin infusion, has progressed to a complete dilation of the cervix. After 3 hours of pushing, the presence of a fever of 101°F, failure of the fetal head to descend adequately into the pelvis and a loss of fetal heart tone variability, the obstetrician has decided to perform a cesarean section.

Description of Procedure (01968)

While monitoring maternal blood pressure and fetal heart rate, the patient is positioned for epidural insertion. In the lumbar area, the skin is prepped with an antiseptic solution, sterile drapes are applied, and the skin is infiltrated with local anesthetic. Using delicate technique, an 18-gauge epidural needle is inserted at the L2-3 interspace and, using a loss of resistance technique, the epidural space is identified. A 20-gauge epidural catheter is passed through the needle and advanced into the epidural space. The introducer needle is then withdrawn, and the catheter is taped into position. A 3-cc test dose is injected through the epidural catheter, and the patient is observed for onset of anesthesia or the development of maternal tachycardia. An initial dose of anesthetic/analgesic is given, and an infusion pump is programmed. Blood pressure, fetal heart rate, and dermatome level of analgesia are regularly checked. A time-based anesthesia record is developed to record expected and unexpected changes in blood pressure and fetal heart rates. The progress of labor is monitored. The patient is visited regularly by the anesthesiologist and the infusion adjusted to meet the analgesic needs of the patient. After 7 hours of epidural infusion, the patient is noted to be completely dilated, though the fetal vertex remains high. The labor nurse reports that there is a moderate amount of meconium staining. Maternal efforts to push the baby out are begun. After 3 hours of excellent maternal efforts at pushing, the fetal heart tones are noted to have increased to 190 beats per minute with a loss of variability, and the fetal vertex remains high in the pelvis. The maternal temperature is 101.6°F. The obstetrician advises the parents that delivery by cesarean section is indicated. The anesthesiologist again reviews the notes of the labor nurse and discusses the alternatives of anesthesia for the planned cesarean section with the patient. Epidural anesthesia, using the already functioning epidural catheter, is recommended.

The consent for surgery having been signed, the epidural infusion and the oxytocin infusion are discontinued, while 30 cc of antacid is given orally to the patient. The surgical suite is checked to ensure proper functioning of the anesthesia machine, the adequacy of the oxygen supply, the presence of suction equipment, and the preparation of anesthesia drugs, especially those to induce general anesthesia should it be necessary. The patient is then transferred to the operating suite, using care to protect against dislodgment of the epidural catheter. The patient moves easily to the operating table, where blood pressure, ECG, and pulse oximetry monitors are applied. Oxygen is provided by mask. Fetal heart tones are checked. Parenteral anesthetic is injected through the epidural catheter to achieve a level of surgical anesthesia. A rolled towel is placed under the patient's right flank to achieve lateral displacement of the uterus from the vena cava. The patient is prepped and draped for surgery. Intravenous fluids are administered in amounts to meet surgical blood loss and maintenance requirements. Lower blood pressure is anticipated due to the sympathetic blockage as a part of the epidural anesthesia. Upon delivery of the baby, intravenous oxytocin and antibiotics are given. Following cessation of surgery, a narcotic analgesic is injected through the epidural catheter to enhance postoperative analgesia. The patient is transferred to a bed and transported to the postanesthesia care unit.

Vital signs, dermatome level of anesthesia, oxygen saturation, and adequacy of ventilation are determined. A verbal report of the patient's condition is provided to the postanesthesia care nurse. Supplemental analgesia is provided with intravenous narcotics. Fluids and vasopressors are administered as necessary to maintain adequate blood pressure and urine output. After the level of epidural anesthesia has subsided, and after stabilization and achievement of adequate analgesia, the patient is discharged to the postpartum unit.

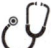 **Clinical Example (01969)**

The patient is a 34-year-old woman who is pregnant for the third time. Her first child was delivered vaginally, but because of dysfunctional labor and a non-reassuring fetal heart rate, the second child was delivered by cesarean section. For both deliveries, she had an epidural. After considering the advantages, disadvantages, and risks, the patient and her obstetrician decide that she is a reasonable candidate for a vaginal birth after cesarean section (VBAC).

Description of Procedure (01969)

The anesthesiologist arrives shortly after being called, and positions and preps the patient for the initiation of an epidural analgesic. After prepping the lumbar area, a local anesthetic is injected at the L3-4 interspace to lessen the discomfort of the epidural needle. A 17-gauge epidural needle is inserted into the epidural space, using the loss of resistance technique to identify the space. A test dose of anesthetic is injected through the needle. When no sign of an intravenous or subarachnoid injection appears, additional anesthetic is injected through the needle. An 18-gauge, bullet-tipped, multi-orifice catheter is then passed through the needle so that approximately 4 cm is in the epidural space. A continuous infusion of anesthetic/analgesic is started. The patient's vital signs are monitored every 5 minutes for 30 minutes; the patient begins to experience pain relief after about three contractions and is quite comfortable within about 12 minutes.

Over the next 3 hours, the patient's labor progresses without incident. However, at about 1300 hours, the character of the contractions changes, the fetal heart rate begins to show late decelerations, and the baseline rate begins to slow. The obstetrician is called, and based on the changes in the monitors, it is decided that an urgent cesarean section is indicated. While awaiting transfer to the labor and delivery operating room, a urinary catheter is inserted, and another large-bore peripheral IV catheter is inserted. The blood bank is called and 4 units of packed red blood cells are ordered. It is decided that since the exact cause of the fetal distress is unclear, and because of the need for delivery as quickly as possible, the epidural will not be "topped up" for delivery but that a general anesthetic will be administered.

The patient is moved to the operating room and placed on the OR table. As the monitors are being placed and the abdomen prepped, supplemental oxygen is administered by mask. When the patient has been draped and the obstetricians are ready to make the incision, general anesthesia is induced and the patient anesthetically paralyzed, while an assistant is applying cricoid pressure. The trachea is intubated and proper placement of the tube ensured by auscultation of both lungs and the presence of a satisfactory end-tidal CO_2 wave form. Volatile anesthetics were given via the endotracheal tube.

The obstetrician, upon entering the abdominal cavity, discovered that there is a tear in the uterus through the previous cesarean scar. The uterine tear is extended and the baby delivered into the wound. The baby's oropharynx is suctioned while the umbilical cord is cut, and the baby is given to the neonatologist in attendance. The baby's 1-minute Apgar score is 6 and the 5-minute score, 9. An additional dose of anesthetic is given. Oxytocin is added to one of the IV solutions that is being rapidly infused.

The uterus remains relatively flaccid, and a blood vessel constrictor is given intramuscularly. The state of the uterus does not change, and the patient is losing significant amounts of blood. The obstetrician, unable to stop the hemorrhage, and with the agreement of the obstetrician who is assisting, decides to do an emergency hysterectomy. The charge nurse, who is in the operating room assisting the circulating nurse, is sent to inform the husband of the problem and the plan to resolve it.

The patient's blood pressure is in the 70-80 mm Hg systolic range. As she is still bleeding, she is given a total of 6 units of PRBCs, in addition to more balanced salt solution. The hysterectomy is accomplished, and the bleeding stops. The hemodynamic status of the patient stabilizes, and there is no further bleeding nor signs of clotting problems. Arterial blood gas analysis shows no problems with oxygenation or ventilation, and the hematocrit is 29%. Blood sent for clotting studies shows only a slightly prolonged PT and PTT; the platelet count is normal. The fluids and blood have been run through a warmer, and the patient's temperature is 36°C.

The abdomen is closed, and the patient emerges from the anesthetic. When her spontaneous respirations are judged adequate and she is able to respond to verbal commands, the endotracheal tube is removed. She is observed in the operating room for approximately 10 minutes, then transferred to the intensive care unit (ICU) for close monitoring.

The anesthesiologist accompanies the patient to the ICU and reports to the ICU staff members the information they need to assume care of the patient. Initial postoperative pain management orders using the indwelling epidural are provided.

Other Procedures

●**01991**   Anesthesia for diagnostic or therapeutic nerve blocks and injections (when block or injection is performed by a different provider); other than the prone position

●**01992**   prone position

▶(Do not report code 01991 or 01992 in conjunction with 99141)◀

Rationale

Codes 01991 and 01992 were established to describe and report anesthesia services for diagnostic or therapeutic nerve blocks and injections with the patient in the prone or other positions, when a block or injection is performed by a different provider.

The anesthesia work involved in delivering this service may differ dramatically from the typical work associated with the currently available codes.

Since the work involved in delivering the typical anesthesia service for nerve blocks or injections differs depending on patient position, with the prone position entailing significantly more work and risk, codes were created to better describe the anesthesia services for the family of surgical services involving nerve blocks and injections.

Clinical Example (01991)

A 47-year-old woman presents to the pain clinic with chronic pain in the left buttock and leg. She has had three previous lumbar spine procedures including microdiscectomy, decompressive lumbar laminectomy, and posterior lumbar interbody arthrodesis and pedicle screw fixation. Her buttock and leg pain persisted and she failed a dorsal column stimulator trial. She also suffers from an anxiety disorder. The pain physician determines that the patient has neuropathic pain and a trial of epidural opioids and/or alpha-2 agonists via indwelling lumbar epidural catheter (CPT code 62319) is indicated. If successful, the physician will recommend implantation of a subarachnoid drug delivery system. The patient had a very unpleasant experience with the dorsal column stimulator and insists upon general anesthesia for the epidural catheter placement. General anesthesia in the lateral position is planned.

Description of Procedure (01991)

The patient is taken to the operating room where she is met by the anesthesiologist, who has already completed the anesthetic machine checkout and prepared the anesthetic medications. After ensuring adequate intravenous access, the anesthesiologist applies monitors, including a non-invasive blood pressure cuff, a pulse oximeter, and a three-lead electrocardiogram. The patient receives oxygen via a face mask for about 5 minutes, followed by a general anesthetic and a short-acting muscle relaxant after the ability to ventilate by mask is confirmed. The anesthesiologist performs direct laryngoscopy and intubates the patient without difficulty. Auscultation of the lungs and monitoring of end-tidal carbon dioxide levels confirms tracheal intubation. After securing the endotracheal tube with tape and taping the eyelids closed, the patient is placed in the lateral decubitus position with an axillary roll.

The anesthesiologist reviews the patient position to ensure that peripheral nerves are adequately protected from injury. A skin temperature probe is applied. The circulating nurse prepares the lumbar region with an iodine-based solution and the operating physician sterilely drapes the field. During the operative phase of the procedure, the anesthesiologist completes the anesthetic record while monitoring the patient's oxygenation, blood pressure, heart rate, temperature, and end-tidal carbon dioxide levels. He adjusts the anesthetic drug delivery to match the level of surgical stimulation. If the surgeon injects any substances before emergence from anesthesia, the anesthesiologist monitors the patient for any adverse sequelae. Once the surgeon successfully places the epidural catheter and a dressing is applied by the circulating nurse, the anesthesiologist supervises repositioning of the patient to the supine position. Anesthetic drug delivery is discontinued and emergence proceeds uneventfully. The anesthesiologist employs a neuromuscular stimulator to determine adequate spontaneous recovery from the non-depolarizing neuromuscular blocker used to facilitate intubation.

Once the anesthesiologist determines that the patient has adequate protective airway reflexes, he removes the endotracheal tube. After a brief period of monitoring in the operating room, the patient is taken to the post-anesthesia care unit in stable condition. The nurse obtains admitting vital signs and the anesthesiologist provides a report to the nurse summarizing the history and anesthetic course. The anesthesiologist prescribes medications to treat pain and post-operative nausea and vomiting on an as-needed basis.

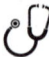

Clinical Example (01992)

A 67-year-old man with lumbar facet syndrome demonstrated by previous diagnostic lumbar facet injections at L4-5 bilaterally presents to the pain clinic for radiofrequency medial branch neurolysis at L3, L4, and L5 bilaterally in the prone position (CPT codes 64622 and 64623). Due to the patient's history of obesity, obstructive sleep apnea, and right heart failure, the pain physician requests anesthesia care from the department of anesthesiology.

Description of Procedure (01992)

The patient is taken to the operating room where he is met by the anesthesiologist, who has already completed the anesthetic machine checkout and prepared the anesthetic medications. After ensuring adequate intravenous access, the anesthesiologist applies monitors, including a non-invasive blood pressure cuff, a pulse oximeter, and a three-lead electrocardiogram. The patient receives oxygen via a face mask for about 5 minutes, followed by a general anesthetic and a short-acting muscle relaxant after the ability to ventilate by mask is confirmed. The anesthesiologist performs direct laryngoscopy and intubates the patient without difficulty. Auscultation of the lungs and monitoring of end-tidal carbon dioxide levels confirms tracheal intubation. After securing the endotracheal tube with tape and taping the eyelids closed, the patient is placed in the prone position. Padding has been pre-placed to provide appropriate positioning for the procedure without impeding respiratory excursion. The anesthesiologist reviews the patient position to ensure that peripheral nerves are adequately protected from injury. In addition, the anesthesiologist confirms the presence of lung sounds and determines that ventilatory pressures are not excessive. A skin temperature probe is applied. The circulating nurse prepares the lumbar region with an iodine-based solution and the operating physician sterilely drapes the field. During the operative phase of the procedure, the anesthesiologist completes the anesthetic record while monitoring the patient's oxygenation, blood pressure, heart rate, temperature, and end-tidal carbon dioxide levels. He adjusts the anesthetic drug delivery to match the level of surgical stimulation. If the surgeon injects any local anesthetics before the patient's emergence from anesthesia, the anesthesiologist monitors the patient for any adverse sequelae. Once the surgeon successfully lesion the medial branch nerves at the desired levels and a dressing is applied by the circulating nurse, the anesthesiologist supervises repositioning of the patient to the supine position. Anesthetic drug delivery is discontinued and emergence from the anesthetic proceeds uneventfully.

The anesthesiologist employs a neuromuscular stimulator to determine adequate spontaneous recovery from the non-depolarizing neuromuscular blocker used to facilitate intubation. Once the anesthesiologist determines that the patient has adequate protective airway reflexes, he removes the endotracheal tube. After a brief period of monitoring in the operating room, the patient is taken to the post-anesthesia care unit in stable condition. The nurse obtains admitting vital signs and the anesthesiologist provides a report to the nurse summarizing the history and anesthetic course. The anesthesiologist prescribes medications to treat pain and post-operative nausea and vomiting on an as-needed basis.

▲ 01996   Daily hospital management of epidural or subarachnoid continuous drug administration

▶(Report code 01996 for daily hospital management of continuous epidural or subarachnoid drug administration performed after insertion of an epidural or subarachnoid catheter placed primarily for anesthesia administration during an operative session, but retained for post-operative pain management)◀

 Rationale

This code descriptor was revised. The parenthetical instruction was added to make a distinction between subsequent day(s) management of an epidural or subarachnoid catheter that primarily served to deliver the anesthetic for a surgical procedure and that same management care for an epidural or subarachnoid catheter that was placed for postoperative pain control. A corresponding instruction has been added to codes 62318/62319.

Surgery

In a return to previous layout conventions for this publication, the codes to be referenced will be found in the numerical order by code. Due to space considerations, the codes affected by the modifier '-63' issue are listed with a reference to page 244, where the rationale for it can be found.

Major changes this year include further refinement of the needle aspiration codes, the Spine (Vertebral Column) subsection guidelines and the guidelines for the Spine/Spinal Cord subsections to include further instructions for the modifier '-62,' the addition and correlating revision of left ventricular pacing codes and Pacemaker or Pacing Cardioverter-Defibrillator guidelines, and addition of a code to report harvest of femoropopliteal vein with the correlating revisions of the guidelines for the coronary bypass procedures. Other changes include many new hematology codes to report apheresis and bone marrow/stem cell services, addition of codes to the CPT code set to represent services previously reported only with HCPCS 'G' codes, and the addition of many new codes to the Urology and Female Genital subsections of the CPT code set.

Surgery

General

10021 Fine needle aspiration; without imaging guidance

10022 with imaging guidance

(For radiological supervision and interpretation, see 76003, 76360, ▶76393,◀ 76942)

(For percutaneous needle biopsy ▶other than fine needle aspiration◀, see ▶20206 for muscle, 32400 for pleura,◀ 32405 for lung ▶or mediastinum, 42400 for salivary gland◀, 47000, 47001 for liver, 48102 for pancreas, 49180 for abdominal or retroperitoneal mass, ▶60100 for thyroid, 62269 for spinal cord)◀

 Rationale

For *CPT 2002*, various cross-references were revised, codes were relocated, and a new subsection was added to clarify that the fine needle aspiration procedures located in the Pathology and Laboratory section were intended to report the actual performance of the biopsy, as opposed to laboratory-based procedures/services, or procedures performed only by pathologists, which placement in this section of the book seemed to indicate. In addition, the descriptor language for the relocated fine needle aspiration codes was refined to delineate fine needle aspiration procedures performed with and without imaging, and appropriate cross-references were added/revised following certain (but not all) anatomically specific percutaneous needle biopsy CPT codes.

At this time, in continuing to refine these codes, the language of the parenthetical note following codes 10021-10022, which references other needle aspiration procedures, was expanded to delineate the intent and use of the fine needle aspiration codes versus the anatomically specific percutaneous needle biopsy codes. The explanatory note following the fine needle aspiration codes 10021 and 10022 has been revised to include "percutaneous needle biopsy for other than fine needle aspiration," referencing codes for core biopsies of the muscle, pleura, mediastinum, salivary gland, thyroid, and spinal cord procedures. The radiological imaging cross-reference following codes 10021-10022 was revised to include a reference to the code for magnetic resonance imaging for fine needle aspiration procedures.

Integumentary System

Skin, Subcutaneous and Accessory Structures

EXCISION—BENIGN LESIONS

Excision (including simple closure) of benign lesions of skin ▶(eg, neoplasm,◀ cicatricial, fibrous, inflammatory, congenital, cystic lesions) ▶includes◀ local anesthesia. See appropriate size and body area below. ▶For shave removal, see 11300 et seq., and for electrosurgical and other methods see 17000 et seq.◀

Excision is defined as full-thickness (through the dermis) removal of ▶a lesion, including margins,◀ and includes simple (non-layered) closure ▶when performed. Report separately each benign lesion excised. Code selection is determined by measuring the greatest clinical diameter of the apparent lesion plus that margin required for complete excision (lesion diameter plus the most narrow margins required equals the excised diameter). The margins refer to the most narrow margin required to adequately excise the lesion, based on the physician's judgment. The measurement of lesion plus margin is made prior to excision. The excised diameter is the same whether the surgical defect is repaired in a linear fashion, or reconstructed (eg, with a skin graft).◀

The closure of defects created by incision, excision, or trauma may require intermediate or complex closure. Repair by intermediate or complex closure should be reported separately. ▶For excision of benign lesions requiring more than simple closure, ie, requiring intermediate or complex closure, report 11400-11466 in addition to appropriate intermediate (12031-12057) or complex closure (13100-13153) codes. For reconstructive closure, see 11400-14300, 15000-15261, 15570-15770. See Integumentary System guidelines for definition of intermediate or complex closure.◀

▲11400   Excision, benign lesion including margins, except skin tag (unless listed elsewhere), trunk, arms or legs; excised diameter 0.5 cm or less

▲11401   excised diameter 0.6 to 1.0 cm

▲11402   excised diameter 1.1 to 2.0 cm

▲11403   excised diameter 2.1 to 3.0 cm

▲11404   excised diameter 3.1 to 4.0 cm

▲11406   excised diameter over 4.0 cm

▲11420   Excision, benign lesion including margins, except skin tag (unless listed elsewhere), scalp, neck, hands, feet, genitalia; excised diameter 0.5 cm or less

▲11421   excised diameter 0.6 to 1.0 cm

▲11422   excised diameter 1.1 to 2.0 cm

▲11423   excised diameter 2.1 to 3.0 cm

▲11424   excised diameter 3.1 to 4.0 cm

▲11426   excised diameter over 4.0 cm

▲11440   Excision, other benign lesion including margins (unless listed elsewhere), face, ears, eyelids, nose, lips, mucous membrane; excised diameter 0.5 cm or less

▲11441   excised diameter 0.6 to 1.0 cm

▲11442   excised diameter 1.1 to 2.0 cm

▲ 11443   excised diameter 2.1 to 3.0 cm

▲ 11444   excised diameter 3.1 to 4.0 cm

▲ 11446   excised diameter over 4.0 cm

EXCISION—MALIGNANT LESIONS

Excision (including simple closure) of malignant ►lesions◄ of skin ►(eg, basal cell carcinoma, squamous cell carcinoma, melanoma) includes◄ local anesthesia. ►(See appropriate size and body area below.)◄ For ►destruction◄ of malignant lesions of skin, see destruction codes ►17260-17286◄.

Excision is defined as full-thickness (through the dermis) removal of ►a lesion including margins, and includes simple (non-layered) closure when performed. Report separately each malignant lesion excised. Code selection is determined by measuring the greatest clinical diameter of the apparent lesion plus that margin required for complete excision (lesion diameter plus the most narrow margins required equals the excised diameter). The margins refer to the most narrow margin required to adequately excise the lesion, based on the physician's judgment. The measurement of lesion plus margin is made prior to excision. The excised diameter is the same whether the surgical defect is repaired in a linear fashion, or reconstructed (eg, with a skin graft).◄

The closure of defects created by incision, excision, or trauma may require intermediate or complex closure. Repair by intermediate or complex closure should be reported separately. ►For excision of malignant lesions requiring more than simple closure, ie, requiring intermediate or complex closure, report 11600-11646 in addition to appropriate intermediate (12031-12057) or complex closure (13100-13153) codes. For reconstructive closure, see 14000-14300, 15000-15261, 15570-15770.◄ See Integumentary System guidelines for definition of intermediate or complex closure.

►When frozen section pathology shows the margins of excision were not adequate, an additional excision may be necessary for complete tumor removal. Use only one code to report the additional excision and re-excision(s) based on the final widest excised diameter required for complete tumor removal at the same operative session. To report a re-excision procedure performed to widen margins at a subsequent operative session, see codes 11600-11646, as appropriate. Append modifier '-58' if the re-excision procedure is performed during the postoperative period of the primary excision procedure.◄

▲ 11600   Excision, malignant lesion including margins, trunk, arms, or legs; excised diameter 0.5 cm or less

▲ 11601   excised diameter 0.6 to 1.0 cm

▲ 11602   excised diameter 1.1 to 2.0 cm

▲ 11603   excised diameter 2.1 to 3.0 cm

▲ 11604   excised diameter 3.1 to 4.0 cm

▲11606   excised diameter over 4.0 cm

▲11620   Excision, malignant lesion including margins, scalp, neck, hands, feet, genitalia; excised diameter 0.5 cm or less

▲11621   excised diameter 0.6 to 1.0 cm

▲11622   excised diameter 1.1 to 2.0 cm

▲11623   excised diameter 2.1 to 3.0 cm

▲11624   excised diameter 3.1 to 4.0 cm

▲11626   excised diameter over 4.0 cm

▲11640   Excision, malignant lesion including margins, face, ears, eyelids, nose, lips; excised diameter 0.5 cm or less

▲11641   excised diameter 0.6 to 1.0 cm

▲11642   excised diameter 1.1 to 2.0 cm

▲11643   excised diameter 2.1 to 3.0 cm

▲11644   excised diameter 3.1 to 4.0 cm

▲11646   excised diameter over 4.0 cm

(For eyelids involving more than skin, see also 67800 et seq.)

MEASURING AND CODING THE REMOVAL OF A LESION

Measuring lesion removal

*A. Example: excision, malignant lesion of the back, 1.0 centimeters. Code 11606.

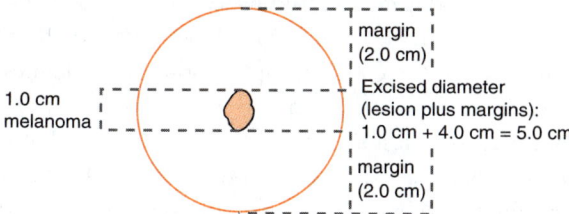

*B. Example: excision of benign lesion of the neck, 1.0 centimeter by 2.0 centimeters. Code 11423.

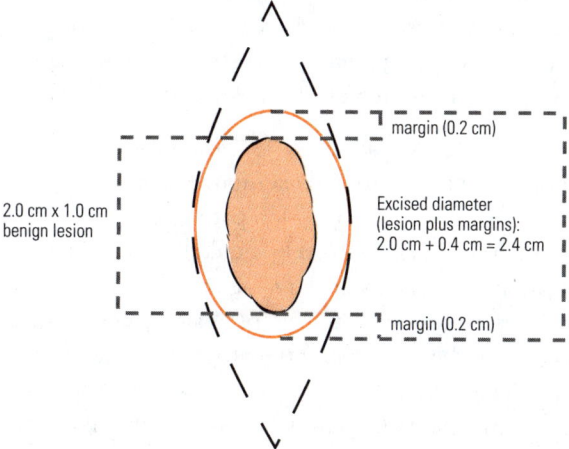

*C. Example: excision, malignant lesion of the nose, 0.9 centimeters with skin margins of 0.6 centimeters. Code 11642.

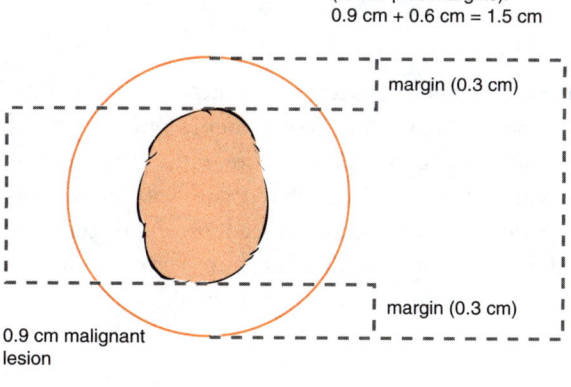

* Please note that these captions have been revised since the *CPT 2003 Professional Edition* was published.

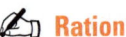 **Rationale**

The excision codes included in this section were revised due to confusion regarding the appropriate use of these codes, including the appropriate method of reporting "re-excision" of a diameter of skin. The codes now reflect a full-thickness (through the dermis) removal of a lesion, including margins, and include simple (non-layered) closure when performed. These codes are reported separately for each benign or malignant lesion excised. To clarify this, language has been included in the code descriptors and the guidelines that precede the section, each identifying inclusion of the margins as part of the measurement. In addition, the word "lesion" was replaced by "excised" to identify that the measurement is not limited to the lesion size alone. Both the Excision—Benign Lesions and the Excision—Malignant Lesions sections also include descriptive language that specifies intended use of these codes. These guidelines and descriptor language identify what is included as part of the excision (the greatest clinical diameter of the lesion and the margins), define what is included as part of the margin (the most narrow margin required to adequately excise the lesion, based on the physician's judgment, which equals the excised diameter), and identify when the measurement is made (prior to excision).

In addition, language was added to the Excision—Malignant Lesions section to identify how to report additional excisions performed as a result of inadequate margin excision. When frozen section pathology reveals margin excisions that are not adequate, a single excision code should be used to report the additional excision and re-excision(s) necessary at the same operative session. Similarly, re-excision procedures performed to widen margins at subsequent operative sessions should be reported by using the code appropriate to identify the size, location, and type of excision performed. The '-58' modifier should be appended if the re-excision is performed during the post-operative period of the primary excision procedure.

Repair (Closure)

OTHER FLAPS AND GRAFTS

▲ **15756** Free muscle or myocutaneous flap with microvascular anastomosis

 Rationale

To provide consistency between the nomenclature for code 15756 and other flap codes that include "cutaneous" components, and to clarify that code 15756 is intended to report a skin flap procedure, rather than a skin graft, code 15756 has been editorially revised to differentiate between the use of skin "flap" (myocutaneous) and skin "graft" procedures. As the code descriptor was previously written, the phrase "with or without skin" was often misinterpreted as describing skin grafts rather than myocutaneous flaps.

Destruction

MOHS MICROGRAPHIC SURGERY

Mohs micrographic surgery, for the removal of complex or ill-defined skin cancer, requires a single physician to act in two integrated, but separate and distinct capacities: surgeon and pathologist. If either of these responsibilities is delegated to another physician who reports his services separately, these codes are not appropriate. If repair is performed, use separate repair, flap, or graft codes. ►If a biopsy of a suspected skin cancer is performed on the same day as Mohs surgery because there was no prior pathology confirmation of a diagnosis, then report diagnostic skin biopsy (11100, 11101) and frozen section pathology (88331) with modifier '-59' to distinguish from the subsequent definitive surgical procedure of Mohs surgery.◄

⊘▲17304 Chemosurgery (Mohs micrographic technique), including removal of all gross tumor, surgical excision of tissue specimens, mapping, color coding of specimens, microscopic examination of specimens by the surgeon, and complete histopathological preparation including the first routine stain (eg, hematoxylin and eosin, toluidine blue); first stage, fresh tissue technique, up to 5 specimens

►(If additional special pathology procedures, stains or immunostains are required, use 88311-88314, 88342)◄

⊘17305 second stage, fixed or fresh tissue, up to 5 specimens

⊘17306 third stage, fixed or fresh tissue, up to 5 specimens

⊘17307 additional stage(s), up to 5 specimens, each stage

+▲17310 each additional specimen, after the first 5 specimens, fixed or fresh tissue, any stage (List separately in addition to code for primary procedure)

►(Use 17310 in conjunction with codes 17304-17307)◄

Rationale

The Mohs microsurgery codes are unique in the CPT code set in that they are the only codes that combine surgical and pathological services by the same provider in the same code. The revisions for *CPT 2003* serve to further clarify the services represented by this unusual series of codes. The Mohs surgery guidelines were revised to clarify that, if a biopsy of a suspected lesion was performed prior to the more definitive Mohs procedure because no pathology confirmation of a diagnosis had yet been performed, then it would be appropriate to report the codes for the diagnostic skin biopsy (11100, 11101) and the frozen section pathology (88331). Modifier '-59' should be appended to distinguish the diagnostic biopsy from the more definitive Mohs procedure. This is occasionally necessary for patients who have never had their suspected cancers biopsied, and a diagnosis is necessary before Mohs surgery is begun. Therefore, a skin biopsy and frozen section (88311) performed on the same date of Mohs surgery to confirm skin cancer are reported separately with modifier '-59' appended.

In addition, code 17304 was revised editorially to clarify that the first routine stain is an inherent component of the Mohs chemosurgery procedure and, therefore, not separately reported. The terminology in the descriptor for code 17304, "complete histopathologic preparation," includes the routine tissue staining with hematoxylin and eosin (H&E) and toluidine blue. Special stains are reported in addition to the routine histopathologic preparation and include add-on codes (88312-88314) for histochemical staining with frozen section (88314) and immunocytochemistry (including tissue immunoperoxidase), each antibody (88342). Other procedures performed at the same session as Mohs surgery, such as decalcification of bone and immunostaining for melanoma, are not included in Mohs surgery and would be separately reported with the appropriate codes (eg, 88311-88314, 88342).

The status of code 17310 was changed to that of an add-on code, and the descriptor was revised to clarify that this code is reported once for each additional specimen excised, prepared, and examined over the first five specimens, reported with codes 17304-17307. This revision provides consistency with the descriptor language currently found in other Surgical Pathology code descriptors, with each additional specimen reported separately to reflect the additional pathology work. Code 17304 is generally performed for the most common skin cancers—those that by size require a standard of up to five specimens to completely examine the tissue. However, occasionally Mohs surgery is performed on larger tumors. The examination of the larger tumor may require that more than five specimens will need to be examined per layer.

Finally, a cross-reference was added to indicate that code 17310 should be reported in addition to codes 17304-17307.

Musculoskeletal System

Cast and strapping procedures ...

The services listed below ...

Definitions

The terms "closed treatment," "open treatment," and "percutaneous skeletal fixation" have been carefully chosen to accurately reflect current orthopaedic procedural treatments. ▶Treatment is used when a fracture is stabilized by an intramedullary implant, as this procedure may be performed either "open" or "closed." In "closed" intramedullary nailing, the fracture fragments are not visualized, but an intramedullary nail is inserted across the fracture site, with the aid of x-ray imaging. As such, a closed nailing procedure is neither open (where the fracture site is visualized and reduced under direct vision) nor is it strictly closed (because the fracture hematoma can communicate with the outside environment.◀

Closed treatment specifically means that the fracture site is not surgically opened (exposed to the external environment and directly visualized). This terminology is used to describe procedures that treat fractures by three methods: 1) without manipulation, 2) with manipulation, 3) with or without traction.

Open treatment is used when the ▶fractured bone is either 1)◀ surgically opened (exposed to the external environment) ▶and◀ the fracture (bone ends) visualized and internal fixation may be used ▶or 2) the fractured bone is opened remote from the fracture site in order to insert an intramedullary nail across the fracture site (the fracture site is not opened and visualized).◀

Percutaneous skeletal fixation ...

 Rationale

The definitions for treatment of fracture care in the Musculoskeletal guidelines and the descriptor terminology in the closed and open femoral fracture codes were revised to more accurately describe the various surgical techniques used in current surgical practice. The text added to the Musculoskeletal guidelines further delineates the terms "open" and "closed" as related to the treatment involving intramedullary fixation to assist in selection of the appropriate code when a combination of these techniques is used. These revisions expand the definition of "open" to include those circumstances where the treatment consists of an incision for placement of an intramedullary implant for treatment of a humeral/femoral/tibial fracture for codes 24516, 27245, 27506 and 27759.

General

INTRODUCTION OR REMOVAL

▲ 20550*   Injection(s); tendon sheath, ligament

   20551   tendon origin/insertion

▲ 20552   single or multiple trigger point(s), one or two muscle(s)

▲ 20553   single or multiple trigger point(s), three or more muscle(s)

(If imaging guidance is performed, see 76003, 76393, 76942)

▲ 20600*   Arthrocentesis, aspiration and/or injection; small joint or bursa (eg, fingers, toes)

▲ 20605*   intermediate joint or bursa (eg, temporomandibular, acromioclavicular, wrist, elbow or ankle, olecranon bursa)

● 20612   Aspiration and/or injection of ganglion cyst(s) any location

▶(To report multiple ganglion cyst aspirations/injections, use 20612 and append modifier '-59')◀

 Rationale

In order to allay confusion and assist in the choice of the most accurate code describing the procedure(s) performed, the code series 20550-20553 has been revised to indicate that codes 20552-20553 are reported one time per session, regardless of the number of injections or muscles injected. These changes were accomplished by appending an "(s)" to the term "Injection" and to the term "muscle."

Contrary to CPT convention, although the parent code for this series, 20550, indicates, "Injection(s)," codes 20550 and 20551 should be reported one time for multiple or single injections to a single tendon sheath, ligament, tendon origin or tendon insertion performed. Thus, multiple injections to the same tendon sheaths, tendon origins, tendon insertion, or ligaments would be reported one time only, while injections to multiple tendon sheaths, tendon origins, tendon insertion, or ligaments are reported one time for each injection.

Prior to this year, ganglion cyst procedures were reported with codes 20550, 20600, and 20605. However, the absence of "aspiration" in these code descriptors was a source of confusion in reporting these procedures. Therefore, these codes have been revised, with the deletion of "ganglion cyst" from the code descriptors and the addition of code 20612 to accurately describe the aspiration or injection of ganglion cysts. A cross-reference has also been added to instruct that multiple ganglion cyst aspirations and/or injections performed at the same session should be reported with code 20612 for the additional cyst, appending modifier '-59' to identify the distinct nature of the additional services.

In addition, the parenthetic note for reporting the imaging guidance with codes 76003, 76393, and 76942, which previously followed code 20550, has been moved. It now follows code 20553, as it applies to codes 20550-20553.

Note: These codes continue to be reviewed through the CPT process.

Head

EXCISION

▲ **21030** Excision of benign tumor or cyst of maxilla or zygoma by enucleation and curettage

▲ **21034** Excision of malignant tumor of maxilla or zygoma

▲ **21040** Excision of benign tumor or cyst of mandible, by enucleation and/or curettage

▶(21041 has been deleted. For enucleation and/or curettage of benign cysts or tumors of mandible not requiring osteotomy, use 21040)◀

▶(For excision of benign tumor or cyst of mandible requiring osteotomy, see 21046-21047)◀

Rationale

Codes 21030 and 21040 have been revised to describe surgical management of benign jaw lesions that only require curettage and enucleation. Descriptor language for code 21034 has also been revised to specify maxilla or zygoma malignant tumor excision as opposed to use of the less specific language " ... facial bone other than mandible...." These changes were necessary since there is a significant difference in the surgical procedure for the aggressive benign lesion as opposed to benign jaw lesions that only require curettage and/or enucleation.

● **21046** Excision of benign tumor or cyst of mandible; requiring intra-oral osteotomy (eg, locally aggressive or destructive lesion(s))

● **21047** requiring extra-oral osteotomy and partial mandibulectomy (eg, locally aggressive or destructive lesion(s))

●**21048** Excision of benign tumor or cyst of maxilla; requiring intra-oral osteotomy (eg, locally aggressive or destructive lesion(s))

●**21049** requiring extra-oral osteotomy and partial maxillectomy (eg, locally aggressive or destructive lesion(s))

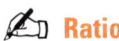
Rationale
A new series of codes (21046-21049) has been added to describe the surgical management of locally aggressive expansile and/or destructive benign lesions of the jaws (ameloblastoma, ameloblastic fibro-odontoma, odontogenic keratocyst, odontogenic myxoma, central giant cell lesions of the jaws). These locally aggressive lesions are classified as benign lesions; however, they require wide radical excisions very comparable to the surgical management of malignant tumors. Usually these defects require stabilization by internal or external fixation systems and reconstruction and simultaneous rehabilitation of the jaws. Code 21041 did not adequately describe the complexity of work involved in the removal of aggressive benign lesions, and thus was deleted with a reference to utilize the new series of codes (21040-21049).

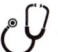
Clinical Example (21046)
A 27-year-old female presents with a 3 x 4-cm radiolucent lesion of the right anterior mandible extending from tooth #26 to #28. Initial biopsy had shown odontogenic myxoma.

Description of Procedure (21046)
Under general anesthesia, utilizing an intra-oral approach, the adjacent teeth #26 and #28 are extracted, and a mandibular osteotomy is performed to resect the lesion with clear 1-cm margins, maintaining continuity of the mandible. The mental nerve is identified and repositioned. Flaps are undermined and advanced to obtain closure. Great attention is used to guarantee hemostasis in the floor of the mouth, after which the defect is packed with iodoform gauze and the flap returned and sutured. Gauze dressing sponges are applied to assist with hemostasis.

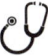
Clinical Example (21047)
A 17-year-old male presents with an abnormal radiodensity in the right mandible, extending from the ramus to the second premolar, from the superior to the inferior border, with displacement of the inferior alveolar nerve to the inferior border of the mandible. He has biopsy-proven juvenile ossifying fibroma. Recent imaging revealed perforation of the lingual and inferior cortices, and displacement of the nerve posteriorly and through the inferior border of the mandible. The lesion extended from the anterior ramus to the mental foramen and involved teeth #29 to #32. Four weeks prior, the teeth in the area were extracted.

Description of Procedure (21047)
Under general anesthesia, a corticocancellous posterior iliac graft with platelet-rich plasma (PRP) is harvested. After bone harvest, the wound is closed in multiple layers and a Jackson Pratte drain is placed. The wound is dressed and the patient is then turned to the supine position, prepped, and draped for the mandibular surgery.

The surgeon and staff re-scrub, re-gown, and re-glove prior to proceeding with the mandibular surgery. Utilizing an extra-oral approach, the mandible is resected from the antegonial notch to the first premolar, with preservation of the nerve. By means of sharp and blunt dissection, access is gained to the inferior border of the mandible, allowing for this resection. Care is taken to identify and preserve the mandibular branch of the facial nerve. Soft tissue specimens are sent for frozen section to guarantee clear margins. After hemostasis and repositioning of the nerve, a mandibular reconstructive plate is applied and the previously harvested cortical cancellous graft is used to reconstruct the defect to give continuity to the mandible. During the surgery, the PRP is prepared and used with the donor bone. The PRP is used in the multiple-layer plastic closure.

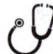

Clinical Example (21048)

A 42-year-old female presents with a "soap bubble" lesion in the anterior maxilla located adjacent to the nasal cavity and the maxillary sinus. Odontogenic keratocyst was diagnosed by biopsy, and medical imaging has shown separation of the cystic lesion from the nasal cavity as well as the maxillary sinus.

Description of Procedure (21048)

Under general anesthesia, a wide surgical excision is made utilizing an intra-oral approach. The excision consists of a peripheral ostectomy and osteotomy to remove the bone adjacent to the lesion to have clear margins. The infra-orbital nerve is identified and great care is necessary to avoid the roots of teeth. The integrity of the maxillary sinus must be maintained. The defect is packed with gauze and the flaps returned and sutured.

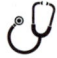

Clinical Example (21049)

A 28-year-old male presents with an expansile lesion of the left maxilla with extension into the infraorbital region. He has biopsy-proven ameloblastic fibro-odontoma. Medical imaging has revealed an 8 x 6-cm radiopaque/radiolucent lesion that originates from the left third molar region and extends into the maxillary sinus with disruption and distortion of the anterior maxillary wall extending above the infraorbital nerve foramen.

Description of Procedure (21049)

Under general anesthesia, utilizing an extraoral approach to access the superior extent of the maxillary tumor, the lesion is resected with a left posterior maxillectomy and appropriate anterior osteotomy to obtain clear margins. Every attempt is made to preserve the infraorbital nerve and reconstruct the maxillary vestibule. A split-thickness skin graft is taken from the lateral thigh, cut, and placed in the defect. The pre-made temporary obturator is loaded with a thermoplastic compound and seated in the defect against the skin graft to customize the superior aspect of the obturator. The appliance is removed and the excess compound is removed. It is heated again and replaced for final contour and to support the skin graft against the surgical defect.

Neck (Soft Tissues) and Thorax

REPAIR, REVISION, AND/OR RECONSTRUCTION

▲21740 Reconstructive repair of pectus excavatum or carinatum; open

●21742   minimally invasive approach (Nuss procedure), without thoracoscopy

●21743   minimally invasive approach (Nuss procedure), with thoracoscopy

 Rationale

Two codes have been added to report the repair of pectus excavatum or carinatum using a minimally invasive approach. The minimally invasive procedure is performed on those children with the most severe conditions and is characterized by two small incisions for access and stabilization and correction of the sternum with a steel bar. The codes are further differentiated to report the performance of the repair with or without thoracoscopy.

Code 21740 is revised to specify that this code is reported for the open approach procedure.

Spine (Vertebral Column)

Cervical, thoracic, and lumbar spine.

Within the Spine section …

To report bone grafts performed after arthrodesis, see codes 20930-20938. Bone graft codes are reported without modifier '-51' (multiple procedure). Do not append modifier '-62' to bone graft codes 20900-20938.

Within the Spine section, instrumentation is reported separately and in addition to arthrodesis. To report instrumentation procedures performed with definitive vertebral procedure(s), see codes 22840-22855. Instrumentation procedure codes 22840-22848 and 22851 are reported in addition to the definitive procedure(s) without modifier '-51.' The modifier '-62' may not be appended to the definitive or add-on spinal instrumentation procedure code(s) 22840▶-22848 and 22850-22852.◀

OSTEOTOMY

To report arthrodesis …

To report instrumentation procedures, see codes 22840-22855. (Report in addition to code(s) for the definitive procedure(s) without modifier '-51.') Do not append modifier '-62' to spinal instrumentation codes 22840-▶22848 and 22850-22852.◀

FRACTURE AND/OR DISLOCATION

To report arthrodesis …

To report instrumentation procedures, see codes 22840-22855. (Report in addition to code(s) for the definitive procedure(s) without modifier '-51.') Do not append modifier '-62' to spinal instrumentation codes 22840-▶22848 and 22850-22852.◀

ARTHRODESIS

Arthrodesis may be performed ...

To report instrumentation procedures, see codes 22840-22855. (Report in addition to code(s) for the definitive procedure(s) without modifier '-51.') Do not append modifier '-62' to spinal instrumentation codes 22840-▶22848 and 22850-22852.◀

POSTERIOR, POSTEROLATERAL OR LATERAL TRANSVERSE PROCESS TECHNIQUE

To report instrumentation procedures, see codes 22840-22855. (Report in addition to code(s) for the definitive procedure(s) without modifier '-51.') Do not append modifier '-62' to spinal instrumentation codes 22840-▶22848 and 22850-22852.◀

SPINE DEFORMITY (EG, SCOLIOSIS, KYPHOSIS)

To report instrumentation procedures, see codes 22840-22855. (Report in addition to code(s) for the definitive procedure(s) without modifier '-51.') Do not append modifier '-62' to spinal instrumentation codes 22840-▶22848 and 22850-22852.◀

SPINAL INSTRUMENTATION

Segmental instrumentation is defined ...

Non-segmental instrumentation ...

Insertion of spinal instrumentation is reported separately and in addition to arthrodesis. Instrumentation procedure codes 22840-22848, 22851 are reported in addition to the definitive procedure(s) without modifier '-51.' Do not append modifier '-62' to spinal instrumentation codes 22840-▶22848 and 22850-22852.◀

 Rationale

In order to further delineate the appropriate use of the modifier '-62' with the spinal instrumentation codes, the Spine (Vertebral Column) subsection guidelines and the guidelines for the Spine/Spinal Cord subsections have been revised to denote that modifier '-62' is appropriately reported with code 22849 for reinsertion of spinal fixation and code 22855 for removal of anterior spinal instrumentation. According to the directions for use of the modifier '-62,' this modifier is appended with:

- any associated add-on code(s) for that procedure as long as both surgeons continue to work together as primary surgeons; and

- additional procedure(s) (including add-on procedure[s]) performed during the same surgical session.

NON-SEGMENTAL SPINAL INSTRUMENTATION (22840)

Fixation at each end of the construct.

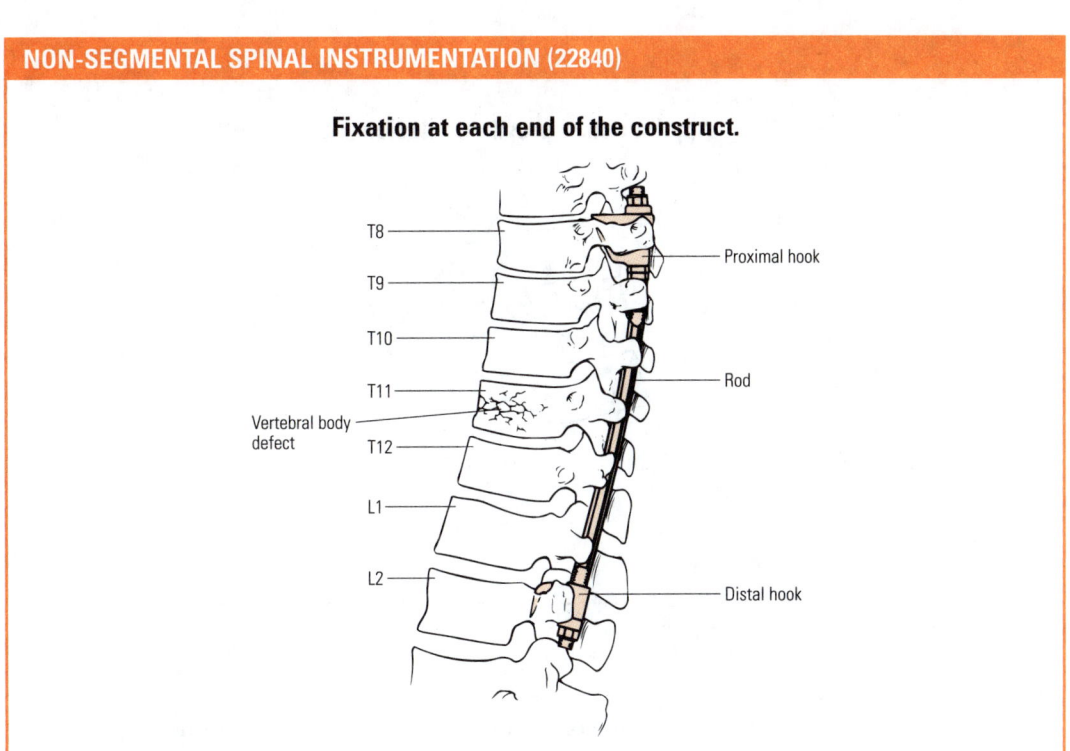

SEGMENTAL SPINAL INSTRUMENTATION (22842-22844)

Fixation at each end of the construct and at least one additional interposed bony attachment.

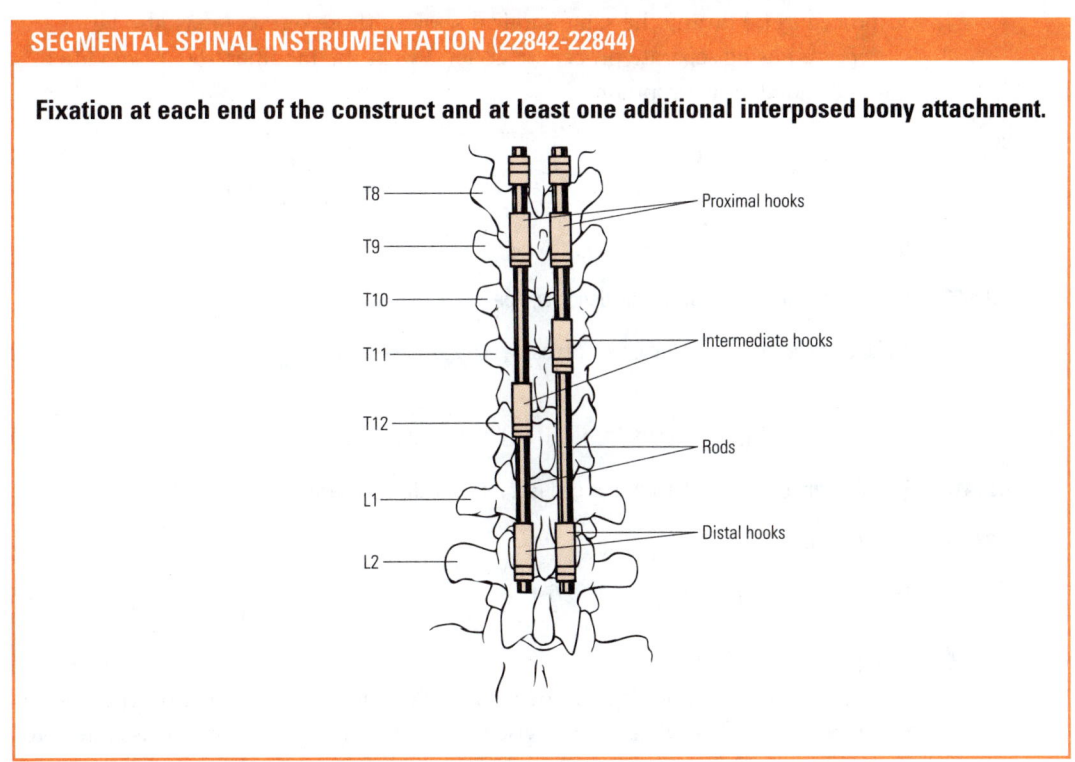

SPINAL PROSTHETIC DEVICES (22851)

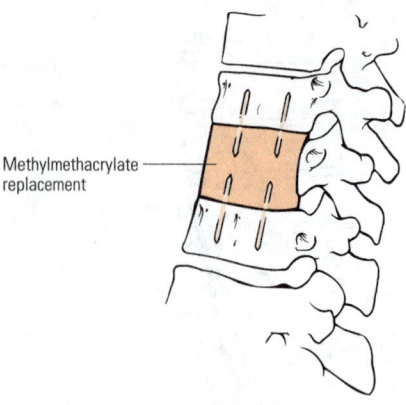

Application of prosthetic device.

Methylmethacrylate replacement

Consistent with previous use of the modifier '-62,' each surgeon should:

- report the co-surgery once using the same procedure code; and
- if a co-surgeon acts as an assistant in the performance of an additional procedure(s) during the same surgical session, those services may also be reported using separate procedure code(s) with the modifier '-80' or modifier '-82' added, as appropriate.

Shoulder

INCISION

23000   Removal of subdeltoid calcareous deposits, open

▶(For arthroscopic removal of bursal deposits, use 29999)◀

REPAIR, REVISION, AND/OR RECONSTRUCTION

▲ **23410**   Repair of ruptured musculotendinous cuff (eg, rotator cuff) open; acute

23412   chronic

▶(For arthroscopic procedure, use 29827)◀

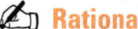 **Rationale**

To accommodate the addition of new code 29827 for reporting arthroscopic rotator cuff repair, code 23410 has been revised to specify that the intent of this code is to report open cuff repair procedures only. A cross-reference has been added to direct users to code 29827 to report the arthroscopic counterpart of this procedure.

Humerus (Upper Arm) and Elbow

FRACTURE AND DISLOCATION

▲24516 Treatment of humeral shaft fracture, with insertion of intramedullary implant, with or without cerclage and/or locking screws

Rationale
Code 24516 was revised to expand the definition of "open" to include those circumstances where the treatment consists of an incision for placement of an intramedullary implant for treatment of a humeral fracture.

Forearm and Wrist

REPAIR, REVISION, AND/OR RECONSTRUCTION

▲25320 Capsulorrhaphy or reconstruction, wrist, open (eg, capsulodesis, ligament repair, tendon transfer or graft) (includes synovectomy, capsulotomy and open reduction) for carpal instability

Rationale
Code 25320 was editorially revised to omit the phrase "any method," and to clarify that this procedure specifically involves an "open" surgical approach. This revision is done as a continuation of the CPT-5 project and specifically addresses the objective to add clarity and precision to CPT code descriptors through more accurate delineation of intent and usage.

Pelvis and Hip Joint

FRACTURE AND DISLOCATION

▲27235 Percutaneous skeletal fixation of femoral fracture, proximal end, neck

▲27244 Treatment of intertrochanteric, pertrochanteric, or subtrochanteric femoral fracture; with plate/screw type implant, with or without cerclage

Rationale
Code 27235 was editorially revised to delete diagnostic references to the displacement severity and the type of fracture for which percutaneous fixation of a femoral fracture is performed. This descriptor is intended for those percutaneous femoral fracture fixation procedures performed with or without exposure of the fracture.

Codes 27244 was editorially revised to more accurately describe the treatment of intertrochanteric, pertrochanteric, or subtrochanteric femoral fractures. This revision expands the definition of "open" to include those circumstances where the treatment consists of an incision for placement of an intramedullary implant for treatment of a femoral fracture.

PERCUTANEOUS TREATMENT OF FEMORAL FRACTURE (27235)

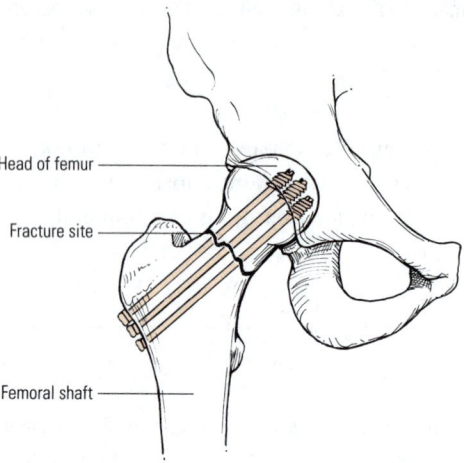

Femoral fracture treatment without fracture exposure.

Femur (Thigh Region) and Knee Joint

REPAIR, REVISION, AND/OR RECONSTRUCTION

▲27425　Lateral retinacular release open

▶(For arthroscopic lateral release, use 29873)◀

Leg (Tibia and Fibula) and Ankle Joint

REPAIR, REVISION, AND/OR RECONSTRUCTION

▲27730　Arrest, epiphyseal (epiphysiodesis), open; distal tibia

27732　　　distal fibula

27734　　　distal tibia and fibula

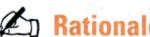 **Rationale**
Codes 27425 and 27730 (the parent descriptor code of 27732, 27734) were editorially revised to omit the phrase "any method" and to clarify that these procedures specifically involve the "open" surgical approach. These revisions are done as a continuation of the CPT-5 project and specifically address the objective to add clarity and precision to CPT code descriptors through more accurate delineation of intent and usage. A cross-reference has been added to code 27425 to instruct appropriate reporting for the arthroscopic counterpart of open approach release of the lateral retinaculum.

FRACTURE AND/OR DISLOCATION

▲27759   Treatment of tibial shaft fracture (with or without fibular fracture) by intramedullary implant, with or without interlocking screws and/or cerclage

Rationale
Code 27759 was revised to expand the definition of "open" to include those circumstances where the treatment consists of an incision for placement of an intramedullary implant for treatment of a tibial fracture.

ARTHRODESIS

▲27870   Arthrodesis, ankle, open

▶(For arthroscopic ankle arthrodesis, use 29899)◀

Rationale
Code 27870 was editorially revised to omit the phrase "any method" and to clarify that this procedure specifically involves an "open" surgical approach. This revision is done as a continuation of the CPT-5 project and specifically addresses the objective to add clarity and precision to CPT code descriptors through more accurate delineation of intent and usage.

Application of Casts and Strapping

LOWER EXTREMITY

Strapping—Any Age

29520   Strapping; hip

29539   knee

▲29540   ankle and/or foot

Rationale
Code 29540 was revised to include strapping procedures of the foot. Prior to this, the CPT book contained codes (29520-29550) to describe casting and strapping procedures for the various anatomical locations of the lower extremity with the exception of the foot. This code is intended to report strapping procedures for treatment of a key area of the lower extremity, for those conditions that require strapping, including strains, sprains, injuries, etc. The procedures for casting and strapping of the foot are contained within the same code as the ankle, because the treatments and the conditions affecting the ankle are often similar in nature.

Endoscopy/Arthroscopy

29806   Arthroscopy, shoulder, surgical; capsulorrhaphy

●29827   with rotator cuff repair

▶(For open or mini-open rotator cuff repair, use 23412)◀

▶(When arthroscopic subacromial decompression is performed at the same setting, use 29826 and append modifier '-51')◀

▶(When arthroscopic distal clavicle resection is performed at the same setting, use 29824 and append modifier '-51')◀

Rationale

Code 29827 was added to describe rotator cuff repair performed using an arthroscopic approach. Three new cross-references were added to instruct the user to appropriate codes for reporting other procedures of the shoulder, including mini-open or open-approach rotator cuff repair and for reporting those procedures that might be performed at the same session, but are not inherent components of rotator cuff repair.

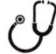

Clinical Example (29827)

A 40-year-old, right-handed stockbroker is an avid tennis player on both weekends and weekdays. He develops insidious pain in the right shoulder, which gradually worsens. He is having problems sleeping on the shoulder and it awakens him if he rolls onto that side. He also complains of significant pain with lifting and overhead work. He visits his orthopedic surgeon and is started on NSAIDs (non-steroidal anti-inflammatory drugs) and physical therapy, which do not provide any relief. A subacromial injection provides short-term relief. A rotator cuff tear is suspected. Surgical intervention is recommended.

Description of Procedure (29827)

A posterior lateral incision is made for the insertion of the arthroscope. Once inserted, the articular surfaces and all intra-articular structures are identified and examined. An anterior portal is created with an inside-out technique after needle localization. A probe is inserted through the anterior cannula and any pathology is confirmed with a probe. Particular attention is given to the subscapularis, the supraspinatus, the infraspinatus and teres minor tendons. If any or all of the above are torn, they are identified and often marked by passing a needle through the anterior cannula and passing a suture through the needle. The suture is grasped and held with a hemostat. A tissue resector is placed through the anterior cannula and the degenerative portion of the tendon(s) is resected. Tendon retraction is addressed by aggressive release of the tethering adhesions. Any repair of the articular portion of the subscapularis is performed at this time. Generally, suture repair, which requires time-consuming and difficult arthroscopic knot tying, is adequate for the subscapularis, and bone anchors are rarely required. The arthroscope is then placed into the subacromial space where the tear is evaluated superiorly. A lateral portal is created after needle localization and one or multiple sutures are placed in the tendon to assure that an adequate release of the adhesions has been performed. Often, a coracohumeral ligament release is required to allow the re-approximation of the supraspinatus tendon back to the greater humeral tuberosity. A fourth arthroscopic portal is needed just off the lateral acromial edge to allow a relatively perpendicular bone anchor placement into a shallow trough, which is created at the lateral humeral articular surface with a bone burr. Margin conversion is performed, which converts an avulsion tear into a vertical tear with a smaller avulsion component. Sutures are placed arthroscopically to recreate the normal anatomy of the tendon and decrease the tendon surface area that is re-attached to the bone. The bone anchors are placed and usually one to four are required. Each bone anchor has two sutures, and the incredibly demanding part of the arthroscopic repair is to pass and tie the sutures. The surgeon's ability to pass and tie arthroscopic sutures accurately and efficiently is the key to the procedure. For large tears, 10 or 12 sutures will be tied. Once the sutures are passed and firmly tied, the cuff is reinspected. The arthroscope is removed and the portals are closed with sutures and a sterile dressing is applied. The patient is transferred to the post-op recovery room.

29871 Arthroscopy, knee, surgical; for infection, lavage, and drainage

●**29873** with lateral release

▶(For open lateral release, use 27425)◀

Rationale
Code 29873 was added to identify surgical arthroscopy of the knee with lateral release. In addition, a cross-reference was added following code 29873 to indicate appropriate reporting for the open-approach counterpart of arthroscopic lateral release.

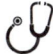
Clinical Example (29873)
A 16-year-old skeletally mature female returns to the office with persistent right knee pain. The knee pain has been persistent for 6 months despite aggressive quadriceps strengthening, hamstring stretching, and activity modification. Physical exam reveals a contracted lateral patellar retinaculum and pain with bent knee and resisted extension exercises. Routine office radiographs reveal a laterally tilted patella. Surgical intervention (lateral release) is recommended.

Description of Procedure (29873)
The patient is taken to the operating room where an examination under anesthesia confirms a tight lateral patellar retinaculum. An anterior lateral portal is created. A comprehensive arthroscopic knee examination is performed. This includes evaluation and probing of the patellar and trochlear articular surfaces, the medial and lateral compartment articular surfaces, the medial and lateral menisci, the anterior and posterior cruciate ligaments, the posterior medial and lateral compartments and the popliteus tendon and hiatus. Once this complete inspection is performed, the abnormally tight lateral patellar retinaculum is addressed. The tight lateral retinaculum causes the patella to tilt throughout the knee range of motion. The medial facet of the patella will not articulate with the trochlea until late in knee flexion, if at all. The arthroscope is transferred to an anterior medial portal and an electrocautery device is introduced through the lateral portal. Care must be exercised to avoid injury to the trochlear and patellar articular cartilage because the tight retinaculum forces the patella against the trochlea. The lateral retinaculum is incised from the inferior edge of the vastus

lateralis, but not to injure the lateral portion of the quadriceps tendon, up to and slightly beyond the lateral portal. Hemostasis is ensured with the electrocautery probe. The incisions are closed.

29894 Arthroscopy, ankle, (tibiotalar and fibulotalar joints), surgical; with removal of loose body or foreign body

●29899 with ankle arthrodesis

▶(For open ankle arthrodesis, use 27870)◀

Rationale
Code 29899 was added to the CPT code set to identify the arthroscopic ankle fusion procedure. In addition, a cross-reference has been added following code 29899 to indicate appropriate reporting for the open-approach counterpart for this procedure.

Respiratory System

Nose

REPAIR

30540 Repair choanal atresia; intranasal

30545 transpalatine

▶(Do not report modifier '-63' in conjunction with 30540, 30545)◀

Rationale
For the codes listed above, see page 244, modifier '-63.'

Larynx

ENDOSCOPY

31515 Laryngoscopy direct, with or without tracheoscopy; for aspiration

31520 diagnostic, newborn

▶(Do not report modifier '-63' in conjunction with 31520)◀

Rationale
For the codes listed above, see page 244, modifier '-63.'

31575 Laryngoscopy, flexible fiberoptic; diagnostic

31576 with biopsy

31577 with removal of foreign body

31578 with removal of lesion

▶(To report flexible fiberoptic endoscopic evaluation of swallowing, see 92612-92613)◀

▶(To report flexible fiberoptic endoscopic evaluation with sensory testing, see 92614-92615)◀

▶(To report flexible fiberoptic endoscopic evaluation of swallowing with sensory testing, see 92616-92617)◀

Rationale
Three new cross-references were added to flexible fiberoptic laryngoscopy codes to instruct appropriate reporting for the endoscopic evaluation of swallowing, evaluation with sensory testing, and evaluation of swallowing with sensory testing.

Cardiovascular System

Heart and Pericardium

TRANSMYOCARDIAL REVASCULARIZATION

33140 Transmyocardial laser revascularization, by thoracotomy; (separate procedure)

+33141 performed at the time of other open cardiac procedure(s) (List separately in addition to code for primary procedure)

(Use 33141 in conjunction with codes 33400-33496, 33510-33536▶, 33542)◀

Rationale
Code 33141 was added to *CPT 2001*, and the procedure it represents is performed as an adjunct procedure to other cardiac procedures, to describe the creation of laser channels through the ventricular wall to relieve angina. Since its addition to the CPT code set, the number of approved procedures with which this procedure may be reported has increased. Previously, the parenthetical note for code 33141 indicated that this code was appropriately reported only in addition to codes 33510-33536 Coronary artery bypass grafts and 33572 Coronary endarterectomy. The list of approved procedures was later expanded to include the valve repair codes 33400-33496. For this year, the cross-reference following add-on code 33141 was editorially revised to indicate that code 33141 is now appropriately reported in conjunction with code 33542 Myocardial resection (eg, ventricular aneurysmectomy) when transmyocardial revascularization is performed at the same session as the myocardial resection procedure.

PACEMAKER/PACING CARDIOVERTER DEFIBRILLATOR

A pacemaker system includes …

A single chamber pacemaker system includes a pulse generator and one electrode inserted in either the atrium or ventricle. A dual chamber pacemaker system includes a pulse generator and one electrode inserted in the right atrium and one electrode inserted in the right ventricle. ▶In certain circumstances, an additional electrode may be required to achieve pacing of the left ventricle (bi-ventricular pacing). In this event, transvenous (cardiac vein) placement of the electrode should be separately reported using code 33224 or 33225.◄

Like a pacemaker system, a pacing cardioverter-defibrillator system includes a pulse generator and electrodes, although pacing cardioverter-defibrillators may require multiple leads, even when only a single chamber is being paced. A pacing cardioverter-defibrillator system may be inserted in a single chamber (pacing in the ventricle) or in dual chambers (pacing in atrium and ventricle). These devices use a combination of antitachycardia pacing, low energy cardioversion or defibrillating shocks to treat ventricular tachycardia or ventricular fibrillation.

Pacing cardioverter-defibrillator pulse generators ...

The electrodes (leads) of a pacing cardioverter-defibrillator system are positioned in the heart via the venous system (transvenously), in most circumstances. ►In certain circumstances, an additional electrode may be required to achieve pacing of the left ventricle (bi-ventricular pacing). In this event, transvenous (cardiac vein) placement of the electrode should be separately reported using code 33224 or 33225.◄

Electrode positioning on the epicardial surface of the heart requires a thoracotomy (codes 33245-33246) ...

When the "battery" of a pacemaker or pacing cardio-defibrillator is changed, it is actually the pulse generator that is changed. Replacement of a pulse generator should be reported with a code for removal of the pulse generator and another code for insertion of a pulse generator.

►Repositioning of a pacemaker electrode, pacing cardioverter-defibrillator electrode(s), or a left ventricular pacing electrode is reported using 33215 or 33226, as appropriate. Replacement of a pacemaker electrode, pacing cardioverter-defibrillator electrode(s), or a left ventricular pacing electrode is reported using 33206-33208, 33210-33213, or 33224, as appropriate.◄

●33215 Repositioning of previously implanted transvenous pacemaker or pacing cardioverter-defibrillator (right atrial or right ventricular) electrode

▲33216 Insertion of a transvenous electrode; single chamber (one electrode) permanent pacemaker or single chamber pacing cardioverter-defibrillator

33217   dual chamber (two electrodes) permanent pacemaker or dual chamber pacing cardioverter-defibrillator

●33224 Insertion of pacing electrode, cardiac venous system, for left ventricular pacing, with attachment to previously placed pacemaker or pacing cardioverter-defibrillator pulse generator (including revision of pocket, removal, insertion and/or replacement of generator)

+●33225 Insertion of pacing electrode, cardiac venous system, for left ventricular pacing, at time of insertion of pacing cardioverter-defibrillator or pacemaker pulse generator (including upgrade to dual chamber system) (List separately in addition to code for primary procedure)

▶(Use 33225 in conjunction with 33206, 33207, 33208, 33212, 33213, 33214, 33216, 33217, 33222, 33233, 33234, 33235, 33240, 33249)◀

●33226 Repositioning of previously implanted cardiac venous system (left ventricular) electrode (including removal, insertion and/or replacement of generator)

 Rationale

To provide more accurate reporting of insertion and repositioning, improve carrier claims data collection, allay confusion regarding the use of these codes, and facilitate hospital outpatient reporting, codes 33216 and 33217 were revised to delete the reference to "repositioning." This correlates with the addition of code 33215, used to report repositioning of a previously transplanted transvenous right atrial or right ventricle pacing electrode.

Prior to this revision, there was no CPT code to describe the utilization of facility/staff resources when the patient was returned to the cardiac catheterization laboratory for electrode repositioning or replacement during the first 14 days post initial or reinsertion. The repositioning/replacement codes were precluded from being reported within a 14-day window. An outpatient reporting issue existed, based on the usage instruction outlined in the introductory notes for these codes. To address this reporting issue, reference to <14-day or >15-day postinsertion repositioning/replacement has been removed from the coding guidelines. This revised nomenclature clarifies both the physician work and the facility resource utilization in those circumstances when electrode repositioning or replacement is performed, regardless of the time frame for the post-insertion. If the insertion or repositioning procedure should occur within the postoperative period assigned by the carrier, then the appropriate CPT modifier (eg, modifier '-78') would be appended. The CPT code(s) for cardiac insertion and repositioning should be used (if within the postoperative period) with the appropriate hospital-approved CPT modifier appended (eg, modifier '-59' for same date, modifier '-76,' '-77,' '-78').

The Pacemaker/Pacing Cardioverter Defibrillator introductory notes have also been revised to indicate appropriate reporting for insertion of electrodes for left ventricular pacing. Two new codes were established, the stand-alone code 33224 and the add-on code 33225 (with a corresponding cross-reference to delineate usage) to describe insertion of a left ventricular lead (ie, electrode) to achieve biventricular pacing. In addition, a new stand-alone code 33226 was established to describe the repositioning of a previously implanted cardiac venous system (left ventricular) electrode 15 days or more after initial insertion. The addition of this code correlates with the action described above, in which code 33215 was added for the repositioning of the transvenous electrode.

The implant procedure for the bi-ventricular pacing systems parallels that of a conventional pacemaker or intracardiac defibrillator (ICD) with the addition of a left ventricular lead and its transvenous placement in a cardiac vein. The additional work involved and complexity of the transvenous placement of the lead in a cardiac vein make this change necessary.

The new codes for left ventricular pacing lead placement were added because the previously existing codes did not adequately reflect the entire procedure being performed with bi-ventricular pacing. Due to the availability of new technology to achieve left ventricular pacing lead placement through the coronary sinus into a cardiac vein, this procedure was not originally encompassed in the existing coding scenarios.

The major procedural differences between insertion of a left ventricular pacing lead and the related procedure codes in the CPT code set for placement of leads in the right ventricle and atrium are indicated here. Placement of a left ventricular pacing lead requires:

- Transvenous left ventricular placement through the coronary sinus into a cardiac vein;

- Access of a different ventricle than conventional pacemaker and defibrillator access;

- The technical skills and tools as described above compared to the existing pacemaker lead placement codes;

- Use of a venogram for placement.

The technique, skill required, and tools are different than those required for placement of leads in the right ventricle and atrium.

The technique used for left ventricular lead placement uses a transcatheter technique requiring access through the coronary sinus into a cardiac vein. The vein must be identified and mapped prior to placement of the lead, and this placement is much more difficult than placement of a right atrial or ventricular lead.

Access to the cardiac veins may be complicated due to variations in cardiac vein anatomy. These differences may include anatomical variations in number, diameter, angulation, and tortuosity.

The tools used to access and guide the placement differ from simple, direct catheter positioning in the right atrium or right ventricle. In addition to using the introducer required for insertion of a catheter into the right atrium or ventricle, the technique for placement of the left ventricular pacing lead requires the use of a coronary guide catheter to access the cardiac vein, a stylet, guide catheter, and a balloon tip catheter. These instruments are unique to the placement of the left ventricular lead.

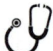

Clinical Example (33215)

Six weeks after pacemaker or pacing cardioverter-defibrillator insertion, a 75-year-old man experiences symptoms of near syncope and intermittent failure to capture, noted on a rhythm strip. The pacemaker or pacing cardioverter-defibrillator evaluation suggests lead dislodgement.

Description of Procedure (33215)

The patient is taken to the procedure room. After preparation and draping of the skin over the existing pulse generator pocket, local anesthetic is injected in the skin and subcutaneous tissues and the pulse generator pocket is entered. The electrode is inspected and evaluated for its pacing and sensing characteristics. The lead is disconnected from the pulse generator and manipulated into a different position. Sensing and pacing thresholds were again evaluated and after being found satisfactory, the electrode is reconnected to the pulse generator. The pocket is closed after hemostasis is achieved. The patient is returned to his room, and the next day, reprogramming is performed and acceptable pacemaker or pacing cardioverter-defibrillator function is confirmed.

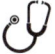

Clinical Example (33224)

A 54-year-old male presents with dilated cardiomyopathy, ejection fraction of 20%, and Class III congestive heart failure. His symptoms persist despite medical treatment with angiotensin converting enzyme (ACE) inhibitors, beta blockers, and diuretic therapy. A left ventricular pacing lead is placed in the coronary sinus to allow biventricular pacing for cardiac resynchronization. The left ventricular pacing lead is then connected to an existing pacemaker or pacemaker-defibrillator generator.

Description of Procedure (33224)

The risks, benefits, and alternatives unique to this procedure (which are in addition to the risks, benefits, and alternatives to the leads already placed) have been discussed with the patient, and informed consent for this additional part of the procedure has been obtained.

The procedure is performed under ECG, intra-arterial blood pressure, and pulse oximetry monitoring. The skin over the generator pocket is prepared and local anesthetic is injected into the insertion site. The generator pocket is opened and the generator and previously placed lead(s) are dissected free from the scar tissue. After achieving venous access, a guide wire is passed into the right atrium under fluoroscopic guidance. A peel-away sheath is passed over the wire, and a guide catheter is placed through the sheath and positioned into the right atrium under fluoroscopic guidance. A steerable catheter is placed within the guide catheter, and the coronary sinus is cannulated. Contrast is injected through the guide catheter to verify engagement of the coronary sinus, the steerable catheter is removed, and a balloon catheter is placed through the guide catheter into the coronary sinus. Contrast venography of the coronary sinus is performed. Following this, the balloon catheter is removed and a left ventricular pacing lead is advanced into the marginal branch of the coronary sinus. Adequate sensing and pacing thresholds are identified. Further manipulation of the lead may be required to attain an adequate location and thresholds. Once the left ventricular lead is in position, the guide catheter is removed. The electrode is then connected to the previously placed pulse generator directly or using an adaptor. The pulse generator pocket is then closed.

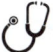

Clinical Example (33225)

A 54-year-old male presents with dilated cardiomyopathy, ejection fraction of 20%, and Class III congestive heart failure. His symptoms persist despite medical

BIVENTRICULAR PACING (33224-33226)

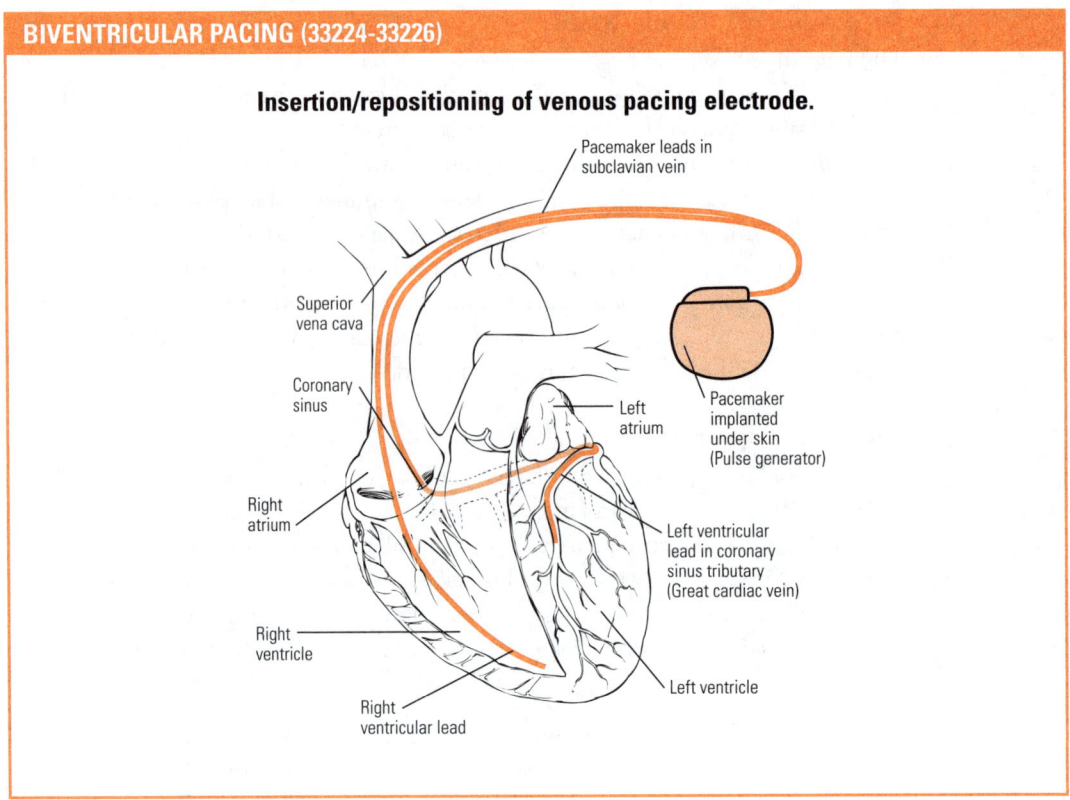

Insertion/repositioning of venous pacing electrode.

treatment with ACE inhibitors, beta blockers, and diuretic therapy. A left ventricular pacing lead is placed in the coronary sinus to allow biventricular pacing for cardiac resynchronization. (Note: The placement of the pacemaker or pacemaker-defibrillator, right atrial pacing lead, and right ventricular pacing lead are coded separately.)

Description of Procedure (33225)

The procedure is performed under ECG, intra-arterial blood pressure, and pulse oximetry monitoring. The insertion site is prepped. Local anesthetic is injected into the insertion site. After achieving venous access, a guide wire is passed into the right atrium under fluoroscopic guidance. A peel-away sheath is passed over the wire, and a guide catheter is placed through the sheath and positioned into the right atrium under fluoroscopic guidance. A steerable catheter is placed within the guide catheter, and the coronary sinus is cannulated. Contrast is injected through the guide catheter to verify engagement of the coronary sinus, the steerable catheter is removed, and a balloon catheter is placed through the guide catheter into the coronary sinus. Contrast venography of the coronary sinus is performed. Following this, the balloon catheter is removed and a left ventricular pacing lead is advanced into the marginal branch of the coronary sinus. Adequate sensing and pacing thresholds are identified. Further manipulation of the lead may be required to attain an adequate location and thresholds. Once the left ventricular lead is in position, the guide catheter is removed.

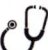 **Clinical Example (33226)**

A 65-year-old man experiences symptoms of progressive heart failure 6 weeks after insertion of a left ventricular pacing electrode to achieve cardiac resynchronization by biventricular pacing. Intermittent capture of the left ventricle is noted on rhythm strip, and pacemaker or pacemaker-defibrillator evaluation suggests lead dislodgement. The left ventricular pacing electrode is repositioned to achieve left ventricular capture.

Description of Procedure (33226)

The patient is taken to the procedure room. After preparation and draping of the skin over the existing pulse generator pocket, local anesthetic is injected in the skin and subcutaneous tissues and the pulse generator pocket is entered. The electrode is inspected and evaluated for its pacing and sensing characteristics. The lead is disconnected from the pulse generator and manipulated into a different position in the coronary venous system. Sensing and pacing thresholds are again evaluated and after being found satisfactory, the electrode is reconnected to the pulse generator. The pocket is closed after hemostasis is achieved. The patient is returned to his room, and the next day, pacemaker reprogramming is performed and confirms acceptable function of the left ventricular lead.

CARDIAC VALVES

Aortic Valves

33400 Valvuloplasty, aortic valve; open, with cardiopulmonary bypass

33401 open, with inflow occlusion

33403 using transventricular dilation, with cardiopulmonary bypass

▶(Do not report modifier '-63' in conjunction with 33401, 33403)◀

 Rationale

For the codes listed above, see page 244, modifier '-63.'

Pulmonary Valves

33470 Valvotomy, pulmonary valve, closed heart; transventricular

▶(Do not report modifier '-63' in conjunction with 33470)◀

33472 Valvotomy, pulmonary valve, open heart; with inflow occlusion

▶(Do not report modifier '-63' in conjunction with 33472)◀

 Rationale

For the codes listed above, see page 244, modifier '-63.'

CORONARY ARTERY ANOMALIES

33502 Repair of anomalous coronary artery; by ligation

33503 by graft, without cardiopulmonary bypass

▶(Do not report modifier '-63' in conjunction with 33502, 33503)◀

33505   with construction of intrapulmonary artery tunnel (Takeuchi procedure)

33506   by translocation from pulmonary artery to aorta

▶(Do not report modifier '-63' in conjunction with 33505, 33506)◀

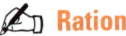

Rationale

For the codes listed above, see page 244, modifier '-63.'

▶ENDOSCOPY◀

▶Surgical vascular endoscopy always includes diagnostic endoscopy.◀

+●33508   Endoscopy, surgical, including video-assisted harvest of vein(s) for coronary artery bypass procedure (List separately in addition to code for primary procedure)

▶(Use 33508 in conjunction with code(s) 33510-33523)◀

▶(For open harvest of upper extremity vein procedure, use 35500)◀

Rationale

33508 was established as an add-on code to describe the endoscopic minimally invasive approach for harvesting of venous conduit for coronary artery bypass procedures. The open approach venous grafting procedures, included within the coronary artery bypass codes (33510-33516), represent the work required for open procurement of vein, but did not accurately reflect the additional work required to complete harvesting of the vein by endoscopic means. In addition to the use of the trocar as an approach tool, this procedure may also be video-assisted for intraoperative visualization of the venous and tissue structures.

The cross-reference following code 35508 is intended to indicate that, when endoscopic harvest of the saphenous vein or other venous conduit is performed for coronary bypass, code 33508 is reported in addition to the appropriate code from the series 33510-33523. An additional cross-reference directs the user to the upper extremity open venous harvest code, which may be reported in addition to the appropriate code from the series 33510-33523 when performed in addition to these procedures.

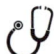

Clinical Example (33508)

This new code is meant to capture the difference in work between a coronary artery bypass graft (CABG) performed where the vein graph is harvested in an open fashion versus using an endoscope. It describes only the additional work related to the use of an endoscope to complete a saphenous vein harvest for a CABG.

Description of Procedure (33508)

A small incision is made over the left saphenous vein at the level of the knee and the vein is identified. The endoscopic dissection system (trocar and camera) is introduced along the anterior surface of the vein. After dissecting the vein for several centimeters, the balloon trocar is introduced, the balloon inflated, and

CO_2 insufflation begun. The saphenous vein is dissected toward the groin, freeing it from surrounding soft tissue. The side branches are ligated. Once the thigh vein is completely dissected free, the trocar and camera are removed and dissection is initiated distally. The trocar is passed along the anterior surface of the vein for several centimeters. The port is introduced and the balloon inflated and CO_2 insufflation again instituted. The distal vein is dissected free of surrounding fatty tissue and side branches are isolated. The camera is removed and the dissection tip removed and replaced with bipolar scissors. The camera is reintroduced and the saphenous vein is carefully inspected. The side branches are ligated using the bipolar scissors beginning at the ankle and working proximally.

Once the calf portion of the saphenous vein is free, the camera and the side port are removed from the knee incision and reinserted, directed toward the groin. The camera is introduced and again the vein inspected and the side branches ligated using the bipolar scissors. The endoscopic equipment is then removed and small incisions made in the groin and ankle. The saphenous vein is ligated proximally and distally; the vein is divided and removed from the leg. The leg wounds are irrigated and closed in layers. Dressings are placed at the conclusion of the procedure.

VENOUS GRAFTING ONLY FOR CORONARY ARTERY BYPASS

The following codes are used ...

Procurement of the saphenous vein graft is included in the description of the work for 33510-33516 and should not be reported as a separate service or co-surgery. ►To report harvesting of an upper extremity vein, use 35500 in addition to the bypass procedure. To report harvesting of a femoropopliteal vein segment, report 35572 in addition to the bypass procedure. When surgical assistant performs graft procurement,◄ add modifier '-80' to 33510-33516.

COMBINED ARTERIAL-VENOUS GRAFTING FOR CORONARY BYPASS

The following codes are used ...

To report combined arterial-venous grafts it is necessary ...

Procurement of the saphenous vein graft is included in the description of the work for 33517-33523 and should not be reported as a separate service or co-surgery. Procurement of the artery for grafting is included in the description of the work for 33533-33536 and should not be reported as a separate service or co-surgery, except when an upper extremity artery (eg, radial artery) is procured. To report harvesting of an upper extremity artery, use 35600 in addition to the bypass procedure(s). ►To report harvesting of an upper extremity vein, use 35600 in addition to the bypass procedure. To report harvesting of a femoropopliteal vein segment, report 35572 in addition to the bypass procedure.◄ When ►surgical assistant performs◄ arterial and/or venous graft procurement, add modifier '-80' to 33517-33523, 33533-33536, as appropriate.

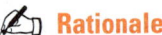 **Rationale**

The Venous Grafting, Combined Arterial-Venous Grafting, and Arterial Grafting subsection guidelines have been revised to instruct users in the additional reporting for add-on codes 35500 and 35572, with addition of text when an upper extremity vein or a femoropopliteal vein is harvested as an adjunct procedure to a coronary bypass procedure using a venous graft.

With this revision, there are now three types of grafts for which procurement is separately reported with the coronary artery bypass graft (CABG) procedures: the upper extremity vein, the femoropopliteal vein, and the upper extremity artery. These procedures are indicated for use in addition to CABG codes 33510-33536 when the saphenous vein supply is inadequate due to prior bypass operations, diseased, or of poor quality. Code 35500 was added for *CPT 2000* to describe harvest of an upper extremity vein. Code 35572 is a new add-on code for *CPT 2003*, describing harvest of the femoropopliteal vein, and would also be additionally reportable with CABG procedures. Code 35600, describing upper extremity artery harvest, is used solely for CABG procedures, which is reflected in the CABG code notes and in the 35600 code descriptor. Procurement of these veins is not included when a coronary bypass graft is reported, and is therefore separately reported.

It should also be noted that for *CPT 2003*, code 33508 has been added for endoscopic minimally invasive vein harvest and is also separately reported with the CABG codes 33510-33523.

ARTERIAL GRAFTING FOR CORONARY ARTERY BYPASS

The following codes are used ...

To report combined arterial-venous grafts it is necessary ...

Procurement of the artery for grafting is included in the description of the work for 33533-33536 and should not be reported as a separate service or co-surgery, except when an upper extremity artery (eg, radial artery) is procured. To report harvesting of an upper extremity artery, use 35600 in addition to the bypass procedure. To report harvesting of an upper extremity artery, use 35500 in addition to the bypass procedure. ▶To report harvesting of an upper extremity vein, use 35500 in addition to the bypass procedure. To report harvesting of a femoropopliteal vein segment, report 35572 in addition to the bypass procedure.◄ When ▶surgical assistant performs◄ arterial and/or venous graft procurement, add modifier '-80' to 33517-33523, 33533-33536, as appropriate.

SINGLE VENTRICLE AND OTHER COMPLEX CARDIAC ANOMALIES

33610 Repair of complex cardiac anomalies (eg, single ventricle with subaortic obstruction) by surgical enlargement of interventricular septal defect

▶(Do not report modifier '-63' in conjunction with 33610)◄

33611 Repair of double outlet right ventricle with intraventricular tunnel repair;

▶(Do not report modifier '-63' in conjunction with 33611)◄

33619 Repair of single ventricle with aortic outflow obstruction and aortic arch hypoplasia (hypoplastic left heart syndrome) (eg, Norwood procedure)

▶(Do not report modifier '-63' in conjunction with 33619)◀

 Rationale

For the codes listed above, see page 244, modifier '-63.'

SEPTAL DEFECTS

33647 Repair of atrial septal defect and ventricular septal defect, with direct or patch closure

▶(Do not report modifier '-63' in conjunction with 33647)◀

33670 Repair of complete atrioventricular canal, with or without prosthetic valve

▶(Do not report modifier '-63' in conjunction with 33670)◀

33690 Banding of pulmonary artery

▶(Do not report modifier '-63' in conjunction with 33690)◀

33692 Complete repair tetralogy of Fallot without pulmonary atresia;

33694   with transannular patch

▶(Do not report modifier '-63' in conjunction with 33694)◀

 Rationale

For the codes listed above, see page 244, modifier '-63.'

TOTAL ANOMALOUS PULMONARY VENOUS DRAINAGE

33730 Complete repair of anomalous venous return (supracardiac, intracardiac, or infracardiac types)

▶(Do not report modifier '-63' in conjunction with 33730)◀

33732 Repair of cor triatriatum or supravalvular mitral ring by resection of left atrial membrane

▶(Do not report modifier '-63' in conjunction with 33732)◀

 Rationale

For the codes listed above, see page 244, modifier '-63.'

SHUNTING PROCEDURES

33735 Atrial septectomy or septostomy; closed heart (Blalock-Hanlon type operation)

33736   open heart with cardiopulmonary bypass

▶(Do not report modifier '-63' in conjunction with 33735, 33736)◀

33750 Shunt; subclavian to pulmonary artery (Blalock-Taussig type operation)

33755   ascending aorta to pulmonary artery (Waterston type operation)

33762 descending aorta to pulmonary artery (Potts-Smith type operation)

▶(Do not report modifier '-63' in conjunction with 33750, 33755, 33762)◀

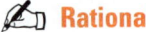 **Rationale**

For the codes listed above, see page 244, modifier '-63.'

TRANSPOSITION OF THE GREAT VESSELS

33778 Repair of transposition of the great arteries, aortic pulmonary artery reconstruction (eg, Jatene type);

▶(Do not report modifier '-63' in conjunction with 33778)◀

Rationale

For the codes listed above, see page 244, modifier '-63.'

TRUNCUS ARTERIOSUS

33786 Total repair, truncus arteriosus (Rastelli type operation)

▶(Do not report modifier '-63' in conjunction with 33786)◀

Rationale

For the codes listed above, see page 244, modifier '-63.'

PULMONARY ARTERY

33918 Repair of pulmonary atresia with ventricular septal defect, by unifocalization of pulmonary arteries; without cardiopulmonary bypass

33919 with cardiopulmonary bypass

▶(Do not report modifier '-63' in conjunction with 33918, 33919)◀

33922 Transection of pulmonary artery with cardiopulmonary bypass

▶(Do not report modifier '-63' in conjunction with 33922)◀

Rationale

For the codes listed above, see page 244, modifier '-63.'

CARDIAC ASSIST

33960 Prolonged extracorporeal circulation for cardiopulmonary insufficiency; initial 24 hours

33961 each additional 24 hours (List separately in addition to code for primary procedure)

▶(Do not report modifier '-63' in conjunction with 33960, 33961)◀

Rationale

For the codes listed above, see page 244, modifier '-63.'

Arteries and Veins

ENDOVASCULAR REPAIR OF ABDOMINAL AORTIC ANEURYSM

▲**34812**   Open femoral artery exposure for delivery of endovascular prosthesis, by groin incision, unilateral

▲**34825**   Placement of proximal or distal extension prosthesis for endovascular repair of infrarenal abdominal aortic or iliac artery aneurysm, false aneurysm, or dissection; initial vessel

+**34826**   each additional vessel (List separately in addition to code for primary procedure)

(Use 34826 in conjunction with 34825)

(Use 34825, 34826 in addition to codes 34800-34808▶, 34900◀, as appropriate)

(For staged procedure, use modifier '-58')

(For radiological supervision and interpretation, use 75953)

●**34833**   Open iliac artery exposure with creation of conduit for delivery of infrarenal aortic or iliac endovascular prosthesis, by abdominal or retroperitoneal incision, unilateral

▶(For bilateral procedure, use modifier '-50')◀

▶(Do not report 34833 in addition to 34820)◀

●**34834**   Open brachial artery exposure to assist in the deployment of infrarenal aortic or iliac endovascular prosthesis by arm incision, unilateral

▶(For bilateral procedure, use modifier '-50')◀

▶ENDOVASCULAR REPAIR OF ILIAC ANEURYSM◀

▶Code 34900 represents a procedure to report introduction, positioning, and deployment of an endovascular graft for treatment of aneurysm, pseudoaneurysm, or arteriovenous malformation or trauma of the iliac artery (common, hypogastric, external). All balloon angioplasty and/or stent deployments within the target treatment zone for the endoprosthesis, either before or after endograft deployment, are included in the work of 34900 and are not separately reportable. Open femoral or iliac artery exposure (eg, 34812, 34820), introduction of guidewires and catheters (eg, 36200, 36215-36218), and extensive repair or replacement of an artery (eg, 35206-35286) should be additionally reported.

For fluoroscopic guidance in conjunction with endovascular iliac aneurysm repair, see code 75954. Code 75954 includes angiography of the aorta and iliac arteries for diagnostic imaging prior to deployment of the endovascular device (including all routine components), fluoroscopic guidance in the delivery of the endovascular components, and intraprocedural arterial angiography to confirm appropriate position of the graft, detect endoleaks, and evaluate the status of the runoff vessels (eg, evaluation for dissection, stenosis, thrombosis, distal embolization, or iatrogenic injury).

Other interventional procedures performed at the time of endovascular aortic aneurysm repair should be additionally reported (eg, transluminal angioplasty outside the aneurysm target zone, arterial embolization, intravascular ultrasound).◀

●**34900** Endovascular graft placement for repair of iliac artery (eg, aneurysm, pseudoaneurysm, arteriovenous malformation, trauma)

▶(For radiological supervision and interpretation, use 75954)◀

▶(For placement of extension prosthesis during endovascular iliac artery repair, use 34825)◀

▶(For bilateral procedure, use modifier '-50')◀

 Rationale

A new heading, subsection, and introductory notes and codes have been added to the Arteries and Veins subsection pertaining to endovascular graft placement repair of iliac artery aneurysms (IAA), and a new treatment option for patients with iliac artery aneurysms/pseudoaneurysms/arteriovenous malformations and trauma. In addition, codes 34812, 34825, and 75953, describing open repair of the femoral artery and endovascular repair of the infrarenal abdominal aorta, were revised to differentiate the technique and anatomy of the specific vasculature from the new codes.

Prior to the addition of these new codes, there were no CPT codes to describe this minimally invasive technique in this specific vasculature. Existing code 35131 describes a direct, open, surgical repair of an iliac aneurysm, using an open transabdominal laparotomy or extended retroperitoneal approach to the external surface of the aneurysm. Subsequent to exposure of the external surface of the aneurysm, the open approach repair technique includes clamping of the arteries proximal and distal to the aneurysm and graft placement by suture techniques. The new code 34900 is similar to endovascular repair codes 34800, 34802, 34804, but the target artery (the aorta) differs.

The endovascular approach described by code 34900 utilizes minimally invasive techniques as opposed to the large incision of the open approach. This approach eliminates the need for a large abdominal or retroperitoneal incision to expose the aneurysm. The endovascular repair technique involves exposure of peripheral arteries with introduction and advancement of a collapsed prosthesis along the inside of the arterial system through arteries in the groin and then advanced into position within the aneurysm using fluoroscopic guidance. Once in the correct location, positioned exactly across the aneurysm, the device is deployed expanding the prosthesis to full size, thereby eliminating the aneurysm from the circulatory system through the inside of the arterial tree. Endovascular IAA repair requires different resources (eg, catheters, endovascular grafts, complex catheter manipulation using high-quality fluoroscopic guidance) than those required by the open approach iliac aneurysm repair procedure described above.

The services that are inherent components of the endovascular IAA repair include balloon dilatation within the endoprosthesis to achieve full expansion of the graft and complete contact of the attachment devices and vascular stents necessary to properly secure the device. Therefore, all balloon angioplasty and/or stent deployments are not separately reportable when performed within the target zone for the iliac endoprosthesis.

The fluoroscopic guidance required for placement of the graft, as well as radiologic supervision for angioplasty/stent deployments in the target zone, is included in code 75954, which is the radiologic supervision and interpretation code for 34900. Therefore, fluoroscopic guidance codes (eg 76000) are not reportable with this procedure.

Three new cross-references were added following code 34900 to instruct users in reporting the appropriate procedure code 75954, which is the radiological supervision and interpretation code specific to the repair of iliac artery aneurysms; to refer to the additional extension codes 34825 and 34826; and to instruct in the appropriate reporting for bilateral iliac aneurysm repair procedures.

As a related issue, cross-references have been added to the Direct Repair of Aneurysm or Excision (Partial or Total) and Graft Insertion for Aneurysm, Pseudoaneurysm, Ruptured Aneurysm, and Associated Occlusive Disease subsections (codes 35001-35162) to indicate the appropriate codes for reporting endovascular repair of iliac and abdominal aortic artery and thoracic aortic aneurysms. In addition, consistent with the revisions made for *CPT 2002*, and based on the Library of Medicine's *Metathesaurus*, the term "false" aneurysm, which formerly appeared in the subsection title preceding codes 35001-35162 has been revised to "pseudoaneurysm."

The revision of code 34812, describing femoral artery exposure, omits "aortic," broadening the application of this code to allow reporting in addition to 34900 for the delivery of the iliac device. The revision of code 34825, adding "iliac" and "false aneurysm and dissection" also broadens the application of this code, and provides consistency in descriptor language with other aneurysm repair codes. The cross-reference below 34825 and 34826 is revised to include code 34900 in the list of codes with which codes 34825 and 34826 would be additionally reported for placement of additional prosthesis extensions.

Codes 34833 and 34834 were added to the Endovascular Repair of Abdominal Aortic Aneurysm subsection to describe creation of iliac conduit to allow introduction of the large carriers and endoprostheses during infrarenal aortic or iliac endovascular prostheses. The stand-alone status of these codes (as opposed to add-on) reflects the fact that exposure of the artery and the attachment and termination of the conduit through which manipulations will be done are not related to the target location of the prosthesis (eg, thoracic aortic, iliac), the prosthesis type, or the artery repair, and therefore are not an included service within these procedures. Code 34833 is intended to report the work of suturing a segment of large-diameter synthetic conduit onto the iliac artery, and the work of subsequently terminating that conduit after completion of endograft deployment.

Since code 34833 includes all the steps of code 34820, Open iliac artery exposure during endovascular therapy, plus the work of creation and termination of the conduit, a cross-reference has been added to indicate that 34820 may not be reported in addition to 34833.

Similarly, code 34834 is created to report creation of a conduit for access through the brachial artery during endovascular therapy. This code is analogous in clinical use and reporting to CPT codes 34812 (Open femoral artery exposure) and 34820 (Open iliac artery exposure). Brachial artery exposure is performed during repair of aortic dissections for the introduction of wires and catheters introduced from the proximal aorta to help find and cannulate the true lumen (eg, during repair of a dissected aorta, or patient with very tortuous iliac arteries).

Clinical Example (34833)

A 65-year-old female smoker with hypertension, chronic obstructive pulmonary disease (COPD), and previous MI has a 7-cm infrarenal aortic aneurysm. Her iliac arteries are very small in caliber and heavily calcified. Placement of an iliac conduit will be required to enable endovascular aortic aneurysm repair.

Description of Procedure (34833)

This procedure begins with a skin incision. Access to the iliac artery is achieved via a transabdominal or retroperitoneal approach. All soft tissue, bowels, ureters, and veins are carefully mobilized as the iliac artery is approached. The artery is cleared for 5-6 cm, and vessel loops are passed around the vessel proximally and distally. Once adequate exposure is achieved and intravenous anticoagulation administered, proximal and distal vascular clamps are applied. A longitudinal arteriotomy is made. The conduit (a large-diameter tubular segment of synthetic bypass graft) is brought onto the field, tailored to appropriate size, and an anastomosis of conduit to iliac artery is sutured. The conduit is clamped and vascular clamps are removed from the iliac artery. The suture line is checked for hemostasis and additional sutures are applied as required.

Endovascular repair (separately reportable) is then undertaken with the prostheses introduced through the newly formed conduit.

Once endovascular repair is complete, closure of the conduit is achieved in one of two ways. The unattached distal end of the conduit may be sewn to the more distal external iliac artery, thereby leaving the conduit in a common place with the external iliac bypass graft. Alternatively, the conduit can be transected close to the iliac artery and oversewn with a suture. Hemostasis is achieved. The wound is irrigated and closed in layers.

Clinical Example (34834)

A 65-year-old female smoker with hypertension, COPD, and previous MI has a 7-cm infrarenal aortic aneurysm. Her iliac arteries are tortuous. Exposure of the brachial artery is performed to insert a guide to enable endovascular aortic aneurysm repair.

Description of Procedure (34834)

This procedure begins with a skin incision. Access to the brachial artery is achieved via an upper arm incision. All soft tissue, nerves, and veins are carefully mobilized as the brachial artery is approached. The artery is cleared for 5-6 cm, and soft vessel loops are passed around the artery proximally and distally. Once adequate exposure is achieved and intravenous anticoagulation administered, proximal and distal vascular clamps are applied/removed as required for subsequent introduction of wires, sheaths, and catheters.

The endovascular procedure is performed (separately reported).

Upon completion of the endovascular procedure, vascular clamps are reapplied. The large hole in the brachial artery is irrigated, edges are trimmed as needed, and it is closed with fine sutures. The suture line is checked for hemostasis and additional sutures are applied as required. The wound is irrigated and closed in layers.

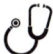

Clinical Example (34900)

A 67-year-old male with coronary artery disease status post MI plus chronic obstructive pulmonary disease has a 5-cm-diameter iliac artery aneurysm. Imaging studies indicate the aneurysm is suitable for endovascular repair.

Description of Service (34900)

This procedure begins after achieving arterial exposure (eg, 34812) and after initial catheter and guidewire placements (typically reported by codes 36200, 36245-36248). These services are separately reportable and subject to multiple procedure payment reduction rules.

The endovascular device is loaded onto the guidewire and advanced into the patient. Depending on the device chosen, this may or may not be done through a large introducer sheath. The device is carefully manipulated through adjacent arteries toward the deployment target. It is carefully positioned such that the proximal edge lies in normal-caliber vessel proximal to the beginning of the aneurysm. Position is confirmed exactly by fluoroscopy, often with injection of contrast. The device is then deployed under exacting fluoroscopic guidance. Fine adjustments in position are made during the deployment to assure accurate deployment. In some patients the mean arterial pressure is transiently reduced by the anesthesiologist to decrease the chance that pressure from flowing blood will push the endograft distally during deployment. After deployment the arterial pressure is normalized. The introducer portion of the main device is removed over the guidewire, leaving the endograft in position.

Some devices require balloon dilatation at the proximal and distal landing zones to help assure proper seating and hemostatic seal with the arterial wall. If this is the case, a large-diameter balloon is advanced over the wire, and using fluoroscopic guidance the balloon is positioned and inflated. This same balloon may be repositioned to fully expand and seat the remainder of the endoprosthesis.

Once the complete endograft is in place, a pigtail catheter or multi-sidehole catheter is repositioned over one of the guidewires, and placed just above the proximal endograft for a final angiographic evaluation. If the graft is in good position and free of endoleaks, the catheters and guidewires are removed.

Closure of the arteriotomy(s) and arterial exposure site(s) is included in the work of the exposure codes.

DIRECT REPAIR OF ANEURYSM OR EXCISION (PARTIAL OR TOTAL) AND GRAFT INSERTION FOR ANEURYSM, ▶PSEUDO◀ ANEURYSM, RUPTURED ANEURYSM, AND ASSOCIATED OCCLUSIVE DISEASE

Procedures 35001-35162 include preparation of artery for anastomosis including endarterectomy.

(For direct repairs associated with occlusive disease only, see 35201-35286)

(For intracranial aneurysm, see 61700 et seq.)

▶(For endovascular repair of abdominal aortic aneurysm, see 34800-34826)◀

▶(For endovascular repair of iliac artery aneurysm, see 34900)◀

(For thoracic aortic aneurysm, see 33860-33875)

▶(For endovascular repair of thoracic aortic aneurysm, see Category III codes 0033T-0034T)◀

35001 Direct repair of aneurysm, pseudoaneurysm, or excision (partial or total) and graft insertion, with or without patch graft; for aneurysm and associated occlusive disease, carotid, subclavian artery, by neck incision

BYPASS GRAFT

Vein

▶Procurement of the saphenous vein graft is included in the description of the work for 35501-35587 and should not be reported as a separate service or co-surgery. To report harvesting of an upper extremity vein, use 35500 in addition to the bypass procedure. To report harvesting of a femoropopliteal vein segment, use 35572 in addition to the bypass procedure. To report harvesting and construction of an autogenous composite graft of two segments from two distant locations, report 35682 in addition to the bypass procedure, for autogenous composite of three or more segments from distant sites, report 35683.◀

+35500 Harvest of upper extremity vein, one segment, for lower extremity or coronary artery bypass procedure (List separately in addition to code for primary procedure)

(Use 35500 in conjunction with codes 33510-33536, 35556, 35566, 35571, 35583, 35587)

(For harvest of more than one vein segment, see 35682, 35683)

▶(For endoscopic procedure, use 33508)◀

+●35572 Harvest of femoropopliteal vein, one segment, for vascular reconstruction procedure (eg, aortic, vena caval, coronary, peripheral artery) (List separately in addition to code for primary procedure)

▶(Use 35572 in conjunction with codes 33510-33516, 33517-33523, 34502, 34520, 35001-35002, 35011-35022, 35102-35103, 35121-35152, 35231-35256, 35501-35587, 35879-35881, 35901-35907)◀

Rationale

A new add-on code and introductory notes have been added to the Bypass Graft/Vein subsection pertaining to the appropriate reporting for harvested vein segments. Code 35572 was established as an add-on code to describe harvest of the main femoropopliteal venous segment for use with vascular reconstruction procedures (eg, coronary bypass arterial occlusion, prosthetic bypass infection of the aorto-iliac or infra-inguinal arterial system). This procedure is designed to treat arterial occlusion requiring bypass with autogenous conduit, prosthetic bypass infection of the aorto-iliac or infrainguinal arterial system. Since every effort is usually made to harvest superficial veins for use as conduits, harvest of the femoropopliteal vein is a last-resort procedure. Typically, procurement of the femoropopliteal venous segment (FPV) is limited to patients in whom virtually all other autogenous conduit has been harvested. Procurement of the FPV has proven particularly effective in the setting where aortic reconstruction is required following removal of an infected aortic synthetic graft.

When the surgical revascularization of legs, arms, and internal organs is performed, the bypass "tubing" or "conduit" of choice is usually autogenous vein or artery. Autogenous conduits remain patent longer at most sites and autogenous conduits are less susceptible to infection. The identification of suitable autogenous conduit becomes an increasingly difficult task as patients undergo multiple bypass operations. As the technology and techniques improve in vascular repair, with wider applications for these procedures, the surgeon must search for other viable, suitable conduits when the more usual superficial sources have been exhausted (eg, lesser saphenous vein, greater saphenous vein). The femoropopliteal vein, which resides deep in the thigh and behind the knee, is harvested for use as bypass tubing and requires extensive dissection with special attention to preservation of surrounding nerves, arteries, and muscles.

A cross-reference was added following code 35572 to indicate applicable procedure codes used in conjunction with the harvest of femoropopliteal vein segment for vascular reconstruction. These procedures include CABG procedures with venous and combined arterial/venous grafting, venous reconstruction procedures (eg, vena cava, vein-to-vein), open aneurysm and ruptured aneurysm artery repairs by various operative approaches, neck vessel repairs utilizing a vein graft, vascular bypass graft repairs utilizing a vein graft, and as replacement graft for infected graft revision procedures. Additional text has been added to the Venous Grafting, Combined Arterial-Venous Grafting, and Arterial Grafting subsection guidelines to instruct users in the additional reporting of this add-on code when a femoropopliteal vein is harvested as an adjunct procedure to a coronary bypass procedure using a venous graft.

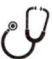 **Clinical Example (35572)**

A 70-year-old male has comorbidities including tobacco abuse, COPD, CAD, and MI, and he is status post revascularization surgeries including CABG using autogenous vein, bilateral lower extremity bypass grafts using autogenous vein, and a synthetic femoral-femoral bypass graft, the latter as treatment for an occluded left iliac artery. He returned to medical attention with complaints of fever, chills, malaise, and a small skin pore in his left groin that is releasing purulent drainage. Diagnostic workup revealed infection of the femoral-femoral graft, requiring surgical removal and extensive debridement. As a result he has severe left leg ischemia, and a new graft must be placed to save his leg. Extensive duplex vein search reveals that he has no remaining autogenous superficial vein suitable for conduit on either lower or upper extremity. Synthetic revascularization is contraindicated due to open groin wounds and significant local infection. Femoral-femoral bypass using vein conduit is recommended (separately reportable as CPT code 35558). Autogenous femoropopliteal vein is harvested for use as conduit.

Description of Procedure (35572)

Intra-service work begins with the skin incision. An incision is extended from the groin along the anterior aspect of the thigh. Soft tissue is dissected with electrocautery. The lateral border of the sartorius muscle is identified and reflected medially to expose the adductor canal. The femoral vein (FV) is identified next to the femoral artery. The branches of the FV are carefully doubly ligated and divided without injuring the vein wall. The dissection is continued distally as the vein and artery travel deep in the thigh. The adductor hiatus is opened by dividing the tendinous insertion of the adductor magnus muscle. The dissection is usually tedious in the distal adductor canal region where there are often multiple large branches that must be carefully ligated, and where the vein is usually in very close apposition to the artery and the aponeurosis of the adductor magnus. At the upper end of the popliteal space the name of the deep vein becomes the popliteal vein. Initial dissection of the popliteal vein follows the same incision and planes as the femoral did, but a separate incision is required to harvest the most distant segment of popliteal vein. When the vein is completely exposed, it is ligated proximally and distally, and divided. The vein segment is removed from the thigh and measured to determine that adequate length has been obtained. Vein valves are disrupted using a valvulotome. Flow through the new conduit is tested by injection of heparinized saline. Any missed branches or rents in the conduit are repaired under loupe magnification using very fine suture.

Once the conduit is proven adequate, it is used in the bypass procedure.

After completion of the bypass, the vein harvest site is irrigated copiously, and hemostasis is achieved with electrocautery and suture ligation as required. The harvest site wound is closed in multiple layers. Drains are inserted as required.

Other Than Vein

35601 Bypass graft, with other than vein; carotid

35606 carotid-subclavian

▶(For open subclavian to carotid artery transposition performed in conjunction with endovascular thoracic aneurysm repair, use Category III code 0037T)◀

35641 aortoiliac or bi-iliac

▶(For open placement of aorto-bi-iliac prosthesis following unsuccessful endovascular repair, use 34831)◀

35646 aortobifemoral

▶(For open placement of aortobifemoral prosthesis following unsuccessful endovascular repair, use 34832)◀

ARTERIAL TRANSPOSITION

35691 Transposition and/or reimplantation; vertebral to carotid artery

35694 subclavian to carotid artery

▶(For open subclavian to carotid artery transposition performed in conjunction with endovascular thoracic aneurysm repair, use Category III code 0037T)◀

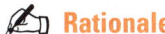 **Rationale**

In order to direct the user to a new series of codes added to the CPT code set describing endovascular thoracic aneurysm repair, requiring at times the concurrent performance of open subclavian to carotid artery transposition, a series of cross-references has been added to the Other Than Vein (codes 35600-35671) and Arterial Transposition (35691-3695) subsections to indicate the appropriate codes for reporting this adjunct procedure. When performing open subclavian to carotid artery transposition in conjunction with endovascular thoracic aneurysm repair, code 0037T from the endovascular repair series of codes is to be reported. It is not appropriate to report a code from the existing, Other Than Vein or Arterial Transposition subsections.

VASCULAR INJECTION PROCEDURES

Venous

▲**36415*** Collection of venous blood by venipuncture

▶(Do not report modifier '-63' in conjunction with 36415)◀

●**36416** Collection of capillary blood specimen (eg, finger, heel, ear stick)

36420 Venipuncture, cutdown; under age 1 year

▶(Do not report modifier '-63' in conjunction with 36420)◀

36450 Exchange transfusion, blood; newborn

▶(Do not report modifier '-63' in conjunction with 36450)◀

36460 Transfusion, intrauterine, fetal

▶(Do not report modifier '-63' in conjunction with 36460)◀

36510* Catheterization of umbilical vein for diagnosis or therapy, newborn

▶(Do not report modifier '-63' in conjunction with 36510)◀

Rationale

Code 36415 was revised and a new code 36416 was added, with the addition of explanatory notes, to instruct in the appropriate assignment of the blood collection codes, to facilitate future transition and subsequent deletion of existing HCPCS Temporary G codes to CPT codes for the services for blood collection. In addition, a parenthetic note regarding inability to append the modifier '-63' has been included after each of the listed codes. Since the codes specify ages in the code descriptor and age has already been included as a factor for use of these codes, use of the modifier '-63' does not apply.

●**36511** Therapeutic apheresis; for white blood cells

●**36512** for red blood cells

●**36513** for platelets

●**36514** for plasma pheresis

●**36515** with extracorporeal immunoadsorption and plasma reinfusion

●**36516** with extracorporeal selective adsorption or selective filtration and plasma reinfusion

▶(36520 has been deleted. To report, see 36511-36512)◀

▶(36521 has been deleted. To report, use 36516)◀

Rationale

Four new codes were added to describe therapeutic apheresis procedures of the components of the blood, two new codes to describe apheresis procedures with plasma reinfusion procedures and codes 36520 and 36521 were deleted to assist in incorporating this new series of codes into the CPT code set.

Prior to this year, the existing apheresis procedure codes 36520 and 36521 described outdated techniques that were no longer widely used. The new series of CPT codes reflects the current clinical practice, and a more specific listing of the various components of the present clinical procedure, allowing more accurate tracking of the frequency of performance of the various therapeutic apheresis procedures. This new series of codes also allows for more accurate coding of the actual work and procedures, and more accurate reporting of the procedures performed for each patient, breaking the apheresis procedure into a number of elements that may or may not be used in a specific patient since the different types of apheresis involve different amounts of work and technique.

These codes are FDA-approved apheresis machines with FDA-approved extracorporeal affinity devices for removal of antibodies for the treatment of patients with immune-mediated disorders such as factor VIII inhibitors. The therapeutic use of these devices is highly specialized and requires expertise in apheresis medicine. The risk to the patient is moderate to high. These procedures may be performed under emergency conditions and may be associated with allergic reactions or other complications requiring physician intervention.

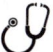
Clinical Example (36511)

The typical patient is a 40-year-old female with acute leukemia who is found to have a leukemic blast count of ≥50,000/µL or a total white blood cell count ≥100,000/µL. At such very high white blood cell or leukemic blast counts there is an unacceptably high risk of cerebral or pulmonary leukostasis, a potentially fatal condition that results from obstruction of small arteries or arterioles by adherent white blood cells. Patients typically suffer strokes or respiratory failure. Emergent lowering of the circulating white blood cell mass, by leukapheresis, is the only viable short-term management option. Under these circumstances, the patient is hospitalized for the apheresis procedure. The physician who is responsible for the procedure must assess the appropriateness of the procedure for the patient, calculate the parameters of apheresis prior to the procedure, and manage the patient during the procedure. The procedure is typically performed emergently.

Description of Procedure (36511)

The procedure is performed using FDA-approved blood processing (apheresis) machines. The machine's tubing system is connected to the patient's venous system either directly using the antecubital veins or, more typically, through a large-bore, dual-lumen dialysis-type central venous catheter. The apheresis physician either operates the machine or attends at the bedside while an apheresis nurse operates the machine. The patient often requires intensive monitoring including cardiac monitoring and continuous pulse oximetry. The patient is assessed at the end of the apheresis procedure.

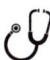
Clinical Example (36512)

The typical patient is a 21-year-old man with sickle cell anemia who has suffered a cerebral infarction and is at very high risk of recurrent stroke. The only effective method for preventing a recurrence is to have his blood chronically replaced with non-sickling blood. Simple red blood cell transfusion therapy is not acceptable or appropriate because it would result in transfusional iron overload, a condition that results in heart failure, liver failure, and death. Red blood cell exchange by apheresis does not result in iron overload. The apheresis physician assesses the patient prior to initiating the procedure and determines the treatment parameters necessary to achieve the targeted substitution of hemoglobin A blood for sickle hemoglobin blood. Automated red blood cell exchange is performed at whole blood flow rates far in excess of typical blood transfusions. The inherent risk of the procedure necessitates frequent attention on the part of the physician during the procedure. A final assessment is performed at the termination of the procedure.

Description of Procedure (36512)

There are four FDA-approved apheresis machines to do this procedure. The patient is connected to the blood processor (apheresis machine) by either the antecubital veins or using a large bore, dual-lumen dialysis catheter. The apheresis procedure exchanges the patient's red blood cells for donor red blood cells. The apheresis physician either operates the machine or attends the patient at the bedside while an apheresis nurse operates the machine. The risk to the patient is moderate. The patient is assessed at the end of the apheresis procedure.

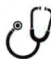
Clinical Example (36513)

The typical patient is a 65-year-old male with a myeloproliferative disorder (essential thrombocythemia, chronic myelogenous leukemia, or polycythemia vera) whose platelet count is unusually high (≥1,000,000/μL). Because of the degree of thrombocytosis, there is a high risk of coronary or cerebral infarction. Therapeutic apheresis often is performed emergently because of altered mental status resulting from the thrombocytosis. The apheresis physician assesses the patient and determines the appropriateness of therapeutic apheresis. The physician also calculates the exchange parameters and writes orders for the procedure. This is a high-acuity setting and the physician is in attendance during the procedure.

Description of Procedure (36513)

The patient is connected to an apheresis machine. The patient's platelets are removed by an apheresis machine. The patient is assessed at the end of the apheresis procedure.

Clinical Example (36514)

The typical patient is a 25-year-old male with thrombotic thrombocytopenic purpura. The universally accepted first-line therapy for this life-threatening condition is therapeutic plasma exchange. The apheresis physician assesses the patient prior to the procedure, paying particular attention to clinical parameters that determine the patient's ability to tolerate exposure to unusually large volumes of allogeneic plasma. The apheresis physician writes orders for the procedure, which often must be performed on a daily basis, determines the appropriate biological replacement fluid, and manages blood product support. These patients are typically treated using a dual-lumen, large-bore dialysis-type catheter. The apheresis physician manages the catheter and monitors the patient for catheter-related complications.

Description of Procedure (36514)

The patient's blood is drawn into the apheresis machine for the purpose of separating blood from plasma. The plasma is diverted to a collection bag and the cells are returned to the patient with a biological replacement fluid such as allogeneic plasma or human serum albumin as determined by the apheresis physician. The apheresis physician manages the central venous dialysis-type catheter on treatment days and on off days. The apheresis physician also must manage allergic reactions to the biological replacement fluids and transfusion reactions that may occur when plasma is the replacement fluid. The patient is assessed at the end of the apheresis procedure.

Clinical Example (36515)

The typical patient has hereditary hemophilia A (factor VIII deficiency) and a high-titer immunoglobulin inhibitor to human factor VIII replacement products. He is acutely and spontaneously hemorrhaging and is unable to respond favorably to infusions of human factor VIII. The apheresis procedure is indicated for removal of the high-titer IgG anti-factor VIII antibodies from the patient's plasma without removing other plasma proteins such as clotting factors and fibrinogen. The apheresis machine is used to separate the patient's plasma from the cellular components of whole blood so that the plasma can be adsorbed on a special affinity column which removes the IgG but allows the rest of the plasma constituents to pass through unadsorbed. The factor VIII inhibitor titer is thus lowered sufficiently to permit the patient to respond to infused human factor VIII.

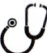
Clinical Example (36516)
The typical patient is a homozygote or heterozygote with familial hypercholesterolemia whose serum lipids have not been satisfactorily controlled with maximum medical therapy. Often these patients will have had a myocardial infarction or other manifestations of coronary artery disease before age 40 years. Weekly or semi-monthly lipid apheresis is the only effective method for controlling symptomatic hyperlipidemias in these patients. The apheresis physician is responsible for assessing the appropriateness of this therapy for the individual patient, for writing appropriate orders, and for managing the patient during treatments. If a venous access device or catheter is required, the apheresis physician is responsible for managing the catheter or venous device as well.

Description of Procedure (36516)
Plasma separation is performed and LDL cholesterol is selectively removed. Depending on the specific device used, the patient's treated plasma may require post-adsorption treatment prior to being reinfused into the patient. The patient is monitored for allergic reactions and for thrombocytopenia. The risk to the patient is above moderate. The patient is assessed at the end of the apheresis procedure.

36533   Insertion of implantable venous access device, with or without subcutaneous reservoir

(For refilling and maintenance of an implantable pump or reservoir for ▶intravenous or intra-arterial drug delivery,◀ use 96530)

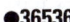
●**36536**   Mechanical removal of pericatheter obstructive material (eg, fibrin sheath) from central venous device via separate venous access

▶(Do not report 36550 in addition to 36536)◀

▶(For venous catheterization, see 36010-36012)◀

▶(For radiological supervision and interpretation, use 75901)◀

●**36537**   Mechanical removal of intraluminal (intracatheter) obstructive material from central venous device through device lumen

▶(Do not report 36550 in addition to 36537)◀

▶(For venous catheterization, see 36010-36012)◀

▶(For radiological supervision and interpretation, use 75902)◀

Rationale
CPT 2003 has added two new codes (36536, 36537) to describe mechanical or manual removal of obstructive material from central venous devices with cross-references to indicate that code 36550 would not be reported separately in addition to these procedures. Additional cross-references have been added to direct the user to the venous catheter codes and appropriate imaging guidance codes to report in conjunction with these newly created codes.

Advances in device technology have allowed for long-term venous access for patients undergoing chemotherapy, dialysis, etc. Occasionally, fibrin will collect at the distal end of these devices or within the lumen. As well, thrombus may form inside the device, thus creating an obstruction. If an injection of a small amount of a thrombolytic agent is unsuccessful, other interventions will often allow continued use of the existing device rather than removing and introducing a new device. This is of far less potential risk and morbidity to the patient. Treatment options include stripping the fibrin sheath from/about the existing catheter by use of either a transcatheter snare or balloon under imaging guidance, or alternatively, clearing the intraluminal obstructive material with a guidewire, brush, or other mechanical device under imaging guidance. While the CPT code set currently contains codes for introducing, revising, and removing some of these devices, the physician work associated with their maintenance goes unrepresented.

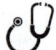
Clinical Example (36536)
A 68-year-old male with gastric cancer and a subcutaneous port presents with a poorly functioning port. Infusion/injection can be made but blood cannot be aspirated.

Description of Procedure (36536)
After venous access (work of access is separately billable and not included in code 36536), a vascular snare is placed in the cava through the catheter, and the tip of the central venous catheter is engaged with the snare. The fibrin sheath and thrombus are stripped from the catheter.

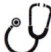
Clinical Example (36537)
A 68-year-old male with gastric cancer and a subcutaneous port presents with a poorly functioning port. Infusion/injection can be made but blood cannot be aspirated.

Description of Procedure (36537)
A ureteral brush is inserted into the catheter lumen and pushed toward the distal tip of the catheter, through the distal end hole, and then retracted into the catheter. The maneuver is repeated several times to "brush" the multiple side holes and the distal end hole. The ureteral brush is removed. The catheter is flushed with appropriate amounts of saline and heparin and the ports are clamped. A sterile dressing is reapplied on the chest wall at the catheter entry site.

▲36540   Collection of blood specimen from a completely implantable venous access device

▶(Do not report 36540 in conjunction with 36415, 36416)◀

▶(For collection of venous blood specimen by venipuncture, use 36415)◀

▶(For collection of capillary blood specimen, use 36416)◀

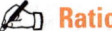 **Rationale**

Code 36540 was revised, and explanatory notes were added to instruct users in the appropriate assignment of the blood collection codes in order to facilitate transition and subsequent deletion of existing HCPCS Temporary G codes to CPT codes for the services for blood collection.

Arterial

36660 Catheterization, umbilical artery, newborn, for diagnosis or therapy

▶(Do not report modifier '-63' in conjunction 36660)◀

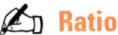 **Rationale**

For the code listed above, see page 244, modifier '-63.'

INTERVASCULAR CANNULIZATION OR SHUNT

36825 Creation of arteriovenous fistula by other than direct arteriovenous anastomosis (separate procedure); autogenous graft

▲**36830** nonautogenous graft (eg, biological collagen, thermoplastic graft)

PORTAL DECOMPRESSION PROCEDURES

▲**37140** Venous anastomosis, open; portocaval

37181 splenorenal, distal (selective decompression of esophagogastric varices, any technique)

▶(For percutaneous procedure, use 37182)◀

●**37182** Insertion of transvenous intrahepatic portosystemic shunt(s) (TIPS) (includes venous access, hepatic and portal vein catheterization, portography with hemodynamic evaluation, intrahepatic tract formation/dilatation, stent placement and all associated imaging guidance and documentation)

▶(Do not report 75885 or 75887 in conjunction with code 37182)◀

▶(For open procedure, use 37140)◀

●**37183** Revision of transvenous intrahepatic portosystemic shunt(s) (TIPS) (includes venous access, hepatic and portal vein catheterization, portography with hemodynamic evaluation, intrahepatic tract recanulization/dilatation, stent placement and all associated imaging guidance and documentation)

▶(Do not report 75885 or 75887 in conjunction with code 37183)◀

 Rationale

Two new codes (37182, 37183) were added to describe portosystemic shunt insertion and shunt revision procedures. The descriptors indicate that the insertion and revision procedures are inclusive of venous access and all associated imaging guidance and documentation. These procedures are therefore not reported separately in addition to the shunt codes. While the shunt insertion and revision procedures may be performed via jugular and transjugular access, these procedures do not limit access to these vessels, specifying instead transvenous insertion. In addition, cross-references were added to instruct the inherent radiological procedures within these procedures. Previously, these procedures were reported using existing codes that approximated the various aspects of the procedure (dilation, stenting).

In keeping with the primary objectives of the CPT-5 project for the development and implementation of guidelines, policies, and procedures to add clarity and precision to CPT coding, certain code descriptors have been revised to omit the use of phrases "any method"; "any approach"; and "any technique." As a result, the portocaval anastomosis code descriptor 37140 was revised to include the term "open," and cross-references were added following code 37140 to refer to the percutaneous procedure, and following code 37182 to refer to the open procedure, code 37140.

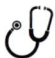

Clinical Example (37182)

A 57-year-old male with cirrhosis is admitted with his third episode of bleeding esophageal varices in 14 days. The patient is referred for diagnostic portography with hemodynamic evaluation to ascertain whether he is a plausible candidate for TIPS. If diagnostic portography with hemodynamics confirms the patient's candidacy for TIPS, the procedure will be performed. When the initial venography and/or portography (including imaging and access) confirms the need for TIPS and TIPS is performed, code 37182 is inclusive of these services. If TIPS is not indicated, then the appropriate codes for venography and/or portography would be reported in lieu of code 37182.

Description of Procedure (37182)

Following anesthesia, the skin is prepared with appropriate antiseptic. Under sterile technique, the right internal jugular vein is entered and a guidewire advanced into the superior vena cava. A large sheath is placed. A curved catheter is used to cannulate the hepatic vein and hepatic venography is performed to assess the adequacy of the vein for TIPS placement. The catheter is advanced deeply into the distal hepatic vein and wedged hepatic venography with carbon dioxide is then performed to assess the position and size of the portal vein. The diagnostic catheter is withdrawn and a sheathed cannula is placed into the hepatic vein over a heavy-duty guidewire. The cannula is positioned in the central portion of the hepatic vein and brought into contact with the inferior wall of the vein. A sharp stylet is advanced into the hepatic parenchyma in the direction of the portal vein and withdrawn slowly until blood return is seen. Contrast is injected to confirm intraportal position and a guidewire is carefully threaded into the portal vein. A pigtail catheter is placed over the wire into the portal vein and portal venous pressures and IVC/right atrial pressures are obtained. A diagnostic portogram is performed and filmed.

After confirming the adequacy of the puncture site into the portal vein for TIPS placement, the hepatic parenchymal tract between the hepatic vein and portal vein is dilated. A balloon angioplasty catheter is placed over the wire and the tract created with serial balloon inflations. A large sheath is advanced into the portal vein.

Stent placement is carried out. Following tract dilation, a self-expanding stent is positioned in the tract and deployed under careful fluoroscopic control to place appropriate amounts of stent within both the portal and hepatic veins. The stent is fully expanded with a second balloon dilation and a portogram performed to check adequacy of the result. A second stent may need to be deployed to ensure adequate coverage of the tract and/or the portal or hepatic veins. Portal pressures are remeasured and compared with pre-TIPS values.

Following repeat intra-operative portography with or without additional hemodynamics, the stent delivery catheter and sheath are withdrawn. Hemostatis is achieved. Patient is sent to the ICU or recovery room.

Clinical Example (37183)

A 62-year-old male with alcoholic cirrhosis who had TIPS performed 6 months ago for treatment of variceal hemorrhage presents with recurrent GI bleeding. Endoscopy confirms the presence of gastric varices and TIPS stenosis or occlusion is suspected. The patient is referred for TIPS revision. When the initial venography and/or portography (inlcuding imaging and access) confirms the need for TIPS revision and TIPS revision is performed, code 37183 is inclusive of these services. If TIPS is not indicated then the appropriate codes for venography and/or portography would be reported in lieu of code 37183.

Description of Procedure (37183)

Following anesthesia, the skin is prepared with appropriate antiseptic. Under sterile technique, the right internal jugular vein is entered and a guidewire advanced into the superior vena cava. A large sheath is placed. A curved catheter is used to cannulate the hepatic vein and hepatic venography is performed. The TIPS shunt is catheterized and a wire and catheter are advanced into the portal vein. A portogram and shunt study of the TIPS tract are performed along with portal pressure measurements.

If thrombus in the TIPS tract or portal vein clot is present, either pharmacological and/or mechanical removal of the thrombus is performed and the tract and portal vein are restudied. If TIPS tract stenosis is present, angioplasty and/or repeat stenting of the tract is performed to re-establish a widely patent tract and normalize pressures.

A portogram is performed to check adequacy of the result. Portal pressures are remeasured and compared with pre-revision values. The catheter and sheath are removed from the puncture site and hemostasis is achieved. The patient is sent to the ICU or recovery room.

▶ENDOSCOPY◄

▶Surgical vascular endoscopy always includes diagnostic endoscopy.◄

●37500 Vascular endoscopy, surgical, with ligation of perforator veins, subfascial (SEPS)

▶(For open procedure, use 37760)◄

●37501 Unlisted vascular endoscopy procedure

Rationale

A new heading, notes, and a new vascular endoscopy CPT code (37500) were established to report as the minimally invasive approach for endoscopic ligation of incompetent perforator veins of the lower extremity subfascial endoscopic perforator surgery (SEPS).

Perforating veins cross the muscular fascia of the leg, connecting the deep venous system with the subcutaneous veins. One-way valves in these veins block the flow of blood from the deep compartments to the subcutaneous soft tissue. Incompetence of the one-way valves has been implicated in the formation of venous stasis condition as venous blood is allowed to engorge the subcutaneous space. In early stages, this condition leads to leg swelling and pain with standing or sitting for protracted periods of time. As it progresses, the symptoms become more severe and include skin induration and discoloration, pruritus, and increased pain. In advanced stages venous stasis ulcers develop, and these are extremely difficult to treat. This is an incapacitating condition leading to chronic disability. Patients with advanced disease may require nearly constant bedrest and leg elevation.

Prior to 2003, only code 37760 was available to describe the open perforator surgery procedure technique first described by Linton to interrupt the incompetent perforators and therefore decrease subcutaneous venous pressure. This operation, known as subfascial perforator interruption, includes a long incision and a large subfascial flap elevation in the lower leg, elevation of the fascia, and ligation of all perforator veins.

Using endoscopic equipment, the new surgical technique for subfascial ligation of perforators can be performed using a few small incisions wherein the subfascial space is entered with an endoscope through a small incision rather than a very long one. The subfascial dissection during SEPS is carried out using an inflatable balloon that pushes the fascia away from the muscle, thereby exposing the perforator veins that cross from muscle to fascia. The endoscopic approach minimizes operative wound morbidity and is especially important in legs that already have major chronic skin changes. Code 37500 would not be reported with 37760.

A cross-reference has been added to instruct that open surgical approach for ligation of subfascial perforator veins should be reported with code 37760.

Consistent with the structure of the CPT book to delineate endoscopic/laparoscopic/arthroscopic procedures, a new code was established to describe unlisted endoscopic vascular procedures to provide greater granularity in the unlisted codes for vascular procedures.

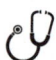 **Clinical Example** (37500)

A 70-year-old patient presents with stasis dermatitis and ulceration of the right lower extremity. Duplex scan of his veins corroborates the clinical diagnosis of perforator vein valvular insufficiency with identification of several large incompetent perforating veins and many smaller ones. To limit skin deterioration and help prevent recurrent ulcers, subfascial endoscopic perforator surgery (SEPS) is performed.

Description of Procedure (37500)

The first incision is made over the medial compartment, through the subcutaneous tissue and through the fascia for introduction of the "space maker" balloon. This device is introduced to the subfascial compartment, expanded with saline, then insufflated with CO_2 to develop the subfascial work area. Two additional incisions are made for port entry. Dissection and identification of perforators is carried out one at a time. CO_2 re-insufflation is performed as necessary. As each suspected perforator is identified it is cleared of soft tissue, absolutely identified as a vein, then clipped and divided with endoscopic instrumentation. A thorough search is made to identify and divide all perforators. The endoscopic spoon dissector is introduced through the port to identify difficult-to-find perforators. Additional incisions and scope insertions are performed as necessary to find and divide all perforators. Once completed the endoscopic equipment is removed.

Very low perforators not amenable to endoscopic visualization are approached through separate small skin incisions. They are identified, ligated, and divided under direct vision. All incisions are irrigated with saline and closed with sutures or Steri-strips.

LIGATION AND OTHER PROCEDURES

37600   Ligation; external carotid artery

37606   internal or common carotid artery, with gradual occlusion, as with Selverstone or Crutchfield clamp

▶(For transcatheter permanent arterial occlusion or embolization, see 61624-61626)◀

▶(For endovascular temporary arterial balloon occlusion, use 61623)◀

 Rationale

Two cross-references were added following codes 37600 and 37606 to direct users to the appropriate codes to report for temporary arterial balloon occlusion (61623) and permanent arterial occlusion or embolism (61624-61626).

▲**37760**   Ligation of perforator veins, subfascial, radical (Linton type), with or without skin graft, open

▶(For endoscopic procedure, use 37500)◀

 Rationale

In keeping with the primary objectives of the CPT-5 project for the development and implementation of guidelines, policies, and procedures to add clarity and precision to CPT coding, certain code descriptors have been revised to omit the use of phrases "any method"; "any approach"; and "any technique." As a result, and in conjunction with the creation of a new endoscopic procedure code, the Linton procedure code descriptor 37760 was revised to include the term "open," and a cross-reference was added to refer to the endoscopic procedure code 37500.

Hemic and Lymphatic Systems

General

BONE MARROW OR STEM CELL SERVICES/PROCEDURES

●38204   Management of recipient hematopoietic progenitor cell donor search and cell acquisition

●38205   Blood-derived hematopoietic progenitor cell harvesting for transplantation, per collection; allogeneic

●38206   autologous

●38207   Transplant preparation of hematopoietic progenitor cells; cryopreservation and storage

▶(For diagnostic cryopreservation and storage, see 88240)◀

●38208   thawing of previously frozen harvest

▶(For diagnostic thawing and expansion of frozen cells, see 88241)◀

●38209   washing of harvest

●38210   specific cell depletion within harvest, T-cell depletion

●38211   tumor cell depletion

●38212   red blood cell removal

●38213   platelet depletion

●38214   plasma (volume) depletion

●38215   cell concentration in plasma, mononuclear, or buffy coat layer

●38220   Bone marrow aspiration only

▲38221   biopsy, needle or trocar

▶(38231 has been deleted. To report, use 38205-38206)◀

38240   Bone marrow or blood-derived peripheral stem cell transplantation; allogenic

38241   autologous

●38242   allogeneic donor lymphocyte infusions

 Rationale

The existing code 38231 for reporting stem cell harvesting has been deleted, with the accompanying revision of the existing bone marrow aspiration and biopsy codes, and 13 new codes have been added to describe the services for management of a bone marrow donor search, stem cell harvesting, and preparation of the marrow for transplant, including depletion of various marrow components and cellular concentration.

Bone marrow transplant procedures are used to treat leukemia, lymphomas (Hodgkin's disease, non-Hodgkin's disease), breast cancer, multiple myeloma, renal cell cancers, neuroblastoma, ovarian cancer, aplastic anemia, inherited inborn errors of metabolism, and immunodeficiencies (eg, DiGeorge's syndrome, Hurler's disease, Gaucher's disease).

The services previously described by code 38231 have been expanded to more accurately describe allogenic and autologous harvest with codes 38205 and 38206.

Codes 38207 and 38208 have been added to describe freezing and thawing of bone marrow harvest after the harvest procedure, for preservation prior to the transplant or re-infusion procedures. Cross-references have been added to these codes to instruct that codes 88240 and 88241 should continue to be reported for performance of diagnostic cryopreservation and storage and diagnostic thawing and expansion of frozen cells procedures. Cytogenetic code 88240 describes freezing a small aliquot of cells to be sent to another facility for diagnostic testing. Code 88241 describes the thawing of the diagnostic samples subsequent to their shipment to another facility. These codes are intended to report procedures performed in the clinical laboratory setting utilizing a technique involving very small amounts of tissue.

Codes 38231 and 86915 are deleted, as these codes did not adequately reflect current technology and had no relevance to the present stem cell harvesting and processing work and procedures.

The harvest and modification procedures vary depending upon the type of cell being sought. A new series of harvest codes was added to provide greater granularity in available codes for these procedures. Codes 38210-38214 describe the depletion of T-cells in the context of an allogeneic graft to reduce the risk of graft versus host disease and include the different types, work, and techniques now used for different types of cell harvesting and transplant preparation, as well as the critical work and techniques involved in stem cell processing prior to a bone marrow transplant.

The newer techniques for transplant preparation of hematopoietic progenitor cells are performed in a transplant laboratory under physician supervision to achieve a pure cell population.

The present bone marrow transplant preservation and thawing techniques for the large amount of cells involve many new techniques, not all of which are used for every patient. The new series of codes provides greater granularity to code properly for the work performed in the specific patient.

The editorial revision of codes 38220 and 38221 serves to further differentiate these codes from the bone marrow harvest procedure codes.

Code 38242 was added to describe allogeneic lymphocyte infusions. Previously, lymphocyte infusions were reported with code 38240, which was typically reported as a second allogeneic bone marrow transplant and is inadequate for donor lymphocyte infusions. Lymphocyte infusion differs from the extender allogeneic transplant infusion in that there is no preparative regimen, there is no immunosuppression monitoring, and patients are not immediately pancytopenic. This procedure includes ordering the amount of cells to be infused, supervision of the infusion of those cells, and monitoring the patient for a transfusion reaction due to frequent crossing of the ABO blood group barrier. Patient monitoring is necessary as there is a high risk for pancytopenia and death due to cytopenia for four weeks after the infusion of the donor lymphocytes. There is also a severe risk of graft versus host disease since this is done as a T-cell infusion without graft versus host disease prophylaxis. The quantity of cells infused is at the discretion of the physician. 1×10^5 cells are used to treat any Epstein-Barr virus lymphoproliferative syndrome developing post-allogeneic transplant. The cellular material for the lymphocyte infusion is provided for the treatment of various viral infections post-allogeneic transplant.

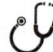

Clinical Example (38204)

The typical patient is a 35-year-old female with acute leukemia who lacks a human leukocyte antigen (HLA) identical sibling. Because of the need for treatment of the leukemia, a search for an unrelated donor is required. The patient's acute leukemia is in relapse.

The unrelated donor registry has 30 potential donors who are AB matched and 5 who are AB DR matched but are molecular subtype mismatched. It is necessary to select potential donors for further HLA typing, review the HLA typing to determine which donor is the best possible match, and select that donor as the potential donor. While a search coordinator orders the testing, the review of which prospective donors are tested and ultimate selection of a prospective donor are done by a physician. Criteria include the patient's age, the donor's age, the patient's controlled mechanical ventilation (CMV) status, the donor's CMV status, and the patient's HLA typing and subtyping. The urgency of transplantation determines how closely the donor must match the recipient to be acceptable and how long the search continues. Once a potential unrelated donor is identified, requests are made for information from the unrelated donor registry to help decide whether to acquire unrelated bone marrow or stem cells from a prospective donor. The donor size, HLA match, and status of patient's leukemia (ie, in remission or relapse) are used to make this decision. If the source of hematopoietic progenitors is umbilical cord blood, the ordering physician reviews how many cells are in the umbilical cord and, if possible, how many CD34(+) cells, before making a decision to order that particular cord blood. The physician managing the unrelated donor search then writes a prescription requesting that hematopoietic progenitor cells be collected from the prospective donor and by either a bone marrow harvest or a blood-derived peripheral blood progenitor cell collection. The requesting physician requests that the progenitor cells be collected to meet the recipient's needs. The bone marrow, stem cells, or umbilical cord blood is collected, local to the donor. The physician responsible for the donor's collection then informs the physician ordering the hematopoietic progenitor what the donor is capable of donating. The recipient's physician determines if this is acceptable to meet the needs of the patient or if the search needs to continue to find a donor able to meet the recipient's needs. The donor's physician tries to balance all donor safety needs with recipient needs for the organ.

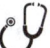
Clinical Example (38205)

The typical patient has acute myeloblastic leukemia (AML) in first relapse with an HLA identical sibling. Allogeneic bone marrow/stem cell transplant is the only curative procedure.

First, the physician evaluates whether the donor is a good donor, hepatitis types (if any), HLA type of the donor, transmissible diseases, and donor size versus recipient size to make a decision about using an allogeneic stem cell harvest. Then the actual peripheral mononuclear stem cells are harvested from the allogeneic donor using an FDA-approved apheresis device. Prior to starting the procedure that day the physician checks donor electrolytes, creatinine, CBC, and ECG. The physician monitors the amount of RBCs removed by the machine continuously if donor and recipient are ABO mismatched. The physician continuously monitors donor safety by evaluating blood pressure, pulse, and replaces electrolytes, especially calcium, as determined by patient symptoms and ECG monitoring. Post-procedure the donor CBC is checked if platelets need to be added from the product. Quality assessment of the collection procedure is performed by the physician using cell counts, cell differentials, flow cytometry, infection control cultures, etc.

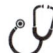
Clinical Example (38206)

The typical patient is a 35-year-old female with Hodgkin's disease in second relapse with no marrow involvement. Bone marrow transplant (BMT) is curative. Autologous peripheral stem cell collection is the treatment of choice. Recipient needs to be assessed for risk of myelodysplasia.

First, the patient's bone marrow cellularity is assessed. The hematopoietic progenitor cells are assessed for any cytogenetic defects and for any blood transmissible diseases. Blood-derived hematopoietic progenitor cells are harvested. Prior to starting the procedure that day the physcian checks patient electrolytes, creatinine, CBC, and ECG. The physician continuously monitors patient safety by evaluating blood pressure, pulse, and replaces electrolytes, especially calcium, as determined by patient symptoms and ECG monitoring. Post-procedure the donor CBC is checked if platelets need to be added from the product. Quality assessment of the collection procedure is performed by the physician using cell counts, cell differentials, flow cytometry, infection control cultures, etc.

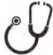
Clinical Example (38207)

Peripheral blood stem cells or bone marrow have been collected. These cells are to be cryopreserved for later use as part of an autologous transplant where hematopoietic progenitor cells first have to be cryopreserved for a later autologous hematopoietic progenitor cell transplant. In many cases, the bone marrow or peripheral blood progenitor cells are also cryopreserved for allogeneic transplants. This ensures that the cells are ready and available when the patient needs them. The physician writes separate prescriptions for cryopreservation and thawing of the product. A physician supervises both cryopreservation and thawing of the product and in an emergency performs these procedures himself/herself as a patient's life is in jeopardy.

The cryopreservation process is begun. It is important to make sure the freezing process is performed correctly to ensure that the cells have been frozen in a safe manner to be acceptable for transplantation. This requires following validated standard operating procedures. Cryopreservation data are reviewed and quality assessment of the procedure is performed. Cells are stored at a low temperature under controlled monitored conditions until needed for transplant. The quality of the cryopreserved transplantation product (bone marrow, blood-derived, or umbilical cord blood-derived hematopoietic progenitor cells, allogeneic T-lymphocytes) must be assessed prior to release of product. Examples of quality assurance are nucleated cell count, differential, viability, sterility, and/or immunophenotyping by flow cytometry for CD34(+) progenitor cells, T-lymphocytes, or tumor cells. The physcian then judges if this product remains suitable for transplantation or if new product needs to be collected.

Clinical Example (38208)

The previously cryopreserved marrow and stem cells are thawed in a heated water bath. A sample is obtained for post-thaw quality assessment such as nucleated cell count and viability. The quality of the thawed transplantation product (bone marrow, blood-derived, or umbilical cord blood-derived hematopoietic progenitor cells, allogeneic T-lymphocytes) must be assessed prior to release of product. Examples of quality assurance are nucleated cell count, differential, viability, sterility, and/or immunophenotyping by flow cytometry for CD34(+) progenitor cells, T-lymphocytes, or tumor cells. These parameters are recognized by two accreditation agencies (FAHCT and AABB) as necessary and are included in the regulations recently proposed by the FDA. The physician then judges if this product remains suitable for transplantation or if new product needs to be collected.

Clinical Example (38209)

Blood-derived hematopoietic progenitor cells have been harvested but the patient mobilizes very poorly with few stem cells. Thus, it is necessary to freeze them in multiple aliquots. Such harvest material contains a significant number of neutrophils or mature granulocytes, which are not capable of restoring hematopoiesis. Only the primitive cells are able to do this. Dimethyl sulfoxide (DMSO) is necessary for the cryopreservation. Because the cells have been frozen in multiple aliquots (multiple bags of these products were frozen over many days and then thawed later), the total content of DMSO is large and the patient gets a large exposure to DMSO. Such large amounts of DMSO in the transplant can potentially cause projectile vomiting and other injury to the patient. Thus, it is necessary to wash the harvest cells to minimize the DMSO content. A physician writes a prescription for this procedure based on the review of the cryopreserved product and whether the recipient needs to maximize cell dose or minimize DMSO toxicity.

The thawed cells are washed using an automated cell washer. During the wash process, cells are concentrated and resuspended in infusible-grade solutions such as saline/albumin. Quality assessment of the washed product is performed. The quality of the thawed transplantation product (bone marrow, blood-derived, or umbilical cord blood-derived hematopoietic progenitor cells) must be assessed prior to release of product. Examples of quality assurance are nucleated cell count, differential, viability, sterility, and/or immunophenotyping by flow cytometry for CD34(+) progenitor cells, T-lymphocytes, or tumor cells. The physcian then judges if this product remains suitable for transplantation or if new or additional product needs to be collected.

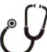
Clinical Example (38210)

The typical patient is a 10-year-old boy with DiGeorge's syndrome who needs a bone marrow/peripheral blood progenitor stem cell transplant from his father. The marrow has to be T-cell depleted for this allogeneic graft to reduce the risk of graft versus host disease.

T-cell depletion is performed using various methods. This instrument enriches the stem cells (CD34+) and passively removes unwanted cells such as T-cells. Quality assessment of the product is performed. The quality of the T-lymphocyte-depleted hematopoietic progenitor cell product (bone marrow or blood-derived) must be assessed prior to release of product. Examples of quality assurance are nucleated cell count, differential, viability, sterility, and/or immunophenotyping by flow cytometry for CD34(+) progenitor cells and T-lymphocytes. The physician then judges if this product remains suitable for transplantation or if new product needs to be collected.

Clinical Example (38211)

The typical patient is a 25-year-old female with B-cell lymphoma or breast cancer metastatic to the bone marrow. The patient needs an autologous peripheral blood stem cell harvest with later transplant but there is known tumor contamination in the bone marrow.

Tumor cell depletion is performed using various methods. This enriches the stem cells (CD34+) and passively removes unwanted cells such as tumor cells. Quality assessment of the product is performed. The quality of the tumor cell-depleted hematopoietic progenitor cell product (bone marrow or blood-derived hematopoietic progenitor cells) must be assessed prior to release of product. Examples of quality assurance are nucleated cell count, differential, viability, sterility, and/or immunophenotyping by flow cytometry for CD34(+) progenitor cells and/or tumor cells. The physician then judges if this product remains suitable for transplantation or if new product needs to be collected.

Clinical Example (38212)

A 35-year-old female with leukemia is blood type O and requires a peripheral blood stem cell transplant. The donor is blood type A. With such a stem cell harvest, ABO blood group barriers are routinely crossed. If fresh bone marrow containing Type A red blood cells is given to the patient, those type A cells will be immediately hemolyzed. This would cause renal failure and ultimately death to the patient because they could not receive post-transplant immunosuppression therapy. Because of the different blood types, red blood cell depletion is required from the harvest. The stem cell harvest is then performed. A physician writes an order for this procedure and supervises it.

The red cell depletion can be done by various methods such as mononuclear cell concentration using an apheresis device and a mononuclear cell enrichment using density gradient solution. Quality assessment of the product is performed. The quality of the hematopoietic progenitor cells (bone marrow, blood-derived, or umbilical cord blood-derived hematopoietic progenitor cells) must be assessed prior to release of product. Examples of quality assurance are hematocrit, red cell count, nucleated cell count, differential, viability, sterility, and/or immunophenotyping by flow cytometry for CD34(+) progenitor cells. The physician then judges if this product remains suitable for transplantation or if new product needs to be collected.

Clinical Example (38213)

The typical patient is a 35-year-old female with leukemia who requires an allogeneic peripheral blood stem cell transplant. The donor is much smaller than the intended recipient, thus requiring multiple days of harvesting. Because multiple successive days of stem cell collection causes the donor's platelets to become severely depleted, prior platelet depletion of the donor is required. The physician assesses both donor needs and recipient needs as this procedure will deplete some of the hematopoietic progenitors collected. A physician writes a prescription for a platelet add back to be obtained and separated from the blood-derived hematopoietic progenitor cell product.

The collected apheresis product is depleted of platelets using a centrifugation method. The separated platelets are infused back to the donor and the stem cells are used for transplantation for the patient. Quality assessment on both products is performed. It is critical to be sure that the donor is not harmed by an excessively low platelet count as part of the transplant process. The physician has to ascertain whether there is a quality platelet product obtained from the donor with minimal risk to the transplant product. The quality of the platelets (bone marrow or blood-derived) must be assessed prior to release of product. Examples of quality assurance are platelet count, hematocrit, nucleated cell count, viability, and sterility. The physician then judges if this product is suitable for infusion.

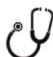

Clinical Example (38214)

The typical patient is a 35-year-old female with leukemia who is type A and requires a bone marrow transplant. The only available donor is type O. The donor's type O plasma has sufficient anti-A that it may cause hemolysis with infusion of the marrow product. The plasma needs to be depleted from this product so that there can be a safe transplant.

Plasma/volume depletion can be done by various methods (ie, centrifugation or nucleated cell concentration). In this process, stem cells are concentrated and plasma/excess volume are removed. In an emergency a physician does this procedure. Quality assessment of the product is performed. The quality of the plasma-depleted hematopoietic progenitor cell transplantation product (bone marrow-derived hematopoietic progenitor cells) must be assessed prior to release of product. Examples of quality assurance are nucleated cell count, differential, viability, sterility, and/or immunophenotyping by flow cytometry for CD34(+) progenitor cells or T-lymphocytes. The physician then judges if this product remains suitable for transplantation or if the procedure needs to be repeated.

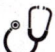
Clinical Example (38215)

The typical patient is a 35-year-old female with leukemia who is type B and requires a peripheral blood stem cell transplant. The only available donor is type A. Thus, to prevent transplant problems, a purified hematopoietic progenitor cell population (with minimal red cell and plasma contamination) is needed for the graft.

In this scenario, to avoid hemolytic transfusion reaction, both the red blood cells (RBCs) and plasma must be removed. This can be achieved by various methods such as mononuclear cell concentration using an apheresis device or density gradient solutions. In this process, stem cells are concentrated and plasma/excess volumes are removed. Quality assessment of the product is performed. The quality of the mononuclear cell preparation of the hematopoietic progenitor cell transplantation product (bone marrow, blood-derived, or umbilical cord blood-derived hematopoietic progenitor cells) must be assessed prior to release of product. Examples of quality assurance are hematocrit, nucleated cell count, differential, viability, sterility, and/or immunophenotyping by flow cytometry for CD34(+) progenitor cells and T-lymphocytes. The physician then judges if this product remains suitable for transplantation or if the procedure needs to be repeated or if new product needs to be collected.

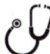
Clinical Example (38242)

The typical patient is a 35-year-old female who has previously received an allogeneic bone marrow transplant for chronic myelogenous leukemia. Post-transplant, the patient relapses with the return of the Philadelphia chromosome-positive cells. A lymphocyte infusion transplant procedure is recommended because of this relapse. An allogeneic donor is found for the lymphocyte infusion and the donor has undergone one day of pheresis to produce the transplant material.

Allogeneic lymphocytes are collected using an apheresis device. The T-cell content of the product is determined by flow cytometry. The precise dose of T-cells depends on the type of donor and whether the patient is being treated for infection or relapsed malignancy. Quality assessment of the product is performed.

Mediastinum and Diaphragm

Diaphragm

REPAIR

39503 Repair, neonatal diaphragmatic hernia, with or without chest tube insertion and with or without creation of ventral hernia

▶(Do not report modifier '-63' in conjunction with 39503)◀

Rationale

For the above listed code, see page 244, modifier '-63.'

Digestive System

Salivary Gland and Ducts

EXCISION

42400* Biopsy of salivary gland; needle

▶(For fine needle aspiration, see 10021, 10022)◀

▶(For evaluation of fine needle aspirate, see 88172, 88173)◀

(If imaging guidance is performed, see 76003, 76360, 76393, 76492)

42405 incisional

 Rationale

In the continued refinement of the fine needle aspiration procedure codes, a series of cross-references has been added to code 42400 to instruct appropriate reporting for the various procedures required for the acquisition and examination of tissue and specimen samples. These cross-references offer specific instruction to delineate the intent and use of the fine needle aspiration codes versus the anatomically specific percutaneous needle biopsy codes. A cross-reference to the fine needle aspiration codes instructs the appropriate reporting for samples from the salivary gland acquired by a method other than percutaneous needle biopsy. The cross-reference to codes 88172 and 88173 is intended to instruct the user in the appropriate reporting for evaluation of fine needle aspirate. The cross-reference to the imaging codes is intended to indicate the appropriate reporting for fluoroscopic, computerized tomography, magnetic resonance, and ultrasound imaging guidance modalities for evaluation of fine needle aspirate.

Esophagus

ENDOSCOPY

For endoscopic procedures, code appropriate endoscopy of each anatomic site examined.

Surgical endoscopy always includes diagnostic endoscopy.

43200 Esophagoscopy, rigid or flexible; diagnostic, with or without collection of specimen(s) by brushing or washing (separate procedure)

●**43201** with directed submucosal injection(s), any substance

▶(For injection sclerosis of esophageal varices, report 43204)◀

43235 Upper gastrointestinal endoscopy including esophagus, stomach, and either the duodenum and/or jejunum as appropriate; diagnostic, with or without collection of specimen(s) by brushing or washing (separate procedure)

●**43236** with directed submucosal injection(s), any substance

▶(For injection sclerosis of esophageal and/or gastric varices, report 42343)◀

Rationale
Coinciding with the two new codes (45335, 45340) added to the rectum endoscopy section, two new codes have been added to the esophagus endoscopy section for directed submucosal injection(s) of any substance. Code 43201 has been added to the esophagoscopy code series and code 43236 has been added to the upper gastrointestinal endoscopy indented series of codes. Prior to the addition of these codes, there were no codes in the CPT code set that adequately described the additional time, work involved, and risk to the patient of the submucosal injection, as typically this is a more difficult and lengthy endoscopic procedure. The code descriptor is generic in stating "any substance" and is to be reported only once for each procedure regardless of the number of injections performed.

Examples of substances that may be injected include india ink, which permits marking of a lesion allowing easier surgical or endoscopic identification of the involved segment of the gastrointestinal tract in the future. Other examples of submucosal injected substances are botulinum toxin, saline, and corticosteroid solutions.

In addition, cross-references now follow the two new codes directing the user to the appropriate code to report when performing injection sclerosis of esophageal and gastric varices, as these procedures should be reported with existing codes 43204 and 43243 and not with the new submucosal injection codes 43201 and 43236.

Clinical Example (43201)
A 75-year-old man with a history of lung cancer that had been previously treated with radiation therapy has been identified to have a radiation-induced benign stricture of his mid-thoracic esophagus. A previous barium esophagogram demonstrates the smooth nature of the stricture and prior endoscopic biopsies demonstrated the benign nature of the lesion. The stricture has been refractory to repetitive balloon dilations and therefore a request has been made to inject the strictured segment with steroids after performing dilation.

Description of Procedure (43201)
The physician explains the procedure to the patient and obtains informed consent. The patient is taken to the endoscopy suite, and an intravenous line is started. After the physician administers intravenous conscious sedation, with monitoring, a video upper endoscope is advanced via the mouth into the esophagus to the level of the stricture. The degree of stenosis precludes passage of the scope beyond the strictured segment.

A through-the-scope balloon dilator is passed through the endoscope and positioned across the stricture. The stricture is dilated to 12 mm. Satisfactory dilation is achieved. The balloon dilator is then withdrawn. With the intent of preventing repeat stricture formation at the site of the previous scarring, a sclerotherapy needle is passed through the endoscope and positioned at the level of the stricture. An assistant prepares the sclerotherapy needle with sterile steroid solution.

With careful manipulation of the needle tip, the endoscopist injects steroid solution into the strictured segment in a four-quadrant fashion. The assistant then withdraws the sclerotherapy needle. The physician monitors the stricture site for signs of bleeding. If stable, the endoscope is then carefully withdrawn. The physician records a post-procedure note, prepares post-procedure orders, dictates a note to the referring physician, assesses the patient's vital signs and status post-procedure, and discusses the findings with the family.

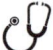

Clinical Example (43236)

A 75-year-old female is referred with complaints of weight loss and difficulty swallowing. Her physician ordered a barium swallow and upper GI x-ray, which revealed a markedly dilated esophagus with a "bird's beak" tapering near the gastroesophageal junction consistent with a diagnosis of achalasia. No other abnormality was seen. The patient would not consent to open surgical myotomy nor high-pressure balloon dilation with an attendant risk of perforation. She has agreed to endoscopic injection of botulinum toxin type A for chemical treatment of the achalasia. After two days of a clear liquid diet, the patient is prepared for upper endoscopy.

Description of Procedure (43236)

The physician explains the procedure to the patient and obtains informed consent. The patient is brought to the endoscopy suite, and an intravenous line is started. Intravenous conscious sedation, with monitoring, is administered by the physician and the video upper endoscope is advanced through the mouth and upper esophageal sphincter into an extremely dilated upper and middle esophagus. A "rosette" of folds is encountered that yields with a "popping" sensation. The endoscope is then able to traverse through the lower esophageal sphincter and complete the remainder of the entire upper gastrointestinal examination.

After inspecting the remainder of the stomach and proximal duodenum, confirming the absence of any co-existing mucosal abnormality, botulinum toxin type A is carefully loaded into a sclerotherapy needle. The sclerotherapy needle is then advanced through the endoscope by the physician, and injections of botulinum toxin type A are placed submucosally into the esophageal wall in each of four quadrants of the lower esophageal sphincter. After observation to confirm the absence of bleeding, the endoscope is then withdrawn. The physician records a post-procedure note, assesses the patient's vital signs and status post-procedure, prepares post-procedure orders, dictates a note to the referring physician, and discusses the findings with the family.

43245   with dilation of gastric outlet for obstruction (eg, balloon, guide wire, bougie)

▶(Do not report 43245 in conjunction with 43256)◀

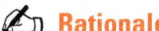 **Rationale**

A new cross-reference now follows code 43245 stating not to use 43245 Upper gastrointestinal endoscopy including esophagus, stomach, and either the duodenum and/or jejunum as appropriate; with dilation of gastric outlet for obstruction (eg, balloon, guide wire, bougie) with 43256 Upper gastrointestinal endoscopy including esophagus, stomach, and either the duodenum and/or jejunum as appropriate; with transendoscopic stent placement (includes predilation). This cross-reference was added to prevent code 43245 from being used for dilation for transendoscopic stent placement. As stated in the code descriptor, predilation is already included in code 43256.

REPAIR

43313 Esophagoplasty for congenital defect (plastic repair or reconstruction), thoracic approach; without repair of congenital tracheoesophageal fistula

43314 with repair of congenital tracheoesophageal fistula

▶(Do not report modifier '-63' in conjunction with 43313, 43314)◀

 Rationale

For the above listed codes, see page 244, modifier '-63'.

Stomach

INCISION

43520 Pyloromyotomy, cutting of pyloric muscle (Fredet-Ramstedt type operation)

▶(Do not report modifier '-63' in conjunction with 43520)◀

 Rationale

For the above listed code, see page 244, modifier '-63.'

OTHER PROCEDURES

43830 Gastrostomy, open; without construction of gastric tube (eg, Stamm procedure) (separate procedure)

43831 neonatal, for feeding

▶(Do not report modifier '-63' in conjunction with 43831)◀

 Rationale

For the above listed code, see page 244, modifier '-63.'

Intestines (Except Rectum)

INCISION

44055   Correction of malrotation by lysis of duodenal bands and/or reduction of midgut volvulus (eg, Ladd procedure)

▶(Do not report modifier '-63' in conjunction with 44055)◄

 Rationale

For the above listed code, see page 244, modifier '-63.'

EXCISION

44126   Enterectomy, resection of small intestine for congenital atresia, single resection and anastomosis of proximal segment of intestine; without tapering

44127   with tapering

+44128   each additional resection and anastomosis (List separately in addition to code for primary procedure)

(Use 44128 in conjunction with codes 44126, 44127)

▶(Do not report modifier '-63' in conjunction with 44126, 44127, 44128)◄

 Rationale

For the above listed codes, see page 244, modifier '-63.'

44140   Colectomy, partial; with anastomosis

(For laparoscopic procedure, use 44204)

44143   with end colostomy and closure of distal segment (Hartmann type procedure)

▶(For laparoscopic procedure, use 44206)◄

44145   with coloproctostomy (low pelvic anastomosis)

▶(For laparoscopic procedure, use 44207)◄

44146   with coloproctostomy (low pelvic anastomosis), with colostomy

▶(For laparoscopic procedure, use 44208)◄

44150   Colectomy, total, abdominal, without proctectomy; with ileostomy or ileoproctostomy

▶(For laparoscopic procedure, use 44210)◄

44152   with rectal mucosectomy, ileoanal anastomosis, with or without loop ileostomy

▶(For laparoscopic procedure, use 44211)◄

44153   with rectal mucosectomy, ileoanal anastomosis, creation of ileal reservoir (S or J), with or without loop ileostomy

▶(For laparoscopic procedure, use 44211)◄

44155   Colectomy, total, abdominal, with proctectomy; with ileostomy

▶(For laparoscopic procedure, use 44212)◀

 Rationale

In correlation with the addition of new codes to report the performance of laparoscopic colectomy procedures, seven new cross-references now follow several open colectomy procedures (44143-44155) directing the user to these new laparoscopic codes if the colectomy procedure is performed laparoscopically.

LAPAROSCOPY

44200   Laparoscopy, surgical; enterolysis (freeing of intestinal adhesion, (separate procedure)

44204   colectomy, partial, with anastomosis

44205   colectomy, partial, with removal of terminal ileum with ileocolostomy

●**44206**   colectomy, partial, with end colostomy and closure of distal segment (Hartmann type procedure)

▶(For open procedure, use 44143)◀

●**44207**   colectomy, partial, with anastomosis, with coloproctostomy (low pelvic anastomosis)

▶(For open procedure, use 44145)◀

●**44208**   colectomy, partial, with anastomosis, with coloproctostomy (low pelvic anastomosis) with colostomy

▶(For open procedure, use 44146)◀

▶(44209 has been deleted. To report, use 44238)◀

●**44210**   colectomy, total, abdominal, without proctectomy, with ileostomy or ileoproctostomy

▶(For open procedure, use 44150)◀

●**44211**   colectomy, total, abdominal, with proctectomy, with ileoanal anastomosis, creation of ileal reservoir (S or J), with loop ileostomy, with or without rectal mucosectomy

▶(For open procedure, see 44152-44153)◀

●**44212**   colectomy, total, abdominal, with proctectomy, with ileostomy

▶(For open procedure, use 44155)◀

●**44238**   Unlisted laparoscopy procedure, intestine (except rectum)

●**44239**   Unlisted laparoscopy procedure, rectum

 Rationale

Six new codes (44206-44212) have been added for laparoscopic colectomy procedures that were not adequately described in the CPT book. New codes 44206-44212 have been added as indents under existing parent code 44200 to allow appropriate coding of these laparoscopic procedures. Cross-references have also been added directing users to the open procedure counterparts of each of the new laparoscopic colectomy codes. In addition, an unlisted laparoscopic code specific to the rectum, 44239, has been added to encompass any laparoscopic procedures of the rectum that do not have a specific code. Also, to accommodate further expansion of the laparoscopic colectomy codes, CPT code 44209, Unlisted laparoscopy procedure, intestine (except rectum), has been deleted, relocated, and renumbered as 44238. A cross-reference has been added for deleted code 44209 directing users to the renumbered code 44238.

Clinical Example (44206)

A 56-year-old female presents to the emergency room with a 24-hour history of severe abdominal pain. Evaluation reveals rebound tenderness throughout the entire abdomen, fever to 39°C, and WBC elevation to 24,000. A CT scan of the abdomen is suggestive of perforated diverticulitis. The patient undergoes a laparoscopic evaluation of the abdomen with plans to proceed with a laparoscopic-aided sigmoid colectomy and colostomy if necessary.

Description of Procedure (44206)

The patient is brought to the OR and placed on an electric OR bed and given general anesthesia. She is placed supine with her legs in hydraulic stirrups. All extremities are checked for proper positioning and padding to avoid neuropathy. The abdomen is prepped and draped in a sterile manner. The initial 10-mm trocar is inserted using open technique and pneumoperitoneum is established at 12-mm Hg. Additional trocars are placed under direct vision in the right lower quadrant, right upper quadrant, and then in the left lower quadrant at the same site chosen for the colostomy. Laparoscopic evaluation of the abdomen indicates perforated diverticulitis with considerable free purulence. A single loop of small bowel is adhered to the inflammatory phlegmon and has to be mobilized out of the pelvis. The considerable adhesions between the sigmoid colon and the pelvic sidewall are meticulously taken down and the sigmoid colon mobilized by incising the lateral peritoneal attachments. The distal resection margin is chosen at the rectosigmoid junction and the bowel divided here using an endoscopic linear stapler/cutter. The mesosigmoid is divided with a combination of clips and harmonic scalpel. The left colon is further mobilized to allow enough length of bowel to exteriorize. Because of the peritonitis, a colostomy is elected rather than an anastomosis. The abdominal cavity is thoroughly irrigated. A stoma site is prepared at the left lower quadrant trocar site and the divided end of the sigmoid colon delivered up through the stoma site. All trocars are removed and the fascia closed at these sites. The proximal resection site is chosen, the bowel divided, and a colostomy matured. Sterile dressings and a colostomy appliance are placed. The patient is then transferred to the post-anesthesia care unit (PACU).

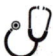

Clinical Example (44207)

The patient is a 62-year-old male who presents with a rectal cancer in the upper rectum. Colonoscopy reveals no other abnormality and CT scan is normal. The patient undergoes a laparoscopic resection of the rectosigmoid with a coloproctostomy.

Description of Procedure (44207)

The patient is brought to the OR and placed on an electric OR bed and given general anesthesia. He is placed supine with his legs in hydraulic stirrups. All extremities are checked for proper positioning and padding to avoid neuropathy. A catheter is placed. The abdomen is prepped and draped in a sterile manner. The initial 10-mm trocar is inserted using open technique and pneumoperitoneum is established at 12-mm Hg. Additional trocars are placed under direct vision in the right lower quadrant, right upper quadrant, and then in the left lower quadrant at the same site chosen for the colostomy. Laparoscopic evaluation of the abdomen indicates a mass in the upper rectum. The liver appears normal. The sigmoid colon is mobilized by incising the lateral peritoneal attachments. The superior rectal vessels are identified, dissected up off of the sacral promontory, and then divided using a combination of clips and electrocautery. The rectum is then mobilized by incising along the lateral edges of the mesorectum and entering the presacral space and dissecting distally to the mid-to-distal rectum. Special care is taken to identify and preserve both ureters and the presacral sympathetic chain. The distal resection margin is chosen at 5 cm distal to the mass. The bowel is divided here using a reticulating endoscopic linear stapler/cutter. The mesorectum is divided with a combination of clips and harmonic scalpel. The left colon is further mobilized to allow enough length of bowel to exteriorize. The abdominal cavity is thoroughly irrigated. The left lower quadrant trocar site is enlarged and the divided end of the rectosigmoid colon delivered up through the stoma site. The proximal resection site is chosen, the bowel divided, and a purse-string suture placed around the end of the bowel. A 31-mm anvil is placed in the end of the bowel and then the bowel placed back within the abdominal cavity. The left lower quadrant site is closed in layers. An EEA stapler is passed transanally and the spike advanced out through the rectal stump. The anvil and the stapler are mated and then fired to form an end-to-end anastomosis. The anastomosis is then air-tested under water. All the remaining trocars are removed and all 10-mm and larger trocar sites are closed at the fascial level. A closed suction drain is placed in the pelvis via a separate stab incision. The skin is closed with a subcuticular stitch and sterile dressings are applied. The patient is then transferred to the PACU.

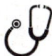

Clinical Example (44208)

A 62-year-old male presents with a large, fixed rectal cancer in the upper rectum. Colonoscopy reveals no other abnormality and CT scan is normal. Following adjuvant radiochemotherapy, the patient undergoes a laparoscopic resection of the rectosigmoid with a coloproctostomy.

Description of Procedure (44208)

The patient is brought to the OR and placed on an electric OR bed and given general anesthesia. He is placed supine with his legs in hydraulic stirrups. All extremities are checked for proper positioning and padding to avoid neuropathy. A catheter is placed. The abdomen and perineum are prepped and draped in a sterile manner. The initial 10-mm trocar is inserted using open technique and pneumoperitoneum is established at 12-mm Hg. Additional trocars are placed under direct vision in the right lower quadrant, right upper quadrant, and then in the left lower quadrant at the same site chosen for the colostomy. Laparoscopic evaluation of the abdomen indicates a mass in the upper rectum. The liver appears normal. The sigmoid colon is mobilized by incising the lateral peritoneal attachments. The superior rectal vessels are identified, dissected up off of the sacral promontory, and then divided using a combination of clips and electrocautery. The rectum is then mobilized by incising along the lateral edges of the mesorectum and entering the presacral space and dissecting distally to the mid- to distal rectum. Special care is taken to identify and preserve both ureters and the presacral sympathetic chain. The distal resection margin is chosen at 5 cm distal to the mass. The bowel is divided here using a reticulating endoscopic linear stapler/cutter. The mesorectum is divided with a combination of clips and harmonic scalpel. The left colon is further mobilized to allow enough length of bowel to exteriorize. The abdominal cavity is thoroughly irrigated. The left lower quadrant trocar site is enlarged and the divided end of the rectosigmoid colon delivered up through the stoma site. The proximal resection site is chosen, the bowel divided, and a purse-string suture placed around the end of the bowel. A 31-mm anvil is placed in the end of the bowel and then the bowel placed back within the abdominal cavity. The left lower quadrant site is closed in layers. An EEA stapler is passed transanally and the spike advanced out through the rectal stump. The anvil and the stapler are mated and then fired to form an end-to-end anastomosis. The anastomosis is then air-tested under water. At the time of testing a small air leak is identified at the anterior border of the anastomosis. This is repaired with interrupted sutures. Because of the air leak and the previous radiotherapy, a diverting ileostomy is placed. The ileostomy site is developed in the right lower quadrant. The ileum is then brought up out through the ileostomy site. A closed suction drain is placed into the pelvis and brought out via a separate stab incision. All the remaining trocars are removed and all 10-mm and larger trocar sites are closed at the fascial level. The skin is closed with a subcuticular stitch and sterile dressings are applied. The ileostomy is matured and a stoma appliance placed. The patient is then transferred to the PACU.

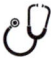 **Clinical Example (44210)**

The patient is a 22-year-old female with known familial polyposis with minimal number of polyps in the rectum. After considering the alternatives, she elects to proceed with a laparoscopic total abdominal colectomy with ileoproctostomy.

Description of Procedure (44210)

The patient is brought to the OR and given general anesthesia. Her legs are placed in hydraulic stirrups. All extremities are checked for adequate padding. A Foley catheter is placed. The abdomen and perineum are prepped and draped in a sterile manner. The initial port is placed in the umbilical port using the open technique and then four additional trocars (two on each side) are placed under direct vision. The bowel is completely mobilized by incising the lateral peritoneal attachments and by separating the omentum from the transverse colon. Starting with the left colon and then proceeding proximally, the mesentery of the abdominal colon is divided using a combination of clips and the harmonic scalpel. The rectosigmoid junction is divided using an endoscopic linear stapler/cutter.

The umbilical port site is then enlarged, allowing the colon to be extracted out through this site. The terminal ileum is divided just proximal to the ileocecal valve and a 28-mm circular stapler anvil is placed in the terminal ileum with a pursestring suture. The terminal ileum is then placed back within the abdominal cavity, the incision closed, and pneumoperitoneum re-established. The circular stapler is passed transanally and the spike brought out through the end of the rectal stump. The anvil in the terminal ileum is fitted to the stapler and the stapler is then fired, forming an end-to-end anastomosis. An air test is performed and then all the trocars are removed. The fascia is closed at the 10-mm trocar sites and all skin incisions are closed with subcuticular stitches. Sterile dressings are applied and the patient is transferred to PACU.

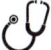 **Clinical Example (44211)**

An 18-year-old female from a known familial polyposis kindred presents with diffuse polyposis. She undergoes a laparoscopic total proctocolectomy, ileoanal anastomosis, creation of ileal reservoir, loop ileostomy, and mucosectomy.

Description of Procedure (44211)

The patient is brought to the operating room and given general anesthesia. Her legs are placed in hydraulic stirrups. All extremities are checked for adequate padding. A Foley catheter is placed. The initial port is placed in the umbilical port using the open technique and then four additional trocars (two on each side) are placed under direct vision. The bowel is completely mobilized by incising the lateral peritoneal attachments and by separating the omentum from the transverse colon. Starting with the left colon and then proceeding proximally, the mesentery of the abdominal colon is divided using a combination of clips and the harmonic scalpel. Dissection is then carried out in the pelvis. The ureters are both identified and the peritoneum incised circumferentially. The presacral space and the rectovaginal plane are entered and dissection is carried out down to the pelvic floor. The rectal dissection is then carried out transanally with a mucosectomy being carried out using a retractor. A low transverse incision is made to gain access to the abdominal cavity. The rectum is divided just above the pelvic floor and the colon and rectum are delivered out through the low transverse incision. The terminal ileum is divided at the ileocecal junction and then a J pouch is constructed using linear stapler/cutters. The J pouch is then placed back inside the abdomen and delivered to the pelvis. A hand-sewn ileoanal anastomosis is completed and then air-tested. A significant air leak is detected and the anastomosis is found to have a small defect that is then repaired. Because of the repair and some moderate tension on the anastomosis, a diverting ileostomy is elected. A proximal loop of ileum is chosen for the diverting ileostomy and a Penrose drain placed around the bowel at this point. The right lower quadrant trocar is removed and this site used for the ileostomy. The skin is excised in a circular fashion and the muscle and fascia split. The ileum is brought out through the stoma site. A closed suction drain is placed into the pelvis and brought out through a separate stab incision. The low transverse incision is closed after irrigating out the abdominal cavity. After removing all the remaining trocars, the fascia is closed at the 10-mm trocar sites and all skin incisions are closed with subcuticular stitches. The ileostomy is matured by incising on the antimesenteric border and then forming a Brooke-type ileostomy. An ileostomy appliance and sterile dressings are applied and the patient is transferred to PACU.

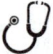

Clinical Example (44212)

The patient is a 32-year-old female who is discovered to have familial polyposis with a large, fixed rectal cancer. Following adjuvant chemoradiotherapy, she elects to proceed with a laparoscopic total proctocolectomy with ileostomy.

Description of Procedure (44212)

The patient is brought to the OR and given general anesthesia. The patient's legs are placed in hydraulic stirrups. A catheter is placed. All extremities are checked for adequate padding. The abdomen and perineum are prepped and draped in a sterile manner. The initial port is placed in the umbilical port using the open technique and then four additional trocars (two on each side) are placed under direct vision. The bowel is completely mobilized by incising the lateral peritoneal attachments and by separating the omentum from the transverse colon. Starting with the left colon and then proceeding proximally, the mesentery of the abdominal colon is divided using a combination of clips and the harmonic scalpel. The terminal ileum is divided just proximal to the ileocecal valve and the rectum is then dissected out. First, both ureters are identified and the peritoneum is incised circumferentially. The presacral space and the rectovaginal plane are entered and dissection is carried out down to the pelvic floor. The operating surgeon then goes to the pelvis and makes an elliptical incision around the anus and incises through the ischiorectal fossa and then the levator muscle to completely free the rectum. The colorectum is delivered out through the perineal wound. The perineal wound is closed in layers and pneumoperitoneum re-established. The terminal ileum is grasped, an ileostomy site is fashioned through all layers in the right lower quadrant, and the terminal ileum is brought out through this opening. All the trocars are removed. The fascia is closed at the 10-mm trocar sites and all skin incisions are closed with subcuticular stitches. The ileostomy is matured in a Brooke-type fashion, sterile dressings and an ileostomy appliance are applied, and the patient is transferred to PACU.

OTHER PROCEDURES

+●44701   Intraoperative colonic lavage (List separately in addition to code for primary procedure)

▶(Use 44701 in conjunction with code 44140, 44145, 44150, or 44604 as appropriate)◀

▶(Do not report 44701 in conjunction with 44300, 44950, 44960)◀

Rationale

A new add-on code (44701) to describe intraoperative colonic lavage performed in conjunction with colectomy procedures has been added to *CPT 2003*. In addition, two new cross-references were added to instruct the user as to the appropriate codes to report in conjunction with this newly established code, and to instruct the user as to which codes not to report in conjunction with new add-on code 44701.

The procedure of intra-operative or on-table colonic lavage is a technique that is gaining widespread acceptance for specific indications. This procedure allows a single-stage colon resection for obstructing lesions, thus avoiding the creation of a colostomy with its associated complication. Furthermore, this procedure avoids a second major operation (colostomy closure) which is associated with morbidity.

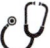

Clinical Example (44701)

The patient is a 65-year-old male who is undergoing emergency surgery for an obstructing sigmoid colon cancer. Intra-operatively it is decided to perform a single-stage procedure.

Description of Procedure

After resection of the cancer a decision to perform on-table colonic lavage is made. Mobilization of both the hepatic and splenic flexures is performed. The cecum is cannulated with a catheter through the base of the newly removed appendix. The distal end of the previously resected colon is opened and cannulated with a piece of sterile corrugated anesthesia tubing. The tubing is secured in place with an umbilical tape. The tube is then passed off the operating table and connected to a plastic container. The colon is then irrigated through the catheter in the appendix with warm normal saline until the effluent is clear. The catcher is removed, and the appendiceal stump is closed. The anesthesia tubing is removed and the distal end of the bowel swabbed with povidone-iodine solution. A one-stage operation is then completed.

44799   Unlisted procedure intestine, except rectum

▶(For unlisted laparoscopic procedure intestine except rectum, use 44238)◀

Rationale

In correlation with the expansion of the laparoscopic colectomy procedures, a cross-reference now follows code 44799 directing the user to renumbered code 44238 for unlisted intestine except rectum procedures performed laparoscopically.

Rectum

ENDOSCOPY

Definitions

Proctosigmoidoscopy ...

Sigmoidoscopy ...

Colonoscopy ...

For an incomplete colonoscopy, ...

Surgical endoscopy always includes diagnostic endoscopy.

45330   Sigmoidoscopy, flexible; diagnostic, with or without collection of specimen(s) by brushing or washing (separate procedure)

●**45335**		with directed submucosal injection(s), any substance
●**45340**		with dilation by balloon, 1 or more strictures

▶(Do not report 45340 in conjunction with 45345)◀

45378   Colonoscopy, flexible, proximal to splenic flexure; diagnostic, with or without collection of specimen(s) by brushing or washing, with or without colon decompression (separate procedure)

●**45381**   with directed submucosal injection(s), any substance

●**45386**   with dilation by balloon, 1 or more strictures

▶(Do not report 45386 in conjunction with 45387)◀

 Rationale

Coinciding with the two new codes (43201, 43236) in the esophagus endoscopy section, two new codes have been added to the rectum endoscopy section for directed submucosal injection(s) of any substance. Code 45335 has been added to the sigmoidoscopy code series and code 45381 has been added to the colonoscopy-indented series of codes. Prior to the addition of these codes, there were no codes in the CPT code set that adequately described the additional time, work involved, and risk to the patient of the submucosal injection, as typically, this is a more difficult and lengthy endoscopic procedure. The code descriptor is generic in stating "any substance" and is to be reported only once for each procedure regardless of the number of injections performed. Examples of substances that may be injected include india ink, which permits marking of a lesion allowing easier surgical or endoscopic identification of the involved segment of the gastrointestinal tract in the future. Other examples of submucosal injected substances are botulinum toxin, saline, and corticosteroid solutions.

Two new codes have also been added for balloon dilation of the sigmoid colon and colon. Code 45340 has been added for sigmoidoscopy with balloon dilation and 45386 has been added for colonoscopy with balloon dilation. As indicated in the code descriptor, these codes can be reported for each stricture that is dilated. This process is under direct visualization via the endoscope where the dilator is distributed uniformly in a radial fashion, avoiding the shearing type of force generated by previous systems. Although codes for this procedure existed in other areas of the CPT code set, there were no codes in the CPT code set that adequately described the new technology associated with "through-the-scope" (TTS) dilation systems for the colon and sigmoid colon. In addition, cross-references now follow these new codes 45340 and 45386 stating not to use these codes with codes 45345 and 45387, respectively. These cross-references were added to prevent new codes 45340 and 45386 from being used for dilation when performing transendoscopic stent placement since, as stated in the code descriptors, predilation is already included in the transendoscopic stent placement codes 45345 and 45387.

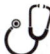
Clinical Example (45335)

A 68-year-old gentleman was previously identified to have a large sessile polyp in his rectum that had been removed endoscopically. The pathology evaluation showed high-grade dysplasia. He now returns for a follow-up surveillance sigmoidoscopy to assess for evidence of recurrence or neoplasm. The patient is prepped for flexible sigmoidoscopy, using enemas.

Description of Procedure (45335)

The physician explains the procedure to the patient and obtains informed consent. The patient is brought to the endoscopy suite and is prepared for endoscopy. A digital exam is performed, which is unremarkable. The flexible sigmoidoscope is inserted through the anus and advanced into the rectum where a stellate scar is identified in the mid-rectum. The instrument is advanced into the descending colon and careful inspection of the mucosa is made on withdrawal. No other abnormalities are identified. Due to the location of the polypectomy site behind one of the Valves of Houston, and to facilitate future identification of this site, india ink injection is undertaken. A sclerotherapy needle is prepared with sterile india ink and passed by the physician through the flexible sigmoidoscope to the site of the stellate scar. At the site of scarring from the previous polypectomy site, sterile india ink is injected to facilitate future identification of the previously removed lesion. The sclerotherapy needle is withdrawn, and the physician observes the site for signs of bleeding. The sigmoidoscope instrument is then withdrawn. The physician records a post-procedure note, assesses the patient's post-procedure vital signs and status, prepares post-procedure orders, dictates a note to the referring physician, and discusses the findings with the family.

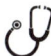
Clinical Example (45340)

A 72-year-old gentleman who previously underwent a low anterior resection for a sigmoid colon cancer has developed symptoms of constipation and difficulty defecating at 8 weeks postoperatively. The patient's surgeon had performed a barium enema that demonstrated a stricture at the anastomotic site. Before the patient's surgery a colonoscopy had been performed, and the only lesion that was identified was that which was surgically removed. The surgeon has requested that balloon dilation of the surgical anastomosis be performed in an attempt to improve the patient's symptoms.

Description of Procedure (45340)

The physician explains the procedure to the patient and obtains informed consent. The patient undergoes a full colon preparation with a lavage solution to facilitate completion of the examination. The patient is brought to the endoscopy suite and is prepared for endoscopy. A digital rectal examination is performed and is unremarkable. The flexible sigmoidoscope is advanced through the anus into the rectum and at 10-cm from the anal verge, the surgical anastomosis is identified with significant luminal narrowing. The sigmoidoscope is able to traverse the narrowing with some degree of resistance. No mass lesions are identified, and the stricture is typical to that of a postoperative nature. A 15-mm through-the-scope balloon is prepared. The balloon is passed by the physician through the flexible sigmoidoscope channel into the rectum and placed across the strictured segment. An assistant carefully inflates the balloon using a special gauge and pressure set to a previously designated value, while the balloon is held in place by the physician under direct visualization. The balloon is deflated and is removed from the endoscope. Another attempt is made by the physician to traverse the stricture. No evidence of perforation is identified. The physician records a post-procedure note, assesses the patient's vital signs and status post-procedure, prepares post-procedure orders, dictates a note to the referring physician, and discusses the findings and expected treatment with the family. The patient is again re-examined after awakening to assess for the development of complications such as perforation.

Clinical Example (45381)

A 55-year-old male with occult blood-positive stool has been previously identified to have an adenomatous sessile polyp in the transverse colon. Colonoscopy has been requested in an attempt to remove the lesion.

Description of Procedure (45381)

The physician explains the procedure to the patient and obtains informed consent. The patient is prepared for colonoscopy using a full colon prep. The patient is brought to the endoscopy suite, and an intravenous line is started. The physician administers intravenous, conscious sedation, and the patient is carefully monitored. The colonoscope is inserted through the anus into the rectum and advanced to the mid-transverse colon where a nodular, flat polyp approximately 2 x 3-cm is encountered. The polyp is too flat to be excised with routine snare technique. A decision is made that the lesion will be carefully marked for future surgical removal, using submucosal injection of india ink. A biopsy forceps is passed through the colonoscope, and biopsies are taken by the physician. The biopsy forceps is withdrawn, and a sclerotherapy-type sheathed needle is then advanced through the colonoscope. The endoscopist carefully maneuvers the needle to the edge of the polyp and positions the needle into the submucosa. Upon the endoscopist's command, an assistant, who has previously loaded the sclerotherapy needle, injects sterile india ink into the four quadrants of the submucosal tissue surrounding the polyp to adequately mark the lesion. The sclerotherapy needle is then withdrawn. The colonoscope is then advanced into the proximal colon and cecum and then withdrawn; the procedure is completed without other findings and the colonoscope is removed. The physician records a post-procedure note, assesses the patient's vital signs and status post-procedure, prepares post-procedure orders, dictates a note to the referring physician, and discusses the findings with the family.

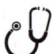

Clinical Example (45386)

A 65-year-old female is found to have occult blood-positive stool and crampy abdominal pain. The primary physician orders a barium enema, which reveals a transverse colon stricture at a prior colonic anastomosis. She also has a history of multiple medical problems including coronary artery disease, hypertension, and diabetes mellitus. After examining the patient, it is decided that colonoscopy would provide the best evaluation for the patient's signs and symptoms.

Description of Procedure (45386)

The physician explains the procedure to the patient and obtains informed consent. The patient is prepared for colonoscopy using a full colon prep. The patient is brought to the endoscopy suite, where an intravenous line is started. The physician administers intravenous, conscious sedation, while the patient is carefully monitored. The video colonoscope is inserted through the anus into the rectum and advanced to the distal transverse colon, where a narrowing of the colon is found that does not permit further passage of the adult-diameter colonoscope. The colonoscope is withdrawn and a smaller-diameter scope is then inserted through the anus into the rectum and advanced to the area of stricture. This colonoscope easily traverses the narrowed area, revealing only a benign stricture. A 15-mm dilating balloon is passed through the colonoscope and positioned across the area of narrowing in the distal transverse colon. An assistant carefully inflates the balloon using a special gauge and pressure set to a previously designated value, while the balloon is held in place by the physician with direct visualization. The stricture is dilated, the balloon is deflated, and the smaller-caliber colonoscope is removed. The adult colonoscope is introduced through the anus into the rectum, and another attempt to traverse the stricture with the adult colonoscope is made, which is successful.

Subsequently, the physician is able to reach the cecum using the adult colonoscope. The colonoscope is then withdrawn, examining all areas. No other lesions are identified and the colonoscope is withdrawn. The physician then records a post-procedure note, assesses the patient's vital signs and status post-procedure, prepares post-procedure orders, dictates a note to the referring physician, and discusses the findings and expected treatment with the family. The patient is again re-examined after awakening to assess for the development of complications such as perforation.

OTHER PROCEDURES

45999 Unlisted procedure, rectum

▶(For unlisted laparoscopic procedure rectum, use 44239)◀

 Rationale

Coinciding with the addition of new code 44239 for unlisted laparoscopic rectum procedures, a cross-reference now follows code 45999 directing the user to this code for unlisted rectum procedures when performed laparoscopically.

Anus

INCISION

46070 Incision, anal septum (infant)

▶(Do not report modifier '-63' in conjunction with 46070)◀

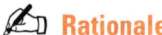 **Rationale**

For the above listed code, see page 244, modifier '-63.'

REPAIR

46700 Anoplasty, plastic operation for stricture; adult

46705   infant

▶(Do not report modifier '-63' in conjunction with 46705)◀

●**46706** Repair of anal fistula with fibrin glue

46715 Repair of low imperforate anus; with anoperineal fistula (cut-back procedure)

46716   with transposition of anoperineal or anovestibular fistula

▶(Do not use modifier '-63' in conjunction with 46715-46716)◀

46730 Repair of high imperforate anus without fistula; perineal or sacroperineal approach

46735   combined transabdominal and sacroperineal approaches

▶(Do not use modifier '-63' in conjunction with 46730-46735)◀

46740 Repair of high imperforate anus with rectourethral or rectovaginal fistula; perineal or sacroperineal approach

46742   combined transabdominal and sacroperineal approaches

46744 Repair of colloquial anomaly by anorectovaginoplasty and urethroplasty, sacroperineal approach

▶(Do not use modifier '-63' in conjunction with 46740-46744)◀

 Rationale

CPT code 46706 has been added to allow a reporting mechanism for anal fistula repair with fibrin glue.

For the above listed codes, see page 244, modifier '-63.'

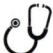 **Clinical Example (46706)**

The patient is a 24-year-old female with an anterior fistula-in-ano from a perirectal abscess. After considering the alternatives, the patient and the surgeon opt for treatment of the fistula by fibrin glue application. This was chosen to minimize the complications of fecal incontinence and rectovaginal fistula associated with anterior division of the anal sphincter muscle.

Description of Procedure (46706)

The patient is brought to the OR and given a spinal anesthetic. The patient is then positioned on the operating table in either lithotomy position or prone jackknife position. She is checked for adequate padding. The perineum is prepped and draped in a sterile fashion. Digital rectal exam is performed. Anoscopic evaluation is performed. A probe is passed from the internal fistula opening to the outer opening. After establishing the course of the tract, all granulation tissue is curetted away. Utilizing a flexible catheter, a bead of fibrin glue is placed at the internal fistula opening. A stream of fibrin glue is utilized to fill the fistula tract. Dry dressing is applied.

Biliary Tract

EXCISION

47700 Exploration for congenital atresia of bile ducts, without repair, with or without liver biopsy, with or without cholangiography

▶(Do not report modifier '-63' in conjunction with 47700)◀

47701 Portoenterostomy (eg, Kasai procedure)

▶(Do not report modifier '-63' in conjunction with 47701)◀

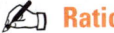 **Rationale**
For the above listed codes, see page 244, modifier '-63.'

Abdomen, Peritoneum, and Omentum

EXCISION, DESTRUCTION

▲**49200** Excision or destruction, open, intra-abdominal or retroperitoneal tumors or cysts or endometriomas;

49201   extensive

49215 Excision of presacral or sacrococcygeal tumor

▶(Do not report modifier '-63' in conjunction with 49215)◀

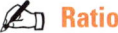 **Rationale**
For the above listed code, see page 244, modifier '-63.'

INTRODUCTION, REVISION, AND/OR REMOVAL

●**49419** Insertion of intraperitoneal cannula or catheter, with subcutaneous reservoir, permanent (ie, totally implantable)

▶(For removal, use 49422)◀

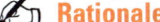 **Rationale**
New code 49419 was added to describe the insertion of a permanent indwelling, totally implantable catheter without external access ports. This procedure requires the work of a separate incision and creation of a pocket for the reservoir and is not inserted for the performance of diagnostic peritoneal lavage (49080). A cross-reference has been added to instruct the user to report 49422 for device removal and revision.

Intraperitoneal chemotherapy is commonly used for the treatment of intraperitoneal carcinomatosis, especially ovarian cancer and primary peritoneal cancer in women. This type of chemotherapy typically is administered through a cath, which is sutured in the subcutaneous tissue of the abdominal wall and connected to the peritoneal cavity by a semi-permanent or permanent catheter. The only CPT code which exists for insertion of a permanent device for intraperitoneal treatment, 49421, does not include the surgical placement of a port to which the intraperitoneal catheter is attached.

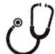

Clinical Example (49419)

A 42-year-old woman with stage IIIC ovarian cancer undergoes initial surgery followed by multi-agent chemotherapy, after which a second-look laparotomy reveals microscopic foci of residual carcinoma limited to the peritoneal cavity. The patient is counseled about treatment options and is advised to undergo intraperitoneal chemotherapy administration. To accomplish this procedure, the patient is advised that she will need to have an intraperitoneal catheter inserted with a subcutaneous reservoir.

Description of Procedure

A 6- to 7-cm incision is made in the upper abdomen. The incision is carried down to the peritoneum, and the peritoneal cavity is entered. Dissection of bowel and adhesions may be required to achieve a completely open peritoneal cavity. A subcutaneous pocket is created on top of the rectus fascia. The Portacath is then sutured to the rectus fascia. The Portacath is filled with heparinized saline. The catheter of the Portacath is then tunneled into the peritoneal cavity lateral to the fascia and peritoneal incision. The Portacath is arranged in a manner that will allow it to have free flow into the peritoneal cavity. The incision in the peritoneum and rectus fascia and skin are then closed in layers.

REPAIR

Hernioplasty, Herniorrhaphy, Herniotomy

49491 Repair, initial inguinal hernia, preterm infant (less than 37 weeks gestation at birth), performed from birth up to 50 weeks post-conceptual age, with or without hydrocelectomy; reducible

49492   incarcerated or strangulated

▶(Do not report modifier '-63' in conjunction with 49491, 49492)◀

49495 Repair, initial inguinal hernia, full term infant under age 6 months, or preterm infant over 50 weeks post-conceptual age and under age 6 months at the time of surgery, with or without hydrocelectomy; reducible

49496   incarcerated or strangulated

▶(Do not report modifier '-63' in conjunction with 49495, 49496)◀

49600 Repair of small omphalocele, with primary closure

▶(Do not report modifier '-63' in conjunction with 49600)◀

49605	Repair of large omphalocele or gastroschisis; with or without prosthesis
49606	with removal of prosthesis, final reduction and closure, in operating room

▶(Do not report modifier '-63' in conjunction with 49605, 49606)◀

49610	Repair of omphalocele (Gross type operation); first stage
49611	second stage

▶(Do not report modifier '-63' in conjunction with 49610, 49611)◀

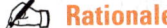 **Rationale**

For the codes listed above, see page 244, modifier '-63.'

OTHER PROCEDURES

●**49904** Omental flap, extra-abdominal (eg, for reconstruction of sternal and chest wall defects)

▶(Code 49904 includes harvest and transfer. If a second surgeon harvests the omental flap, then the two surgeons should code 49904 as co-surgeons, using modifier '-62')◀

+▲**49905** Omental flap, intra-abdominal (List separately in addition to code for primary procedure)

▶(Do not report 49905 in conjunction with 47700)◀

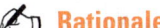 **Rationale**

New code 49904 describes extra-abdominal reconstruction of sternal and chest wall defects using an omental flap. In concert with the addition of code 49904, CPT add-on code 49905 was revised to describe intra-abdominal reconstruction procedures. A cross-reference has been added instructing the user to append modifier '-62' to code 49904 if a second surgeon harvests the omental flap.

Clinical Example (49904)

A 67-year-old man developed a sternal wound infection two weeks after open-heart surgery for coronary artery bypass. He is referred to the plastic surgeon for repair of the sternal wound defect following two extensive debridement procedures by the thoracic surgeon. The plastic surgeon reviews the patient's medical history and laboratory values, examines the sternal wound, chest, and abdomen, and confers with the referring thoracic surgeon. After the surgeon discusses the present problem and treatment alternatives with the patient and his family, the patient chooses to proceed with an omental flap reconstruction of the sternal wound defect.

Description of Procedure (49904)

At operation, the patient is prepared for general anesthesia. The abdomen and chest are prepped with prep solution and sterile draping is done. The abdomen is entered through an upper midline incision that extends to just below the umbilicus. The skin, subcutaneous layer, and linea alba of the midline fascia are incised. The peritoneum is incised and the abdominal cavity is entered. A nasogastric tube is inserted and its position is checked from within the abdomen.

After a brief exploration of the abdominal organs, attention is turned to assessing the omentum and its vessel pattern. By temporary digital occlusion of the left and right gastroepiploic vessels and Doppler flow measurements, a determination is made as to which vessels are dominant and which vessel pedicle would provide the best omental flap length, arc of rotation, and robust vascular supply. The omentum is carefully lifted up from the colon, and any adhesions are isolated and sharply divided while protecting the viscus from which they are liberated. After the omentum is freed, its attachment to the transverse colon is isolated and carefully divided. Care is taken to avoid injury to the middle colic vessels within the transverse mesocolon. Small blood vessels are individually clamped and ligated with fine silk ties. The short vessels between the gastroepiploic arch and the greater curvature of the stomach are individually clamped and ligated close to the gastric serosa. The omentum is lifted from the abdomen and over the chest to ascertain its reach. To provide more length, the left gastroepiploic vessels are divided at a convenient point along the greater curvature, without entering the region of the splenic hilum. Dissection at an area of the anterior diaphragm is enlarged to allow passage of the omental flap into the sternal wound without tension. The omental flap is transposed into the chest. It is carefully placed so as to fill the sternal defect in all directions. Care is taken to ensure that the omental pedicle is lying unobstructed and without compression and does not cause tethering of the right gastroepiploic vessels, which could cause gastric outlet obstruction or vascular compromise. The omental flap is secured to the surrounding structures with several interrupted sutures of 3-0 Vicryl. A Jackson-Pratt drain is placed over the flap and is brought out through a separate exit wound and anchored to the skin with a 2-0 silk suture. The abdominal peritoneum is closed with 2-0 Vicryl and the fascia is closed with 1-0 PDS suture. The skin of both the recipient and donor sites is closed with interrupted and running subcuticular 3-0 Vicryl sutures. The wounds are cleansed and sterile dressings are applied. The patient is taken to the recovery area.

Urinary System

Kidney

EXCISION

(For excision of retroperitoneal tumor or cyst, see 49200, 49201)

▶(For laparoscopic ablation of renal mass lesion(s), use 50542)◀

50200* Renal biopsy; percutaneous, by trocar or needle

(For radiological supervision and interpretation, see 76003, 76360, 76393, 76942)

50240 Nephrectomy, partial

▶(For laparoscopic partial nephrectomy, use 50543)◀

LAPAROSCOPY

50541 Laparoscopy, surgical; ablation of renal cysts

●**50542** ablation of renal mass lesion(s)

▶(For open procedure, see 50220-50240)◀

●**50543** partial nephrectomy

▶(For open procedure, use 50240)◀

Rationale

Two new renal procedure codes (50542, 50543) have been added to describe laparoscopic renal procedures. Code 50542 represents a retroperitoneal laparoscopic approach that allows the renal lesions (ie, small peripheral renal cell cancers and nonfunctioning obstructed renal moieties) to be visualized and destroyed by radiofrequency or cryosurgery without surgical removal. Code 50543 similarly utilizes a retroperitoneal laparoscopic approach and enables removal of renal tumors without an open incision utilizing technologies such as a beam coagulator. These two procedures involve a completely different operative approach and work effort when compared to the open nephrectomy procedures 50220-50240.

Clinical Example (50542)

A 59-year-old male has a routine abdominal CT performed for evaluation of abdominal pain. The CT demonstrates gallstones; however, an incidental 2-cm solid mass consistent with a renal cell carcinoma is discovered involving the posterior hilum of the left kidney. Due to the size and location of the tumor, it is elected to proceed with laparoscopic ablation.

Description of Procedure (50542)

The patient is taken to the operating room, positioned, padded, and secured to the operating table in a modified left flank position. His left flank is prepped and draped in the normal sterile fashion. A pneumoperitoneum is achieved in the standard manner and three trocars are placed: a trocar above the umbilicus, another trocar lateral to the rectus muscle half way between the umbilicus and ribcage, and a another trocar halfway between the umbilicus and xiphoid. All trocars are placed under direct vision and secured to the skin with sutures. The laparoscope is placed into the abdominal cavity through the port. Utilizing sharp dissection, the colon is reflected medially. The left kidney is identified and dissected away from the Gerota's fascia. The renal artery and vein are identified and freed up. Once the kidney is free, an ultrasound probe is utilized and demonstrates a solitary lesion at the posterior hilum consistent with the CT scan. The ablation device is deployed into the lesion, under ultrasound guidance, and the tumor is ablated in two cycles of up to 90 watts power. Once the lesion appears to be completely ablated, the device is removed. A small drain is placed in the retroperitoneum on the left side and sutured to the skin. All bleeding points are thoroughly coagulated. The trocar sites are removed and closed with sutures after all gas has been removed from the abdomen. The skin is closed with sutures and sterile adhesive strips.

Clinical Example (50543)

A 49-year-old female is noted to have microscopic hematuria on a routine visit to her internist and is referred to a urologist for further evaluation. An abdominal CT is performed which demonstrates a 3.0-cm solid mass consistent with a renal cell carcinoma involving the lower pole of her right kidney. Because of the size and location of the tumor, it is elected to perform a nephron-sparing procedure via a laparoscopic approach.

Description of Procedure (50543)

The patient is taken to the operating room and positioned in the modified right flank position. She is adequately padded and taped to the table and the flank is prepped and draped in a sterile fashion. A pneumoperitoneum is achieved and then three trocars are placed: a trocar roughly 6 cm above the umbilicus in the midline, a trocar two finger breadths off the xiphoid in the midline, and a trocar at the level of the first trocar in the midclavicular line. All trocars are placed under direct vision and secured to the skin with sutures. The liver is retracted anteriorly by placing a port to the left of the midline, halfway between the midline trocars. A paddle retractor is used to retract the liver anteriorly. Then the peritoneum over the kidney is circumscribed and using blunt and sharp dissection the kidney is dissected out within the Gerota's fat. Inspection of the kidney confirms a pedunculated 3-cm solid mass originating from the lower pole that is easily visualized. The renal artery and vein are dissected free by fulgurating lymphatic channels in the hilum. There are two renal arteries and one renal vein. The ureter is preserved and the periureteric tissue is preserved. The surface of the kidney is scored and bulldog clamps are placed on the arteries and veins. The tumor is excised, placed in the lap sac and removed. Biopsies are taken of the base of the kidney resection margin and frozen sections are reported as negative. The tumor is also sent for frozen section and good margins are also confirmed. All blood vessels are sutured. The collecting system is seen and closed with figure-of-eight sutures. A beam coagulator is used to fulgurate the parenchyma. Fibrin glue is applied over where the collecting system is closed and over the hilum of the incision. Pledgets are placed in the base and then the capsule is reapproximated with sutures. The bulldogs are removed. Total ischemic time is 25 minutes. The kidney pinks up nicely and papaverine is placed on the arteries. There appears to be good perfusion at the end of the procedure. A drain is placed through a lateral stab incision and placed posterior to the kidney and sutured to the skin with a suture. Prior to leaving the abdomen, the abdomen is inspected for bleeding, with no bleeding being noted. The trocar sites are closed with sutures. All trocars are removed under direct vision. All gas is removed prior to removing the last trocar. The skin is closed with sutures and sterile adhesive strips.

Endoscopy

50551	Renal endoscopy through established nephrostomy or pyelostomy, with or without irrigation, instillation, or ureteropyelography, exclusive of radiologic service;
50561	with removal of foreign body or calculus
●50562	with resection of tumor

Rationale

Code 50562 describes a renal endoscopy procedure for transpelvic resection of renal pelvic tumors through an established nephrostomy or pyelostomy. Previously no code existed to capture the technical aspect and work involved in this procedure. A renal endoscopy involves a completely different operative approach and work effort compared to performing a cystoscopic resection of a bladder tumor (52234-52235) or a ureteroscopic resection of a ureteral tumor (52355). Codes 52234 and 52235 describe resection of bladder tumors through a transurethral approach, whereas code 50562 describes resection of a renal pelvis tumor through a nephrostomy site. Code 52355 describes resection of a ureteral tumor through a ureteroscope passed transurethrally, whereas code 50562 utilizes a nephrostomy approach.

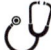 **Clinical Example** (50562)

A 69-year-old female with a solitary left kidney is referred to a urologist for gross painless hematuria. An intravenous pyelogram (IVP) demonstrates a papillary filling defect involving the medial aspect of the renal pelvis just above the ureteropelvic junction (UPJ). A voided cytology is positive for transitional cell carcinoma and confirms the neoplastic nature of the visualized lesion. Because the patient has only one kidney and the tumor involves the renal pelvis, it is elected to endoscopically resect the tumor.

Description of Procedure (50562)

The patient is taken to the operating room and placed in the left flank position. The field is sterilized, prepped, and draped. Under fluoroscopic guidance the left kidney is identified and a percutaneous guidewire placed into the left renal pelvis. A percutaneous tract is then established and segmentally dilated to accept an appropriate resectoscope. Renal endoscopy is performed with a flexible nephroscope and confirms a low-grade papillary transitional cell cancer on the medial wall of the renal pelvis. The nephroscope is removed and a resectoscope is then passed into the renal pelvis. The tumor is carefully resected, being careful not to perforate the thin wall of the renal pelvis or injure the renal pedicle. The tumor is then irrigated out of the pelvis with an evacuator and all bleeding points fulgurated. The resectoscope is removed and a temporary nephrostomy tube is placed to allow for drainage. The tube is secured to the patient's skin with a suture.

Bladder

INTRODUCTION

▶(Codes 51701-51702 are reported only when performed independently. Do not report 51701-51702 when catheter insertion is an inclusive component of another procedure.)◄

●**51701**   Insertion of non-indwelling bladder catheter (eg, straight catheterization for residual urine)

●**51702**   Insertion of temporary indwelling bladder catheter; simple (eg, Foley)

●**51703**   complicated (eg, altered anatomy, fractured catheter/balloon)

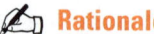 **Rationale**

The catheterization codes 53670 and 53675 listed in the CPT code set that represent procedures performed on the urethra have been deleted and replaced with anatomically specific codes that are reclassified as procedures on the bladder. Three types of catheters are described in the new codes. Code 51701 describes catheterization of a patient for residual urine. Code 51702 describes insertion of Foley catheter for patients with chronic problems, such as neurogenic bladder, and insertion of catheters in patients with acute retention in the hospital setting. Code 51703 describes a complicated insertion with examples of possible complications (eg, altered anatomy, fractured catheter/balloon). These new codes were developed to replace HCPCS code G0002, Office procedure, insertion of temporary indwelling catheter, Foley type (separate procedure). Codes 51701 and 51702 should not be reported when performed in association with another procedure.

URODYNAMICS

●**51798** Measurement of post-voiding residual urine and/or bladder capacity by ultrasound, non-imaging

 Rationale

A new code has been created (51798), located in the urinary section that describes a non-invasive procedure involving ultrasonic technology. This procedure involves use of a hand-held Doppler ultrasonic device to measure post-voiding residual urine and bladder capacity. The procedure represents only technical involvement, with no associated physician work involvement and was developed to replace HCPCS code G0050 Measurement of post-voiding residual urine and/or bladder capacity by ultrasound code.

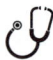 **Clinical Example (51798)**

A 70-year-old man complains of progressive decrease in force of urinary flow, urgency, frequency, and nocturia times five. As a part of his urologic evaluation a residual urine volume needs to be determined. With the patient supine on the exam table a dedicated ultrasound machine is used to measure the residual urine immediately after the patient voids. The residual urine volume is measured at 655 mL, therefore the patient is asked to go to the bathroom again to try to empty more completely. He is then rescanned and the urine volume is measured at 608 mL.

Description of Procedure (51798)

The patient's abdominal area is palpated to identify the pubic bone, and ultrasound jelly is applied to the suprapubic area. The suprapubic area is repeatedly scanned, typically three to six times. If the volume is high, the patient is asked to void again and the procedure is repeated. The jelly is cleaned off of the patient's abdominal area.

ENDOSCOPY—CYSTOSCOPY, URETHROSCOPY, CYSTOURETHROSCOPY

▲**52001** Cystourethroscopy with irrigation and evacuation of multiple obstructing clots

Ureter and Pelvis

52351 Cystourethroscopy, with ureteroscopy and/or pyeloscopy; diagnostic

▲**52354** with biopsy and/or fulguration of ureteral or renal pelvic lesion

▲**52355** with resection of ureteral or renal pelvic tumor

Rationale

An editorial revision to code 52001 has been made to clarify the use of this code for evacuation of large clots that are obstructing the bladder neck and causing urinary retention. Additionally, two other editorial revisions to clarify the use of codes 52354 and 52355 were made to more precisely describe the location of the ureteral or renal pelvic lesion/tumor.

Clinical Example (52001)

A 65-year-old male presents to the emergency room with lower abdominal pain and voiding small amounts of grossly bloody urine with clots. On physical examination, his bladder is tender and distended. Several urethral catheters are placed; however, they rapidly obstruct secondary to clots. Due to inadequate bladder drainage, the patient is taken to the OR.

Description of Procedure (52001)

After anesthetic is administered, a cystoscope is passed into the bladder and reveals diffuse prostatic bleeding with massive clots within the bladder. The cystoscope is removed. A resectoscope is passed into the bladder and the clots are evacuated with an evacuator. Inspection of the bladder shows no residual clots, stones, or tumors. The resectoscope is removed and a catheter is inserted to provide continuous bladder irrigation and tamponade any prostatic bleeding. After observation for 15 minutes, the irrigate appears clear and flows freely. The patient is taken to the recovery room.

Clinical Example (52354)

A 59-year-old male presents with a two-day history of gross, painless hematuria. An IVP demonstrates an area of narrowing in the left mid-ureter. A urine cytology is suspicious for transitional cell cancer.

Description of Procedure (52354)

The patient is taken to the OR and, after adequate anesthesia is achieved, a cystoscope is passed into the bladder. Inspection of the bladder with 30 and 70 degree lenses reveals normal mucosa. A guidewire is then passed up the left ureter to the region of the narrowing and the cystoscope is removed. A semi-rigid ureteroscope is passed over the guidewire into the bladder. Utilizing the wire as a guide, the ureteroscope is then passed through the left orifice and up the left ureter to the level of the narrowing. The area of narrowing is identified and appears suspicious for possible cancer. The guidewire is removed and the ureteroscopic biopsy forceps passed through the ureteroscope to the level of the lesion. A biopsy is taken and the biopsy forceps removed. A small electrocautery electrode is passed up to the biopsy site and the site fulgurated. The ureteroscope is removed and the bladder is emptied. The patient is taken to the recovery room.

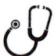 **Clinical Example (52355)**

A 48-year-old male with a solitary left kidney presents with intermittent gross hematuria for several weeks. An intravenous pyelogram (IVP) demonstrates a 1-cm filling defect in the left renal pelvis. A urine cytology test is positive for transitional cell cancer.

Description of Procedure (52355)

The patient is taken to the OR and, after adequate anesthesia is achieved, a cystoscope is passed into the bladder. Inspection of the bladder with 30 and 70 degree lenses reveals normal mucosa. A guidewire is passed up the left ureter into the left renal pelvis. The cystoscope is removed and a semi-rigid ureteroscope is passed over the guidewire into the bladder. Utilizing the wire as a guide, the ureteroscope is then passed through the left orifice and up the left ureter to the level of the left renal pelvis. The cancer is identified and the guide wire removed. A contact laser fiber is passed through the ureteroscope into the renal pelvis. Utilizing a holmium laser power source, the tumor is vaporized at its base. The mass is then removed with a grasping forceps. The edges are then lasered, vaporizing all margins. The laser fiber is pulled back 1 mm from the base and lasering is continued to coagulate the base. Further inspection demonstrates that the lesion is fully resected down to the muscle of the renal pelvis. The base of the lesion is inspected and there is no evidence of bleeding. The laser fiber is retracted and the ureteroscope is removed. The bladder is emptied and the patient is taken to the recovery room.

Urethra

INCISION

53020   Meatotomy, cutting of meatus (separate procedure); except infant

53025   infant

▶(Do not report modifier '-63' in conjunction with 53025)◀

 Rationale

For the code listed above, see page 244, modifier '-63.'

REPAIR

▲**53440**   Sling operation for correction of male urinary incontinence (eg, fascia or synthetic)

▲**53442**   Removal or revision of sling for male urinary incontinence (eg, fascia or synthetic)

 Rationale

Codes 53440 and 53442 were revised to differentiate male urinary sling procedures apart from artificial urethral sphincter prosthesis procedures (53431-53449).

Codes 53440 and 53442 are intended to describe treatment of male urinary incontinence, myelodysplasia, bladder extrophy, post-radical prostatectomy, incontinence, sphincter incompetence, spinal cord injury, and post-transurethral resection of prostate (TURP) incontinence. Urologists can treat these conditions/disorders either by insertion of an artificial urinary sphincter or by creation of a male periurethral sling utilizing synthetic or autologous fascia. With the advent of new synthetic materials, male sling procedures have become an important alternative to artificial sphincters in the treatment of male urinary incontinence.

Code 53442 is intended to describe the removal or revision of a sling in the instance where a sling may become infected, erode, or fail.

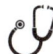

Clinical Example (53440)

A 62-year-old male status post radical retropubic prostatectomy has a 1-year history of severe urinary incontinence uncontrolled by medication. He currently soaks five pads per day and is embarrassed by his incontinence. Urodynamic studies reveal external sphincteric dysfunction. The patient is advised that there are two methods of treatment for his incontinence: a sling procedure or an artificial sphincter. He elects to have a sling procedure.

Description of Procedure (53440)

The patient is placed in the lithotomy position and a catheter passed into the bladder. First, a transverse incision is made in the suprapubic area and carried down to the rectus fascia. The rectus fascia is opened and the retropubic space entered. Then a second U-shaped perineal incision is made in the perineum under the scrotum and carried down to the bulbospongiosus muscle. The urethra is carefully dissected and the retropubic space is entered on both sides lateral to the urethra. A ligature passer is used to traverse the retropubic space through the incision from above, perforating the endopelvic fascia and exiting in the perineum on the left of the urethra. A sling graft (fascia or synthetic) is soaked and placed under the urethra. One end of the sling is attached to the ligature passer and then pulled up through the endopelvic fascia into the retropubic space on the left side. The ligature passer is then passed again from above, this time exiting on the right of the urethra. The other side of the sling is then pulled up through the retropubic space on the right. The sling is seated underneath the urethra and the tension is adjusted to provide support but not obstruction. The perineal wound is closed in a layered fashion. The abdominal fascia is closed with a suture. The sling sutures are tunneled through the inferior leaf of the rectus fascia and tied down firmly over the closed rectus fascia. The subcutaneous and skin layers are then closed.

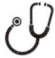

Clinical Example (53442)

A 70-year-old male had a periurethral prolene sling placed 8 months ago for post-radical prostatectomy urinary incontinence. He now presents with swelling and pain in the perineal region and pyuria. An office cystoscopy reveals erosion of the sling into the urethra. Removal of the sling is planned.

Description of Procedure (53442)

The patient is placed in the lithotomy position and a catheter placed into the bladder. A perineal incision is made under the scrotum and carried down to the bulbospongiosus muscles. The urethra and surrounding sling are identified. The sling is freed up from the surrounding urethra, being careful not to further injure the urethra or its vasculature. The sling is then mobilized laterally at its exit through the endopelvic fascia and into the retropubic space. A second incision is then made suprapubically and the abdominal ends of the sling are identified. The sling is mobilized through the abdominal fascia into the retropubic space from above. The sling is then removed by pulling it downward from the perineal wound. The urethral erosion is debrided and closed with interrupted sutures. The abdominal and perineal wounds are irrigated with antibiotic solution and individually closed with sutures. A drain is placed in the perineum and the abdominal wound before closure is complete.

MANIPULATION

▶(53670 has been deleted. To report, see 51701, 51702)◀

▶(53675 has been deleted. To report, use 51703)◀

Rationale
For rationale, see p. 132.

Male Genital System

Penis

INCISION

54000 Slitting of prepuce, dorsal or lateral (separate procedure); newborn

▶(Do not report modifier '-63' in conjunction with 54000)◀

54001 except newborn

Rationale
For the code listed above, see page 244, modifier '-63.'

EXCISION

54150 Circumcision, using clamp or other device; newborn

▶(Do not report modifier '-63' in conjunction with 54150)◀

54152 except newborn

54160 Circumcision, surgical excision other than clamp, device or dorsal slit; newborn

▶(Do not report modifier '-63' in conjunction with 54160)◀

54161 except newborn

Rationale
For the codes listed above, see page 244, modifier '-63.'

Prostate

EXCISION

55840   Prostatectomy, retropubic radical, with or without nerve sparing;

55842   with lymph node biopsy(s) (limited pelvic lymphadenectomy)

55845   with bilateral pelvic lymphadenectomy, including external iliac, hypogastric, and obturator nodes

(If 55845 is carried out on separate days, use 38770 with modifier '-50' and 55840)

▶(For laparoscopic retropubic radical prostatectomy, use 55866)◀

▶LAPAROSCOPY◀

▶Surgical laparoscopy always includes diagnostic laparoscopy. To report a diagnostic laparoscopy (peritoneoscopy) (separate procedure), use 49320.◀

●**55866**   Laparoscopy, surgical prostatectomy, retropubic radical, including nerve sparing

▶(For open procedure, use 55840)◀

Rationale

Code 55866 for laparoscopic, surgical radical retropubic prostatectomy has been added. This procedure is a less invasive alternative when compared to open retropubic prostatectomy procedures (55840, 55842, 55845).

Improved retroperitoneal laparoscopic access techniques have permitted surgeons to easily visualize, manipulate and remove the prostate without resorting to an open incision. Laparoscopy for a radical retropubic prostatectomy involves a completely different approach and work effort compared to an open prostatectomy, and thus a new code was warranted.

Clinical Example (55866)

A 48-year-old male with a PSA of 3.5 undergoes a prostate biopsy which reveals Gleason 7 adenocarcinoma of both lobes. He is counseled on the risks and benefits of surgery versus radiation and chooses laparoscopic radical prostatectomy.

Description of Procedure (55866)

The patient is taken to the operating room and placed in the modified lithotomy position. The lower abdomen is prepped and draped in the standard fashion. A pneumoperitoneum is achieved in the standard fashion and four trocars are placed. The laparoscope is introduced and attention is turned to first dissecting the seminal vesicles and vas deferens. The peritoneum at the reflection point of the anterior rectum and posterior bladder is incised. The vas deferens is identified on each side and then divided. The seminal vesicles are carefully dissected out using the harmonic scalpel to divide all bleeding vessels until the structures are completely freed. The space just posterior to the seminal vesicles is dissected in order to open Denonvilliers fascia, thereby revealing a pre-rectal fat plane.

Attention is then turned to complete mobilization of the opening of the peritoneum and mobilization of the bladder. The median umbilical ligaments and urachus are divided close to the umbilicus. Careful blunt dissection is used to reflect the bladder away from the abdominal wall. This exposes the endo-pelvic fascia. The fat overlying the endo-pelvic fascia is then cleared off and the endo-pelvic fascia is incised bilaterally to free the prostate away from the lateral pelvic side wall. The dorsal vein complex is developed and suture ligated. The bladder neck is then opened. The catheter is removed and a curved urethral sound is placed to aid in traction of the prostate. This allows identification of the posterior bladder neck, which is then carefully dissected away from the base of the prostate. The area of the pedicles of the prostate is then taken down. The tissue is opened overlying the seminal vesicles, these structures are then withdrawn into the area of dissection and used as traction. Both lateral pedicles are then taken down, up to the level near the apex. The dorsal vein complex is then divided. Careful sharp dissection is used around the apex of the prostate. The prostate is rocked back and forth and dissection continues along the lateral pedicle plane to define the apex of the prostate posteriorly. The urethra is then identified and sharp dissection is used to divide the anterior and posterior urethra and the rectourethralis muscle.

Then the final attachments are undone and the specimen is withdrawn in the endo-cath sac. Hemostasis is assured. The vesicourethral anastomosis is performed with interrupted suture. A catheter is placed through the anastomosis. A drain is placed through one of the abdominal side ports. All of the four trocar sites are inspected, and all surgical sites are inspected at 5 mm Hg pressure before removing the trocars under direct vision.

Female Genital System

Vulva, Perineum and Introitus

▶ENDOSCOPY◀

● **56820**   Colposcopy of the vulva;

● **56821**   with biopsy (s)

▶(For colposcopic examinations/procedures involving the vagina, see 57420, 57421; cervix, 57452-57461)◀

Rationale
For the codes listed above, see Cervix Uteri section, p. 141.

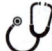
Clinical Example (56820)
A 44-year-old female presents with a one-year history of vulvar irritation and itching. She has a past history of human papilloma virus (HPV) changes to Pap smear and has previously undergone cryotherapy of the cervix. Her family

physician has tried antifungal as well as antibiotic cream preparations and yet her symptoms persist. She presents now for further evaluation of the vulva to exclude the process.

Description of Procedure (56820)

Colposcopic examination is performed employing a 5% acetic acid staining of the entire vulva. After adequate time for the acetic acid effect, the colposcope is then directed at the vulva under appropriate magnification. As no suspicious lesions are found, the patient is reassessed and biopsies are not performed.

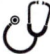

Clinical Example (56821)

A 55-year-old woman with a history of vulvar intraepithelial neoplasia complains of vulvar itching. Physical examination does not reveal an obvious lesion. She is advised to undergo vulvar colposcopy with biopsies of colposcopically abnormal areas of the vulva.

Description of Procedure (56821)

The vulva is cleansed several times with 5% acetic acid. Colposcopic examination is done at 7-15 magnification. Abnormal area suspicious for cancer is identified. The area is cleansed and locally infiltrated with lidocaine. A 3-mm punch biopsy instrument is used to obtain a biopsy. The biopsy site is treated with silver nitrate or Monsel's solution.

Vagina

ENDOSCOPY

▶(For speculoscopy, see Category III codes 0030T, 0031T)◀

●57420   Colposcopy of the entire vagina, with cervix if present;

●57421   with biopsy(s)

▶(For colposcopic visualization of cervix and adjacent upper vagina, use 57452)◀

▶(When reporting colposcopies of multiple sites, use modifier '-51' as appropriate. For colposcopic examinations/procedures involving the vulva, see 56820, 56821; cervix, 57452-57461)◀

Note: The cross-reference above 57420 is incorrect and will be corrected in CPT 2004 to reference codes 0031T and 0032T.

Rationale

For the codes listed above, see Cervix Uteri section, page 141.

Clinical Example (57420)

A 42-year-old female has a Pap smear test result showing atypical cells of undetermined significance. The physician cannot rule out dysplasia. Three years ago she was treated with a radical hysterectomy and adjuvant radiation therapy for Stage IB squamous carcinoma of the cervix. She now presents for colposcopic evaluation of the entire vagina.

Description of Procedure (57420)

Acetic acid is applied to the entire vagina. After adequate time for acetic acid effect, all vaginal surfaces are evaluated with a colposcope at several magnifications. Colposcopic evaluation shows no evidence of neoplastic or pre-neoplastic changes, and the abnormal cytologic changes are interpreted as being due to radiation effect. Accordingly, biopsies are not performed.

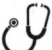

Clinical Example (57421)

A 42-year-old female has a Pap smear showing a high-grade squamous intraepithelial lesion. Three years ago she had a radical hysterectomy for Stage IB squamous cell carcinoma of the cervix.

Description of Procedure (57421)

Acetic acid is applied to the entire vagina. All surfaces of the vagina are evaluated with the colposcope at several magnifications. Colposcopic evaluation reveals a suspicious lesion at the vaginal cuff and a second area in the mid-vagina. Both areas are injected with local anesthetic, biopsies are taken, and bleeding is controlled with Monsel's solution or silver nitrate.

Cervix Uteri

(For cervicography, see Category III code 0003T)

▶ENDOSCOPY◀

▶For colposcopic examinations/procedures involving the vulva, see 56820, 56821; vagina, see 57420, 57421◀

▲57452*   Colposcopy of the cervix including upper/adjacent vagina;

▶(Do not report 57452 in addition to 57454–57461)◀

▲57454*   with biopsy(s) of the cervix and endocervical curettage

●57455   with biopsy(s) of the cervix

●57456   with endocervical curettage

▲57460   with loop electrode biopsy(s) of the cervix

●57461   with loop electrode conization of the cervix

▶(Do not report 57456 in addition to 57461)◀

Rationale

Prior to 2003, only three codes existed for pelvic endoscopy: 57452, 57454 and 57460. These three codes were included under the Vagina section of the CPT code set, although in practice the focus of these codes was based primarily on procedures involving the cervix. Thus, codes 57452, 57454, and 57460 have been revised and relocated under the Cervix Uteri section and two new codes, 57420 and 57421, have been added to the Vagina section.

The new series of pelvic endoscopy codes was added to reflect the focus of the specific anatomical site involved. The endoscopy codes are included in three subsections of the CPT code set, under Vulva (56820, 56821), Vagina (57420, 57421), and Cervix Uteri (57452, 57454, 57455, 57456, 57460, 57461).

The vulva endoscopy codes 56820, 56821 are limited to the vulva. Additional endoscopic examinations of other sites should be reported separately with modifier '-51' appended. Examination and magnification of the vulva are used to evaluate patients with symptoms or physical findings suggestive of vulvar human papilloma virus (HPV), vulvar intraepithelial neoplasia or vulvar malignancy. Some symptoms or physical findings may be pruritus, irritation, pain, hyperkeratosis, hyperpigmentation, or ulceration of the vulva, especially with a prior history of HPV infection.

The focus of the endoscopic examination included in new codes 57420 and 57421 is the entire vagina. However, when the cervix is viewed adjunctively, then it is also included in codes 57420 and 57421. If the primary examination is focused on the cervix, then the endoscopy codes within the Cervix Uteri section (57452, 57454) should be used instead. Examination and magnification of the vagina are used to evaluate patients with abnormal Pap smears in whom either a prior hysterectomy including removal of the cervix has been performed or an abnormal Pap smear is associated with no clinical evidence of cervical pathology in a woman whose cervix is still present. The work involved with endoscopic examination of the vagina includes a larger and more irregularly marked surface area compared with that of the cervix, and constant refocusing and change of speculum to visualize the entire vaginal wall. Thus, a distinction in the amount of work needed to visualize the vagina compared with the cervix necessitated separate endoscopy codes for the cervix and the vagina.

The endoscopy codes in the Cervix Uteri section (57452-57461) include examination of the entire cervix and may also include the upper/adjacent portion of the vagina when examined or when a cervical lesion extends into the vagina. These codes in this section reflect procedures used to evaluate women with abnormal Pap smear test results to detect cervical intraepithelial neoplasia and cervical cancer. This new section includes existing codes 57452, 57454, and 57460 as discussed above, and three new codes to reflect various procedures including endocervical curettage (57455), biopsy of the cervix (57456), and loop electrode conization of the cervix (57461). If colposcopic examinations involving the vulva and entire vagina are also performed, these procedures should be reported separately with modifier '-51' appended.

The revision of code 57460 and addition of code 57461 differentiate between two different cervical loop electrode excision procedures. Code 57460 does not include removal of a portion of the endocervix and does not typically include removal of the transformation zone (area at risk for cervical cancer), hence the loop excision procedure is not a conization. This procedure is used to obtain a large tissue specimen from patients with abnormal Pap smears where a discrete colposcopic lesion is identified on the exocervix.

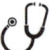
Clinical Example (57452)
A 30-year-old woman with a mildly abnormal Pap smear result is advised to undergo colposcopic visualization of the cervix. She is advised that a biopsy will be obtained if a lesion is identified.

Description of Procedure (57452)
The cervix including the upper/adjacent vagina is cleaned several times with 3% acetic acid. After adequate time for acetic acid effect, the cervix and vaginal fornices are examined with a colposcope at several magnifications. The transformation zone (area at risk for cervical cancer) is seen completely and no colposcopically abnormal areas are identified. Accordingly, no biopsy procedure is performed.

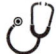
Clinical Example (57454)
A 30-year-old female with an abnormal Pap smear is advised to undergo colposcopic visualization of the cervix. She is advised that a biopsy will be obtained if a lesion is identified.

Description of Procedure (57454)
The cervix including the upper/adjacent vagina is cleaned several times with 3% acetic acid. After adequate time for acetic acid effect, the cervix and vaginal fornices are examined with a colposcope at several magnifications. The transformation zone (area at risk for cervical cancer) is seen completely and abnormal acetowhite areas are noted at 12 o'clock extending into the endocervical canal. An endocervical curettage and a cervical biopsy at 12 o'clock are performed. The biopsy site is treated with Monsel's solution or silver nitrate for hemostasis.

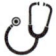
Clinical Example (57455)
A 27-year-old female has a Pap smear test result of epithelial cell abnormality. The descriptive report includes any of the following: atypical squamous cells of undetermined significance (ASCUS), possible HPV, dysplasia; low-grade squamous intraepithelial lesion encompassing HPV, mild dysplasia, CIN I; any reference to moderate or high-grade dysplasia, CIN III, or invasive carcinoma.

Description of Procedure (57455)
The cervix including the upper/adjacent vagina is cleaned several times with 3% acetic acid. After adequate time for acetic acid effect, the cervix and vaginal fornices are examined with a colposcope at several magnifications. An adequate exam views the entire transformation zone (area at risk for cervical cancer). An abnormality consisting of leukoplakia, mosaicism, punctation, or atypical vessels is noted during exam. Abnormal acetowhite areas are noted at 12 o'clock not extending into the endocervical canal. A cervical biopsy at 12 o'clock is done. The biopsy site is treated with Monsel's solution or silver nitrate for hemostasis.

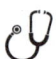
Clinical Example (57456)
A 27-year-old female has a Pap smear test result of epithelial cell abnormality. The descriptive report includes any of the following: ASCUS, possible HPV, dysplasia; low-grade squamous intraepithelial lesion encompassing HPV, mild dysplasia, CIN I; any reference to moderate or high-grade dysplasia, CIN III, or invasive carcinoma.

Description of Procedure (57456)

The cervix including the upper/adjacent vagina is cleaned several times with 3% acetic acid. After adequate time for acetic acid effect, the cervix and vaginal fornices are examined with a colposcope at several magnifications. A suspicious lesion is noted in the endocervical canal. The exocervix is completely normal. An endocervical curettage is done under direct colposcopic visualization.

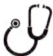

Clinical Example (57460)

A 25-year-old woman with an abnormal Pap smear is advised to undergo colposcopic visualization of the cervix. She is advised that a biopsy will be obtained if a lesion is visualized.

Description of Procedure (57460)

The cervix including upper/adjacent vagina is cleaned several times with 3% acetic acid. After adequate time for acetic acid effect, the cervix and vaginal fornices are examined with a colposcope at several magnifications. A suspicious lesion is noted in the endocervical canal. The exocervix is completely normal. An endocervical curettage is done under direct colposcopic visualization.

Clinical Example (57461)

A 31-year-old female patient previously underwent a colposcopic evaluation following a Class IV Pap smear. She was found to have CIN III, extending into the endocervix.

Description of Procedure (57461)

The cervix is cleansed several times with 3% acetic acid. After adequate time for acetic acid effect, the cervix and vaginal fornices are examined with a colposcope at several magnifications. The size of the lesion is determined. A grounding pad is placed. A Teflon-coated speculum is hooked up to suction. The cervix is infiltrated from 1-12 o'clock with lidocaine. An appropriate-sized loop electrode is then used to ensure excision of the lesion on the ectocervix with adequate margins. A second loop is then utilized to remove the involved portion of the endocervix. At the conclusion of the excision, a curette is used to sample the upper boundary of the excision to assure complete removal of the dysplasia. Homeostasis is achieved with electrocautery and topical Monsel's solution.

Corpus Uteri

EXCISION

▲ 58140   Myomectomy, excision of fibroid tumor(s) of uterus, 1 to 4 intramural myoma(s) with total weight of 250 grams or less and/or removal of surface myomas; abdominal approach

58145   vaginal approach

● 58146   Myomectomy, excision of fibroid tumor(s) of uterus, 5 or more intramural myomas and/or intramural myomas with total weight greater than 250 grams, abdominal approach

▶(Do not report 58146 in addition to 58140-58145, 58150-58240)◀

▲ **58260** Vaginal hysterectomy, for uterus 250 grams or less;

58262 with removal of tube(s) and ovary(s)

58263 with removal of tube(s), and/or ovary(s), with repair of enterocele

58267 with colpo-urethrocystopexy (Marshall-Marchetti-Krantz type, Pereyra type) with or without endoscopic control

58270 with repair of enterocele

● **58290** Vaginal hysterectomy, for uterus greater than 250 grams;

● **58291** with removal of tube(s) and/or ovary(s)

● **58292** with removal of tube(s) and/or ovary(s), with repair of enterocele

● **58293** with colpo-urethrocystopexy (Marshall-Marchetti-Krantz type, Pereyra type) with or without endoscopic control

● **58294** with repair of enterocele

LAPAROSCOPY/HYSTEROSCOPY

● **58545** Laparoscopy, surgical, myomectomy, excision; 1 to 4 intramural myomas with total weight of 250 grams or less and/or removal of surface myomas

● **58546** 5 or more intramural myomas and/or intramural myomas with total weight greater than 250 grams

▲ **58550** Laparoscopy surgical, with vaginal hysterectomy, for uterus 250 grams or less;

▶(58551 has been deleted. To report see 58545, 58546)◀

● **58552** with removal of tube(s) and/or ovary(s)

● **58553** Laparoscopy, surgical, with vaginal hysterectomy, for uterus greater than 250 grams;

● **58554** with removal of tube(s) and/or ovary(s)

 Rationale

Code 58140 has been revised and several new codes, 58146, 58545, 58546 have been added to differentiate between the number and the weight of intramural myomas excised by open abdominal (58140, 58146), and open vaginal (58145), and laparoscopic methods (58545, 58546). A myomectomy is a procedure used to treat women with uterine fibroids. The procedure can be used as an alternative to a hysterectomy for women who wish to preserve or enhance fertility potential and, if necessary, for pregnant women. The laparoscopic approach is an option for women who have conditions that preclude the vaginal route while still enabling them to avoid major abdominal surgery.

Code 58260 has been revised and a series of new vaginal hysterectomy codes have been added to differentiate between the size (weight) of the uterus by excisional methods (58290-58294) and laparoscopic methods (58550-58554). Prior to 2003, there was no distinction between standard and complex vaginal hysterectomy procedures.

An enlarged uterus (defined as a uterus over 250 grams) has been considered a contradiction to vaginal hysterectomy and was often cited as justification for the abdominal and, more recently, the laparoscopic approach. Recent developments have allowed physicians to excise a larger uterus vaginally. Techniques employed by physicians to remove the larger uterus vaginally include bisection, morcellation, myomectomy, and coring when uterine mobility and access are adequate. These techniques are generally not necessary with a uterus less than 250 grams. Employing these techniques results in a modest increase in operative time. Additionally, the excision of the fallopian tube(s) and/or ovary(s) vaginally can be technically more difficult when coupled with removal of an enlarged uterus.

Laparoscopic and open excisional myomectomy is an inherent component of a hysterectomy. The removal/debulking of the uterus of myomas prior to the removal of the uterus is an inclusive component of the complex vaginal and excisional hysterectomy procedure codes (58290-58294), (58553-58554) and the total abdominal hysterectomy and radical pelvic exenteration codes (58150-58240).

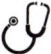
Clinical Example (58140)

A 37-year-old, gravida 1 para 0 woman is referred for abnormal uterine bleeding causing anemia. The patient has been treated pharmacologically and has received a dilatation and curettage during the past year without success. The patient has also experienced heavier and longer menses and dysmenorrhea over the past 6 months. Multiple scattered intramural and subserosal myomata ranging in size from 1 cm to 8 cm were documented by ultrasonography. The patient is given treatment alternatives and still desires childbearing. A myomectomy is indicated and the abdominal approach is recommended because of the location of the fibroids.

Description of Procedure (58140)

Under general anesthesia the abdomen is entered through a midline incision. An exploratory laparotomy is performed. The fibroid is identified. An incision is made in the overlying serosa and myometrium down to the level of the fibroid. The fibroid is dissected free. The myometrial defect is closed in multiple layers. The serosa is closed with fine suture to try to decrease the rise of post operative adhesion formation. The abdominal wall is closed in a routine fashion.

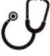
Clinical Example (58146)

A 35-year-old, nulligravid patient is evaluated for menorrhagia with anemia. She is recently married and is anxious to have children. On examination she is found to have a 16-week-size fibroid uterus. Ultrasound confirms a 15-cm uterus with multiple fibroids distorting the endometrium. Management options are discussed with her. The patient expresses a desire to keep fertility options open to her and keep her uterus. The patient elects a myomectomy. An abdominal myomectomy is performed.

Description of Procedure (58146)

Exam under anesthesia is performed. The patient is prepped and draped in a sterile fashion. A catheter is inserted into the bladder. A low transverse abdominal incision is made. This incision provides good exposure and allows good assistance and careful isolation of the tumors. A multi-arm self-retaining retractor is inserted. A rubber tourniquet is applied to the entire uterine mass. As the uterus is approached, the location and direction of the blood supply are assessed. The uterus is also assessed as to how to make as few incisions as possible. Vasopressin is injected into the myometrium overlying the fibroids. An incision is made on the uterus parallel with the course of the vascular bed.

Once the first myoma is exposed, it is grasped with a tenaculum. The myoma is dissected free from the surrounding myometrium using a combination of sharp and principally blunt dissections. The dissection is carried down to the pedicle that contains the main blood supply to the myoma. The pedicle is isolated and clamped before the myoma is removed. The patient is found to have eight myomas ranging from 4-cm to 6-cm in size. Multiple uterine incisions are utilized to remove all of the intramural fibroids. The physician then repairs the multiple uterine incisions that were made during the procedure. Each uterine incision is closed in layers to obtain hemostasis and preserve the anatomic relationship. The tourniquet is removed. The uterus is observed during reperfusion and additional sutures are placed in each incision to assure complete hemostasis.

The physician then closes the layers of the abdominal incision.

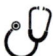

Clinical Example (58260)

A 44-year-old patient, gravida 1 para 1, presents with menorrhagia and dysmenorrhea unresponsive to medical management. She has failed both oral contraceptives and non-steroidal anti-inflammatory drugs (NSAIDs). On examination her uterus is 6-8 weeks' size and boggy. It is somewhat tender to palpation and has limited descensus. The patient feels strongly about maintaining her ovarian function but requests hysterectomy since her quality of life is significantly impaired by her symptoms. She is therefore scheduled for vaginal hysterectomy without removal of the ad nexae.

Description of Procedure (58260)

The speculum is inserted into the vaginal canal. The cervix is visualized and the tenaculum is applied. Following administration of fluid (saline, local anesthesia, vasoconstrictive agents), the uterus and cervix are excised. Following hemostasis, closure and suturing of the vaginal cuff are completed.

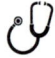

Clinical Example (58290)

A 45-year-old gravida 1 para 1 patient is evaluated for profound menorrhagia with anemia. Her hematocrit is 25% despite daily iron therapy and treatment with oral contraceptives. On physical examination she has an irregular, mobile 14-week-size fibroid uterus. Ultrasound confirms multiple uterine fibroids, several of which impinge on the endometrium. After management options are discussed with her, the patient elects hysterectomy. A vaginal hysterectomy is performed.

Description of Procedure (58290)

As soon as the patient is under anesthesia, a careful bimanual pelvic examination is conducted. Through this examination it is determined that the uterus is clearly mobile; there is surgical accessibility to the lower uterine segment; and the size and configuration of the uterine fibroids are determined.

All of these factors indicate that although it is an enlarged uterus, the conditions are favorable for it to be removed transvaginally.

Since the uterine size greatly limits the surgeon, the surgeon focuses on reducing the uterine size intra-operatively to facilitate the vaginal hysterectomy. Once the pelvic examination is complete, the cervix is grasped by tenaculums bilaterally. A circumferential incision is made at the junction of the vagina and cervix so that the vagina could be reflected upward, thereby freeing the attachments of the bladder to the uterus. The anterior and posterior cul-de-sacs are entered. The uterosacral, cardinal, and broad ligaments are bilaterally clamped, cut and ligated. The uterus is bisected in an antero-posterior direction with a knife with progressive reposition of tenaculums until the fundus is reached. The pedicles are clamped. Bisection assists in reducing the tension on the infundibulopelvic ligament. This allows the descent of the uterus and it also helps in removal of myomas during the course, thus reducing the bulk of the uterus. Once the uterine fundus can be delivered into the vagina, it is removed in multiple separate pieces.

All procedures are now complete. All pedicles are carefully inspected to assure hemostasis. The peritoneum and vaginal cuff are closed.

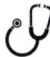

Clinical Example (58291)

A 45-year-old gravida 1 para 1 female is evaluated for profound menorrhagia with anemia. Her hematocrit is 25% despite daily iron therapy and treatment of oral contraceptives. On physical examination she has an irregular, mobile fibroid uterus. Ultrasound confirms multiple uterine fibroids, several of which impinge on the endometrium. After management options are discussed with her, the patient elects hysterectomy. The patient has a strong history of ovarian cancer in her family and does not desire any more children, so she elects to have her tube(s) and ovary(s) removed. An attempt at a vaginal approach is made since the uterus is mobile.

Description of Procedure (58291)

As soon as the patient is under anesthesia, a careful bimanual pelvic examination is conducted. Through this examination the uterus is found to be clearly mobile; surgical accessibility to the lower uterine segment is confirmed; and the size and configuration of the uterine fundus with multiple and discrete predominately posterior fundal myomas are determined.

All of these factors indicate that although it is an enlarged uterus, the conditions are favorable for it to be removed transvaginally.

Since the uterine size greatly limits the surgeon, the surgeon focuses on reducing the uterine size intra-operatively to facilitate the vaginal hysterectomy. Once the pelvic examination is complete, the cervix is grasped by tenaculums bilaterally. A circumferential incision is made at the junction of the vagina and cervix so that the vagina can be reflected upward, thereby freeing the attachments of the bladder to the uterus. The uterus is bisected in an antero-posterior direction with a knife with progressive reposition of tenaculums until the fundus is reached. The pedicles are clamped. Bisection assists in reducing the tension on the infundibulopelvic ligament. This allows the descent of the uterus. It also helps in removal of small myomas during the course, thus reducing the bulk of the uterus. These debulking techniques, which are only necessary with an enlarged uterus, require an experienced surgeon with good manual dexterity. Once the uterine fundus is able to be delivered into the vagina, it is removed in multiple separate pieces.

Once the uterus is removed, it is noted that the tube(s) and ovary(s) are visible and accessible. This indicates favorable conditions to continue with the procedure. The fimbriated end of the fallopian tube is incorporated into the utero-ovarian ligament pedicle. The infundibulopelvic ligament is then double-clamped and tied and the fallopian tube and ovary are then resected. Both procedures are now complete. A peritoneal purse-string suture is done just prior to the vaginal cuff closure.

Clinical Example (58292)

A 45-year-old gravida 1 para 1 patient is evaluated for profound menorrhagia with anemia. Her hematocrit is 25% despite daily iron therapy and treatment with oral contraceptives. On physical examination she has an irregular, mobile fibroid uterus. Ultrasound confirms multiple uterine fibroids, several of which impinge on the endometrium. After management options are discussed with her, the patient elects hysterectomy. The patient has a strong history of ovarian cancer in her family and does not desire any more children, so she elects to have her tube(s) and ovary(s) removed. An attempt at a vaginal approach is made since the uterus is mobile.

Description of Procedure (58292)

As soon as the patient is under anesthesia, a careful bimanual pelvic examination is conducted. Through this examination it is determined that the uterus is clearly mobile; there is surgical accessibility to the lower uterine segment; and the size and configuration of the uterine fundus are multiple with discrete predominately posterior fundal myomas. All of these factors indicate that although it is an enlarged uterus, the conditions are favorable for it to be removed transvaginally.

Since the uterine size greatly limits the surgeon, the surgeon focuses on reducing the uterine size intra-operatively to facilitate the vaginal hysterectomy. Once the pelvic examination is complete, the cervix is grasped by tenaculums bilaterally. A circumferential incision is made at the junction of the vagina and cervix so that the vagina can be reflected upward, thereby freeing the attachments of the bladder to the uterus. The uterus is bisected in an antero-posterior direction with a knife with progressive reposition of tenaculums until the fundus is reached. The pedicles are clamped. Bisection assists in reducing the tension on the infundibulopelvic ligament allowing the descent of the uterus. It also helps in removal of small myomas during the course, thus reducing the bulk of the uterus. These debulking techniques, which are only necessary with an enlarged uterus, require an experienced surgeon with good manual dexterity. Once the uterine fundus can be delivered into the vagina, it is removed in multiple separate pieces.

Once the uterus is removed, it is noted that the tube(s) and ovary(s) are visible and accessible. This indicates favorable conditions to continue with the procedure. The fimbriated end of the fallopian tube is incorporated into the utero-ovarian ligament pedicle. The infundibulopelvic ligament is then double-clamped and tied and the fallopian tube and ovary are then resected.

During the procedure a vaginal enterocele is identified. The enterocele is protruding through the posterior vaginal wall. The physician attempts to repair it. The hernia sac is excised and ligated, and the surrounding tissues are strengthened and sutured.

All procedures are now complete. A peritoneal purse-string suture is done just prior to the vaginal cuff closure.

The bladder is suspended by using the Marshall, Marchetti and Krantz (MMK) technique. First, the retropubic space is assessed via an abdominal incision. The retropubic space is dissected, cleared and sutures are placed through the fibromuscular wall of the paravaginal tissue, lateral to the urethra. The abdomen is closed in layers and dressings are applied. All procedures are now complete. A peritoneal purse-string suture is done just prior to the vaginal cuff closure.

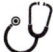

Clinical Example (58293)

A 45-year-old gravida 1 para 1 female is evaluated for profound menorrhagia with anemia. Her hematocrit is 25% despite daily iron therapy and treatment with oral contraceptives. She also complains of urinary incontinence. On physical examination she has an irregular, mobile fibroid uterus. Ultrasound confirms multiple uterine fibroids, several of which impinge on the endometrium. After management options are discussed with her, the patient elects hysterectomy. An attempt at a vaginal approach with bladder suspension is made since the uterus is mobile.

Description of Procedure (58293)

As soon as the female is under anesthesia, a careful bimanual pelvic examination is conducted. Through this examination it is determined that the uterus is clearly mobile; there is surgical accessibility to the lower uterine segment; and the size and configuration of the uterine fundus are multiple with discrete predominately posterior fundal myomas.

All of these factors indicate that although it is an enlarged uterus, the conditions are favorable for it to be removed transvaginally.

Through an incision in the vagina around the cervix, the physician removes the uterus including the cervix. Since the uterine size greatly limits the surgeon, the surgeon will focus on reducing the uterine size intra-operatively to facilitate the vaginal hysterectomy. Once the pelvic examination is complete, the cervix is grasped by tenaculums bilaterally. A circumferential incision is made at the junction of the vagina and cervix so that the vagina can be reflected upward, thereby freeing the attachments of the bladder to the uterus. The uterus is bisected in an antero-posterior direction with a knife with progressive reposition of tenaculums until the fundus is reached. The pedicles are clamped. Bisection assists in reducing the tension on the infundibulopelvic ligament. This allows the descent of the uterus. It also helps in removal of small myomas during the course thus reducing the bulk of the uterus. These debulking techniques, which are only necessary with an enlarged uterus, require an experienced surgeon with good manual dexterity. Once the uterine fundus can be delivered into the vagina, it is removed in multiple separate pieces.

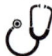

Clinical Example (58294)

A 45-year-old gravida 1 para 1 female is evaluated for profound menorrhagia with anemia. Her hematocrit is 25% despite daily iron therapy and treatment with oral contraceptives. On physical examination she has an irregular, mobile fibroid uterus. Ultrasound confirms multiple uterine fibroids, several of which impinge on the endometrium. After management options are discussed with her, the patient elects hysterectomy. An attempt at a vaginal approach is made since the uterus is mobile.

Description of Procedure (58294)

As soon as the patient is under anesthesia, a careful bimanual pelvic examination is conducted. Through this examination it is determined that the uterus is clearly mobile; there is surgical accessibility to the lower uterine segment; and the size and configuration of the uterine fundus are multiple with discrete predominately posterior fundal myomas. All of these factors indicate that although it is an enlarged uterus, the conditions are favorable for it to be removed transvaginally.

Since the uterine size greatly limits the surgeon, the surgeon focuses on reducing the uterine size intra-operatively to facilitate the vaginal hysterectomy. Once the pelvic examination is complete, the cervix is grasped by tenaculums bilaterally. A circumferential incision is made at the junction of the vagina and cervix so that the vagina can be reflected upward, thereby freeing the attachments of the bladder to the uterus. The uterus is bisected in an antero-posterior direction with a knife with progressive reposition of tenaculums until the fundus is reached. The pedicles are clamped. Bisection assists in reducing the tension on the infundibulopelvic ligament. This allows the descent of the uterus and it also helps in removal of small myomas during the course, thus reducing the bulk of the uterus. These debulking techniques, which are only necessary with an enlarged uterus, require an experienced surgeon with good manual dexterity. Once the uterine fundus can be delivered into the vagina, it is removed in multiple separate pieces.

During the procedure a vaginal enterocele is identified. The enterocele is protruding through the posterior vaginal wall. The physician repairs it. The hernia sac is excised and ligated, and the surrounding tissues are strengthened and sutured.

All procedures are now complete. A peritoneal purse-string suture is done just prior to the vaginal cuff closure.

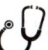
Clinical Example (58545)

A 35-year-old nulligravid patient is evaluated for menorrhagia with anemia. She is recently married and anxious to have children. On examination she is found to have a 16-week-size fibroid uterus. Ultrasound confirms a 15-cm uterus with multiple fibroids distorting the endometrium. Management options are discussed with her. The patient expresses a desire to keep her fertility options open and keep her uterus. The patient elects a myomectomy. An attempt at a laparoscopic myomectomy is made since her physician is trained and experienced in this procedure and the patient wishes to take advantage of the benefits of the laparoscopic approach.

Description of Procedure (58545)

The physician places an instrument transvaginally that will facilitate manipulating the uterus in the forth-coming procedure. A small incision is then made just below the umbilicus and a laparoscope is inserted. Additional incisions are made in the lower quadrants of the abdomen depending on the location of the myomas. Additional instruments are inserted as needed. The physician manipulates the uterine manipulator as well as the laparoscopic instruments so the pelvic organs can be comprehensively inspected. The patient is found to have several myomas ranging from 4 to 6 cm in size. Hemostatic techniques are employed such as the use of a harmonic scalpel or injection of vasopressin to minimize blood loss during the forth-coming myomectomy.

The myomas must then be surgically excised from the body of the uterus. Each of them is tagged to facilitate retrieval. Next, the surgical site from which the myomas have been excised must be repaired. Depending on the depth of the myoma, this may require a multi-layer or single-layer closure. This is performed using a laparoscopic suturing technique. After repair of the uterine sites of myoma excision, the myomas themselves must then be removed from the abdominal cavity. Several techniques can be employed from morcellation to piece meal extraction or vaginal colpotomy and removal. Once the operation is complete, the abdomen is deflated, the trocars are removed, and the abdominal incisions are closed with sutures.

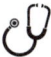
Clinical Example (58550)

A 45-year-old, gravida 1 para 1 female is evaluated for profound menorrhagia with anemia. Her hematocrit is 25% despite daily iron therapy and treatment with oral contraceptives. On physical examination she has an irregular, mobile 12- to 14-week size fibroid uterus. Ultrasound confirms multiple uterine fibroids, several of which impinge on the endometrium. After management options are discussed with her, the patient elects a hysterectomy. Due to previous surgeries that make the vaginal route more risky, an attempt at a laparoscopic-assisted vaginal hysterectomy (LAVH) is made.

Description of Procedure (58550)

The physician first inserts an instrument through the vagina to grasp the cervix and manipulate the uterus during surgery. Next, the surgeon makes a small incision just below the umbilicus through which the fiberoptic laparoscope is inserted. A second incision is made on the left side of the abdomen and additional instruments are placed through this incision. Gas is gently pumped into the abdomen and pelvis to cause it to tent and create a cavity in which the surgeon can operate by viewing through the camera. The myomas are assessed in terms of their size and location to plan sequential removal that would enable a size reduction of the uterus to proceed with the laparoscopic hysterectomy. To protect from intra operative hemorrhage, additional techniques and instrumentation are employed to minimize blood loss that would require increased operative time. As the large myomas are removed, they are either morcellated using special instrumentation or suture tagged for subsequent removal so they are not lost within the abdominal cavity. The uterus itself can either be bisected or sequentially morcellated to reduce its size to the point where it can eventually fit through the colpotomy incision at the level of the vaginal cuff. The various debulking techniques, which are only necessary with such an enlarged uterus, are technically challenging and even with experienced surgeons, operating time is significantly prolonged. Once the uterine fundus can be delivered through the vagina, it too may be removed in multiple or separate pieces. A vaginal incision is sutured closed either through a transvaginal or laparoscopic approach. The abdominal cavity is then deflated and instruments and trocars are removed, with suture closure of the trocar sites both at the level of the fascia and skin.

Nervous System

Skull, Meninges, and Brain

TWIST DRILL, BURR HOLE(S), OR TREPHINE

61105* Twist drill hole for subdural or ventricular puncture;

(61106 has been deleted)

⊘**61107** for implanting ventricular catheter or pressure recording device

▶(For intracranial neuroendoscopic ventricular catheter placement, use 62160)◀

61108 for evacuation and/or drainage of subdural hematoma

61156 Burr hole(s); with aspiration of hematoma or cyst, intracerebral

⊘**61210*** for implanting ventricular catheter, reservoir, EEG electrode(s) or pressure recording device (separate procedure)

▶(For intracranial neuroendoscopic ventricular catheter placement, use 62160)◀

61215 Insertion of subcutaneous reservoir, pump or continuous infusion system for connection to ventricular catheter

▶(For refilling and maintenance of an implantable infusion pump for spinal or brain drug therapy, use 95990)◀

Rationale

Two new cross-references were added following the cerebral catheter insertion codes 61107 and 61210 to instruct that placement of intracranial neuroendoscopic ventricular catheters should be reported with code 62160. In addition, a new cross-reference was added following subcutaneous reservoir insertion code 61215 to instruct that refilling and maintenance of an implantable infusion pump for the spine or brain should be reported with code 95990, Refilling and maintenance of implantable pump or reservoir for drug delivery, spinal (intrathecal, epidural) or brain (intraventricular).

CRANIECTOMY OR CRANIOTOMY

+●61316   Incision and subcutaneous placement of cranial bone graft (List separately in addition to code for primary procedure)

▶(Use 61316 in conjunction with codes 61304, 61312, 61313, 61322, 61323, 61340, 61570, 61571, 61680-61705)◀

●61322   Craniectomy or craniotomy, decompressive, with or without duraplasty, for treatment of intracranial hypertension, without evacuation of associated intraparenchymal hematoma; without lobectomy

▶(Do not report 61313 in addition to 61322)◀

▶(For subtemporal decompression, use 61340)◀

●61323   with lobectomy

▶(Do not report 61313 in addition to 61323)◀

▶(For subtemporal decompression, use 61340)◀

▲61340   Subtemporal cranial decompression (pseudotumor cerebri, slit ventricle syndrome)

▶(For decompressive craniectomy or craniotomy for intracranial hypertension, without hematoma evacuation, see 61322, 61323)◀

+●61517   Implantation of brain intracavitary chemotherapy agent (List separately in addition to code for primary procedure)

▶(Use 61517 only in conjunction with codes 61510 or 61518)◀

▶(Do not report 61517 for brachytherapy insertion. For intracavitary insertion of radioelement sources or ribbons, see 77781-77784)◀

Rationale

Codes 61322, 61323 have been added for treatment of traumatic brain injuries (eg, intracranial hypertension). Refractory intracranial hypertension due to post-traumatic intracranial hypertension may indicate the need for immediate surgical treatment with decompressive craniectomy/craniotomy and duraplasty to permit expansion of the brain and control of intracranial pressure. Prior to the creation of these two codes, there was no code to describe decompressive craniectomy/craniotomy and duraplasty for treatment of traumatic brain injuries. Additionally, code 61340 (other cranial decompression) has been revised to describe its original intent to reflect decompressions for pseudotumor cerebri or slit ventricle syndrome. Code 61313 describes intracerebral craniectomy or craniotomy for evacuation of hematoma. The new codes 61322, 61323 represent craniectomy/craniotomy procedures performed in the absence of hematoma or seizure disorder.

Code 61322 is intended to represent treatment of refractory intracranial hypertension where no focal surgically resectable lesion is identified. The etiologies may include trauma as well as cerebral infarction with mass effect and elevated intracranial pressure.

Code 61323 is intended for treatment of refractory intracranial hypertension where one lobe of the brain is substantially involved with cerebral edema causing local mass and elevated intracranial pressure without associated hematoma formation.

An add-on code, 61316, was created to describe the temporary placement of a cranial bone graft into a distant site for future retrieval. This procedure involves incision and creation of a subcutaneous pocket into a suitable area (usually the abdominal wall) for temporary housing of a cranial bone flap that may be retrieved and subsequently used for cranial repair procedures (ie, 61304, 61312, 61313, 61340, 61570, 61571, 61680-61705). For example, this procedure is often performed at the time of surgical decompressive craniotomy, lobectomy, or evacuation of intracranial hematoma (61322, 61323) where immediate replacement of the cranial bone flap may aggravate intracranial hypertension from brain swelling.

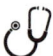

Clinical Example (61316)

A 25-year-old male was taken to the operating room for emergency supratentorial craniotomy and decompressive lobectomy.

Description of Procedure (61316)

While in the operating room, at the time of a primary surgical procedure for the treatment of intracranial hypertension (eg, decompressive craniotomy, lobectomy or evacuation of intracranial hematoma) where immediate replacement of the cranial bone flap may aggravate intracranial hypertension from brain swelling, a suitable area of the abdominal wall is prepped and draped in a sterile manner. An incision is made, and a subcutaneous pocket is created. Hemostasis is achieved. The cranial bone flap is placed into the subcutaneous space. Closure of the subcutaneous tissues and skin is completed. A sterile dressing is applied. Orders appropriate for the primary procedure are written and specific description of the bone graft transplantation is incorporated into the operative report. Postoperative exams of this wound site are made, as necessary, until such time that the graft is used for reconstruction.

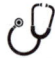

Clinical Example (61322)

A 36-year-old male, involved in a motor vehicle accident, has suffered a severe traumatic brain injury and has been in the Surgical Intensive Care Unit for approximately 24 hours. An intracranial pressure monitor was placed for recording of continuous intracranial pressure (ICP). The patient develops intracranial hypertension uncontrolled by medical therapy. A CT scan revealed multiple non-hemorrhagic supratentorial contusions producing obliteration of the basal cisterns. At operation, a supratentorial decompressive craniotomy/ craniectomy with duraplasty is performed.

Description of Procedure (61322)

Under general anesthesia, the head is positioned and fixed in a pin headholder, using care to protect the intracranial pressure device. A bicoronal incision is made with elevation of a large bifrontal cranial bone flap. Meticulous hemostasis is observed. The frontal sinus opened during the craniotomy is stripped of its mucosa and obliterated with absorbable gelatin sponge. The dura is noted to be extremely tense. The dura is then opened, beginning over the polar areas of the frontal lobes. The dural opening is made very low near the frontal skull base, the sagittal sinus is ligated at its rostral extremity, the falx cerebri is divided, and the dural opening is carried across midline for approximately 10 cm length opening from one temporal to the opposite temporal fossa, allowing the frontal lobes to expand through the dural opening. Hemostasis is ensured and the dura is closed with a cadaveric dural graft in a watertight manner to allow for anterior expansion of the swollen brain. The bifrontal bone flap is not replaced. An epidural drain is left in place to prevent epidural hematoma formation. A two-layer closure of the scalp is then completed. (Placement of the bone flap in the abdominal area through a separate incision for subsequent cranioplasty, if elected, is reported separately.)

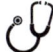

Clinical Example (61323)

A 25-year-old male has suffered a severe traumatic brain injury and has been in the Surgical Intensive Care Unit for several days. An intracranial pressure monitor was placed for recording of continuous intracranial pressure (ICP). The patient develops intracranial hypertension uncontrolled by medical therapy. CT scan reveals a non-hemorrhagic supratentorial, temporal lobe contusion with significant edema and uncal herniation. At operation, a decompressive supratentorial craniectomy and lobectomy and duraplasty are performed.

Description of Procedure (61323)

Under general anesthesia, the head is positioned and fixed in a pin headholder, using care to protect the intracranial pressure device. The neurosurgeon performs a cranial incision and turns a large unilateral bone flap overlying the frontal and temporal lobes. Care is taken to preserve the pericranium, which may be used for a dural expansion graft. Prior to the opening of the dura, close coordination with anesthesia is carried out to maximize medical control of the swollen brain. The dura over the temporal lobe is then opened. The brain is swollen and surgical landmarks are extremely difficult to identify. The anterior 5 cm of the temporal lobe are removed including the mesial structures in order to clearly identify the incisura. The vessels in the sylvian fissure are distorted by the underlying edema and are avoided to prevent disruption of major vascular channels. Adequate mesial temporal lobe resection allows the visualization of the third nerve, posterior cerebral artery and lateral portion of the brain stem. Following adequate decompression and thorough hemostasis, the dura is closed with a pericranial graft to allow for expansion. The bone flap is replaced, if ICP and brain swelling permit (if brain swelling precludes safe replacement of the cranial flap, it can be placed in a subcutaneous pocket in the abdominal area; separately reportable). A layered closure is completed.

+●61517   Implantation of brain intracavitary chemotherapy agent (List separately in addition to code for primary procedure)

▶(Use 61517 only in conjunction with codes 61510 or 61518)◀

▶(Do not report 61517 for brachytherapy insertion. For intracavitary insertion of radioelement sources or ribbons, see 77781-77784)◀

Rationale

Code 61517 was established as an add-on code to describe the implantation of agents for the continuous delivery of interstitial/intracavitary chemotherapy to the brain subsequent to removal of a malignant brain tumor. These devices are implanted as part of a craniotomy for malignant brain tumor procedure. This code is intended to report implantation of chemotherapy agents for the continuous delivery of interstitial chemotherapy to the brain, as part of a craniotomy for removal of a malignant brain tumor implant. Code 61517 is reported as an add-on code with the craniectomy procedures 61510 and 61518 (for excision of brain tumor). Prior to this time, the only codes available for reporting cerebral chemotherapy described chemotherapy when administered intravenously, subarachnoid, or intraventricular via a subcutaneous reservoir. After diagnosis and treatment with tumor resection, chemotherapy of high-grade gliomas consisted of local application of cytostatic drugs that were administered through a number of different modalities, including infusion pumps, catheters, and reservoirs.

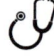

Clinical Example (61517)

A 50-year-old male is diagnosed with a recurrent frontal-parietal brain tumor. The tumor is a glioblastoma multiforme. He undergoes surgery to resect the tumor followed by implantation of brain interstitial/intracavitary chemotherapy wafers.

Description of Procedure (61517)

As part of the base service, the tumor is resected using standard techniques. When the tumor is resected, a sample of the tumor is evaluated by a neuropathologist who determines that the tumor is in fact a glioblastoma multiforme and not radiation necrosis. The neurosurgeon determines that it is appropriate to implant BCNU wafers in the resected tumor bed, which is prepared by inspection for bleeding and any communication with a ventricle.

The neurosurgeon puts on an extra pair of gloves and receives the wafers from the scrub nurse. The number of wafers implanted is dependent on the size and location of the tumor cavity. The wafers are placed against the wall of the tumor cavity by forceps, close together with only slight overlapping. Great care is taken to ensure that the wafers cover the greatest area of the walls of the tumor cavity and yet avoid the ventricles and large vascular structures. Once full coverage of the surgical cavity is achieved, the neurosurgeon applies a topical absorbable haemostatic agent to the area to secure the wafers in place.

ENDOVASCULAR THERAPY

●61623 Endovascular temporary balloon arterial occlusion, head or neck, (extracranial/intracranial) including selective catheterization of vessel to be occluded, positioning, and inflation of occlusion balloon, concomitant neurological monitoring and radiologic supervision and interpretation of all angiography required for balloon occlusion and to exclude vascular injury post occlusion

▶(If selective catheterization and angiography of arteries other than artery to be occluded is performed, use appropriate catheterization and radiologic supervision and interpretation codes)◀

▶(If complete diagnostic angiography of the artery to be occluded is performed immediately prior to temporary occlusion, use appropriate radiologic supervision and interpretation codes only)◀

▲61624 Transcatheter permanent occlusion or embolization (eg, for tumor destruction, to achieve hemostasis, to occlude a vascular malformation), percutaneous, any method; central nervous system (intracranial, spinal cord)

Rationale

New code 61623 has been added to describe procedures involving temporary extracranial/intracranial endovascular balloon occlusion and concomitant neurologic testing.

Code 61624 has been revised to include the word "permanent" to differentiate temporary endovascular balloon occlusion (61623) and permanent endovascular balloon occlusion procedures. The device(s) for "temporary" versus "permanent" occlusion are different in their behavior and usage. The procedure is completely different and the intended outcome is different. Comprehensive neurologic assessment is a mandatory part of extracranial temporary balloon occlusion due to the fact that these vessels supply the brain or other vital neurological structures and there is the risk of stroke from hypoperfusion or cerebral embolization secondary to the procedure.

Two additional cross-references were added following new code 61623 directing the user to separate radiological supervision and interpretation codes for catheterization and angiography of arteries other than the cerebral artery to be occluded and for instances when diagnostic imaging of the artery to be occluded needs further examination outside of the imaging necessary to perform the occlusion. An inclusive list of the radiology codes that may be additionally reported is not specified, due to the large range of possible codes.

Two cross-references following code 37606 have been included in the Cardiovascular System subsection directing users to newly established codes for endovascular approach codes 61623 and revised code 61624.

Endovascular intracranial or extracranial temporary vessel occlusion utilizes radiologic imaging to facilitate the placement of an intravascular occlusion device in the vasculature or the head or neck to reversibly occlude blood flow to the brain to demonstrate the feasibility and safety of intentional blockage or unintentional occlusion of a major vascular supply to the brain. Abrupt permanent surgical ligation of extracranial vessels has been performed for many years, but with unpredictable cerebral tolerance and risk of ischemic sequelae (stroke). Gradual occlusion of the internal or common carotid artery utilizing Selverstone or Crutchfield clamp has been performed as an open surgical procedure for more than 30 years in an attempt to decrease ischemic complications. In an attempt to optimize outcomes and decrease ischemic complications, these open surgical techniques have been abandoned in favor of endovascular-surgical procedures. No viable open surgical technique exists to evaluate temporary vertebral artery occlusion by any means other than utilizing endovascular technique.

Endovascular image-guided temporary balloon occlusion is a procedure that was not described by any single CPT code or combination of CPT codes prior to *CPT 2003*. Existing code 37605 (Ligation, internal or common carotid artery) is not appropriate for a procedure that is performed via endovascular approach where the occlusion is temporary and reversible. Code 37606 (Ligation, internal or common carotid artery, with gradual occlusion) describes gradual occlusion by external screw clamp through the skin and has not been performed for many years. Code 37606 does not describe an endovascular approach, but rather the permanent surgical implantation of a foreign object into the neck.

Code 61626 describes percutaneous permanent (not temporary or reversible) transcatheter occlusion or embolization of an extracranial vessel and is not intended to be used for neurological testing of tolerance to permanent occlusion. The devices utilized for permanent occlusion are different in behavior from temporary balloon occlusion catheters, are incompatible with reversibility, and the intended result of the procedure for 61626 would be considered a major complication for the procedure under discussion.

Temporary occlusion of a cerebral artery requires continuous repetitive neurologic assessment of the patient's cognitive, motor, sensory, visual, memory, and auditory functions, at a minimum, to not only permit safe temporary vessel occlusion, but also to assess the results of the temporary occlusion procedure.

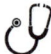
Clinical Example (61623)
A 70-year-old male presents with right retro-orbital pain, headache, and diplopia, progressively worsening over three months. The patient is evaluated by his physician, who finds a right sixth nerve paresis and the physician recommends a brain CT. This excludes a hemorrhage, but suggests a parasellar mass lesion. He is referred to a neurosurgeon who orders an MRI and a cerebral angiogram. These imaging tests demonstrate a wide-necked right cavernous sinus segment internal carotid artery aneurysm measuring 2.5 cm in diameter. The right anterior cerebral artery A1 segment is noted to be hypoplastic and a small right posterior communicating artery is identified. Endovascular trapping with resultant sacrifice of the cavernous right internal carotid artery aneurysm is recommended. Prior to treatment of this aneurysm by endovascular therapy, it is mandatory to ascertain whether occlusion of the internal carotid artery will result in a stroke.

Description of Procedure (61623)
Access to the vascular tree is made via the right common femoral artery. A micropuncture set is used to access the common femoral artery by puncturing with a 22-gauge needle followed by a 0.021-in guidewire. This is then exchanged for

the micropuncture introducer sheath that is then used to introduce the 0.035-in guidewire. A 7 Fr femoral sheath is placed and its tip deployed in the thoracic aorta. Through this, a JB-1 angled diagnostic neuroangiography catheter is used to select the target vessel (in this case, the carotid artery) and confirm the hemodynamic status. Fluoroscopic monitoring is performed for this process.

After catheter placement, diagnostic images are obtained to evaluate possible vessel damage or cerebral embolization. The diagnostic angiogram confirms the suspected aneurysm and is used to evaluate baseline hemodynamics of brain perfusion. If a recent pre-operative diagnostic angiogram of sufficient quality has been performed and is available at the time of this endovascular surgical procedure, and there is no change in the patient's clinical status, a repeat diagnostic angiogram would not be performed or coded at this time. If such a recent high-quality angiogram were not available, a diagnostic angiogram would be performed at this time and the diagnostic angiogram RS&I would be reported separately.

After placement of the diagnostic catheter, baseline arterial blood sampling is obtained for ACT. Intravenous heparin is administered to reach an ACT of approximately 300. A temporary occlusion balloon catheter is carefully prepared in sterile fashion with half-strength contrast to remove all bubbles from the system and balloon. The diagnostic catheter is positioned in the internal carotid artery and a 300-cm neuro-exchange wire is advanced through the catheter and its tip placed within the petrous portion of the internal carotid artery. The diagnostic catheter is removed and replaced with the temporary balloon occlusion catheter over the neuro-exchange wire utilizing fluoroscopic monitoring. The balloon is advanced into the high cervical internal carotid artery and the wire removed. The catheter is double flushed with heparinized saline. The balloon occlusion catheter is attached to a three-way stopcock and the system is then attached to an airless heparinized flush system previously prepared. A baseline neurological examination is performed, consisting of motor function, cognition, sensory function including visual fields, speech, and short- and long-term memory. The system is attached to a separate flush system for baseline measurement of intra-arterial distal occlusion pressure. The temporary balloon occlusion catheter is carefully inflated and the carotid artery is thus occluded under radiographically confirmed roadmap technique utilizing contrast injections and filming to confirm stasis.

A small amount of contrast is gently injected to document stasis distal to the balloon. Occlusion intra-arterial "stump" pressure is then measured. Immediately, neurologic examination is performed for confirmation of neurological stability. This is repetitively performed at three-minute intervals. After 15 minutes of evaluation with no change in neurological status, systemic hypotension is induced by slow administration of pharmaceutical agent (eg, sodium nitroprusside) to a level 30% lower than baseline mean arterial pressure. The patient remains neurologically intact for an additional 30 minutes with confirmation of neurological stability by repeated exams including tests of motor strength, speech, and cognition. Continued monitoring of "stump" pressure is performed. After completion of the process of neurological testing, the occlusion balloon is slowly deflated and withdrawn into the common carotid artery and the nitroprusside is stopped.

Contrast is injected through the catheter and images are obtained to verify the absence of trauma to the internal carotid artery at the location of the balloon and to verify that there is no change in the filling of the distal territory of the internal carotid artery as well as the vessels within the brain. No hemodynamic change or embolus is identified and the patient remains neurologically intact. An arterial blood sample is obtained to measure ACT. The heparin is reversed by means of a slow infusion of protamine over 10 minutes intravenously. The catheter is removed from the groin and hemostasis is obtained utilizing an endovascular suture device.

STEREOTAXIS

61750   Stereotactic biopsy, aspiration, or excision, including burr hole(s), for intracranial lesion;

▲**61751**   with computed tomography and/or magnetic resonance guidance

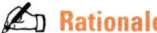 **Rationale**

For *CPT 2003*, in order to update the language, codes containing the phrases "computerized axial tomography" have been revised to state "computed tomography." The term "axial" is misleading since computed tomography may be done in any plane (ie, axial, coronal, sagittal, or multiplanar). Typically, direct acquisition of images are obtained in the axial plane for computed tomographic studies, but in certain instances direct acquisition may be obtained in other planes (eg, coronal plane for sinus studies). Elimination of the term "axial" will clarify to the user that the CT codes are appropriate for reporting CT direct acquisition imaging performed in any plane (ie, axial, coronal, sagittal or multiplanar).

NEUROSTIMULATORS (INTRACRANIAL)

61862   Twist drill, burr hole, craniotomy, or craniectomy for stereotactic implantation of one neurostimulator array in subcortical site (eg, thalamus, globus pallidus, subthalamic nucleus, periventricular, periaqueductal gray)

▶(For intraoperative neurophysiologic recording, see 95961-95962)◀

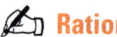 **Rationale**

In the course of review of the series of codes for the neuroendoscopic procedures, code 61862 was identified to be appropriately reported with the intraoperative neurophysiologic recording codes, 95961-95962. These procedures are intended to report the performance of intraoperative functional mapping of both subcortical and cortical sites using depth electrodes to identify vital brain structures by mapping cortical and subcortical areas of the brain. The same electrodes might be used for stimulation of brain tissue or for recording of brain cells during the process of mapping.

REPAIR

+●**62148**   Incision and retrieval of subcutaneous cranial bone graft for cranioplasty (List separately in addition to code for primary procedure)

▶(Use 62148 in conjunction with codes 62140-62147)◀

 Rationale

The retrieval of the cranial bone graft from the temporary subcutaneous site is included in another new add-on code, 62148. This code includes the repair of the temporary site as well. This new add-on code should be used in conjunction with the cranial repair codes (62140-62147).

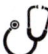 **Clinical Example (62148)**

A 25-year-old male, who is status post-emergency craniotomy for decompression with intraoperative placement of the bone graft into an abdominal subcutaneous pocket presents for elective cranioplasty repair of the skull defect. While in the operating room for elective cranioplasty, the abdominal graft site incision is sterilely prepped and draped. The previous incision is opened sharply, and the bone graft is identified. Using blunt dissection and electrocautery, the graft is freed from the surrounding tissue and temporarily placed in antibiotic solution on the back table, pending cranial implantation. The wound is irrigated, hemostasis is ensured, and the skin is closed and dressed after completion of the cranial procedure.

Description of Procedure (62148)

While in the OR for elective cranioplasty, the abdominal graft site incision is sterilely prepped and draped. The previous incision is opened sharply, and the bone graft is identified. Using blunt dissection and electrocautery, the graft is freed from the surrounding tissue and temporarily placed in antibiotic solution on the back table, pending cranial implantation. The wound is irrigated, hemostasis is ensured, and the skin is closed and dressed after completion of the cranial procedure.

▶NEUROENDOSCOPY◀

▶Surgical endoscopy always includes diagnostic endoscopy.◀

+●62160 Neuroendoscopy, intracranial, for placement or replacement of ventricular catheter and attachment to shunt system or external drainage (List separately in addition to code for primary procedure)

▶(Use 62160 only in conjunction with codes 61107, 61210, 62220, 62223, 62225, or 62230)◀

●62161 Neuroendoscopy, intracranial; with dissection of adhesions, fenestration of septum pellucidum or intraventricular cysts (including placement, replacement, or removal of ventricular catheter)

●62162 with fenestration or excision of colloid cyst, including placement of external ventricular catheter for drainage

●62163 with retrieval of foreign body

●62164 with excision of brain tumor, including placement of external ventricular catheter for drainage

●62165 with excision of pituitary tumor, transnasal or trans-sphenoidal approach

CEREBROSPINAL FLUID (CSF) SHUNT

62200 Ventriculocisternostomy, third ventricle;

▲**62201** stereotactic, neuroendoscopic method

▶(For intracranial neuroendoscopic procedures, see 62161-62165)◀

62220 Creation of shunt; ventriculo-atrial, -jugular, -auricular

▶(For intracranial neuroendoscopic ventricular catheter placement, use 62160)◀

62223 ventriculo-peritoneal, -pleural, other terminus

▶(For intracranial neuroendoscopic ventricular catheter placement, use 62160)◀

62225 Replacement or irrigation, ventricular catheter

▶(For intracranial neuroendoscopic ventricular catheter placement, use 62160)◀

62230 Replacement or revision of cerebrospinal shunt, obstructed valve, or distal catheter in shunt system

▶(For intracranial neuroendoscopic ventricular catheter placement, use 62160)◀

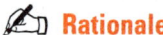 **Rationale**

A new subsection with six new codes (62160-62165) has been added to accurately describe neuroendoscopic procedures, which allows the performance of certain neurosurgical procedures with less invasiveness and trauma to the skull, brain and meninges.

An instructional note was added preceding code 62160 informing the user that surgical endoscopy always includes diagnostic endoscopy. Therefore, when a diagnostic neuroendoscopy is performed at the same session as a surgical neuroendoscopy, the diagnostic neuroendoscopy is not separately reported.

Code 62160 describes intracranial neuroendoscopy for the placement or replacement of a ventricular catheter and attachment to a shunt system or external drainage. Code 62160 is designated as an add-on code, and should be reported only with certain codes. As such, cross-references have been added to direct the user to report code 62160 in addition to codes 61107, 61210, 62220, 62223, 62225, or 62230 when neuroendoscopic placement or replacement of a ventricular catheter and attachment to a shunt system or external drainage is performed in addition to one of these primary procedures. These cross-references specify which primary procedure codes are intended to be reported with code 62160, as the work described by code 62160 is not considered an inclusive component of these codes.

Code 62161 describes intracranial neuroendoscopy with dissection of adhesions, fenestration of septum pellucidum or intraventricular cysts. This code includes placement, replacement, or removal of a ventricular catheter. This procedure is typically performed for patients with complicated hydrocephalus with intraventricular barriers to the free flow of cerebrospinal fluid who need to have these barriers removed.

Code 62162 describes intracranial neuroendoscopy with fenestration or excision of a colloid cyst, including placement of an external ventricular catheter for drainage. This procedure is typically performed for patients with intraventricular colloid cysts.

Code 62163 describes intracranial neuroendoscopy with removal of a foreign body from the brain.

Code 62164 describes intracranial neuroendoscopy with excision of brain tumor, including the placement of an external ventricular catheter for drainage. This procedure is typically performed to excise any type of intracranial neoplasm.

Code 62165 describes intracranial neuroendoscopy with the excision of a pituitary tumor, using a transnasal or trans-sphenoidal approach. This procedure is typically performed for the excision of any pituitary tumor.

Code 62201 in the cerebrospinal fluid (CSF) shunt subsection has been revised to clarify that this code includes neuroendoscopic technique. Cross-references have been added below codes 62220, 62223, 62225, and 62230 to clarify proper use of the new neuroendoscopy codes.

A cross-reference has been added below code 62201 to direct the user to see codes 62161-62165 for intracranial neuroendoscopic procedures. This cross-reference provides clarification for the user that there are other codes for intracranial procedures using neuroendoscopic technique.

Clinical Example (62160)

A 5-year-old boy with hydrocephalus secondary to intraventricular hemorrhage and prematurity develops shunt malfunction. Examination of the shunt system shows very slow refilling and CT scan reveals enlarged ventricles with the ventricular catheter positioned along the choroid plexus in the lateral ventricle. He is admitted for replacement of his ventricular catheter using neuroendoscopy to facilitate removal of the obstructed catheter and accurate placement of a new ventricular catheter.

Description of Procedure (62160)

At operation, the ventricular catheter is replaced (coded separately) using neuroendoscopy. The neuroendoscope is placed through the burr hole into the lateral ventricle and advanced to allow identification of the ventricular catheter, the foramen of Monro, and the choroid plexus. Under direct visualization, the malfunctioning catheter is removed and a new ventricular catheter is placed in a location away from the choroid plexus.

Clinical Example (62161)

A 19-year-old male presents with a history of hydrocephalus complicated in the past by ventriculitis and intraventricular pseudocyst formation, previously treated with two ventriculo-peritoneal shunts, now complicated by infection of the peritoneal catheters. The shunts have been removed for treatment of the infection and a new shunt must be placed with the terminus in the right atrium of the heart. He undergoes neuroendoscopy where the pseudocyst walls are opened so that all the ventricles communicate and are drained by a single ventriculo-atrial shunt catheter.

Description of Procedure (62161)

The skin is incised and hemostasis achieved with retraction and electrocautery. A power perforator is used to make a burr hole and hemostasis is achieved with bone wax. The dura is coagulated with bipolar coagulation and opened with sharp dissection. The cortex is inspected to make sure that there are no large cortical blood vessels directly in the area where a cortical incision will be made. The cortex is coagulated with bipolar coagulation and opened with sharp dissection. A 5-mm peel-away trocar is introduced through the brain into the ventricle. The inner stylet of the trocar is removed and the flexible neuroendoscope is passed through the trocar into the ventricle. The walls of the pseudocyst are identified. Using various micro-instruments through the working channel of the neuroendoscope, the pseudocyst wall is perforated and the opening enlarged. The neurosurgeon then advances the neuroendoscope into the pseudocyst and the back wall of the pseudocyst is opened and enlarged with the micro-instruments. Bleeding is controlled with irrigation and bipolar electrocautery. The neuroendoscope is advanced to inspect the rest of the ventricular system and ensure that there is good communication of spinal fluid throughout the system. The neuroendoscope is carefully backed out until the tip of the endoscope is straight and located in an area free of choroid plexus and loose pseudocyst wall. The trocar sheath is then advanced to the tip of the neuroendoscope and the length of the neuroendoscope relative to the trocar is noted. The neuroendoscope is removed and replaced with a ventricular catheter at exactly the same length as the neuroendoscope. The neurosurgeon takes a small sample of cerebrospinal fluid and sends it to pathology for analysis. The trocar is peeled away. The ventricular catheter is cut to the proper length and secured to the proximal portion of a one-way flow-control valve. The distal shunt tubing is passed from the scalp incision to a new incision in the neck using a shunt passer (coded separately). A branch of the external jugular vein is isolated in the neck and the distal shunt is passed into the venous system toward the right atrium. The location of the tip of the distal catheter is monitored by the neurosurgeon with intra-operative fluoroscopy until it is in the right atrium. The neurosurgeon consults with the anesthesiologist to make sure that there are no cardiac arrhythmias. The proximal portion of the catheter is cut to the proper length and secured to the distal port of the flow-controlled valve. The ventricular catheter is secured to the periosteum. The wounds are closed.

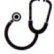

Clinical Example (62162)

A 21-year-old male with acute hydrocephalus secondary to a third ventricular colloid cyst undergoes neuroendoscopic excision of the colloid cyst.

Description of Procedure (62162)

The skin is incised and hemostasis achieved with retraction and electrocautery. A power perforator is used to make a burr hole and hemostasis is achieved with bone wax. The dura is coagulated with bipolar coagulation and opened with sharp dissection. The cortex is inspected to make sure that there are no large cortical blood vessels directly in the area where a cortical incision will be made. The cortex is coagulated with bipolar coagulation and opened with sharp dissection. A 5-mm peel-away trocar is introduced through the brain into the ventricle. The inner stylet of the trocar is removed and the neuroendoscope is passed through the trocar into the ventricle. The choroid plexus, the foramen of Monro, and the colloid cyst are identified. The neuroendoscope is advanced toward the colloid cyst. A small cutting suction catheter is passed through the working channel of the neuroendoscope until it touches the wall of the colloid cyst. While a small amount of suction is applied, the neurosurgeon gently twists the catheter until an opening is made. The contents of the colloid cyst are evacuated with the suction, shrinking the cyst. The cutting suction catheter is removed and the attachment of the cyst is visualized by the neurosurgeon. An electrocautery probe is passed through the working channel of the neuroendoscope. The wall of the cyst near its attachment is coagulated with the electrocautery. The electrocautery probe is removed and a micro-scissor is passed through the working channel of the neuroendoscope. The attachment is cut. The micro-scissor is removed and a micro-grasping forceps is passed through the working channel of the neuroendoscope. The shrunken cyst wall is grasped and the colloid cyst and neuroendoscope are removed together. After the colloid cyst and micro-grasping forceps are removed from the neuroendoscope, the neuroendoscope is passed back into the ventricle and the site of the cyst removal is observed. Bleeding at the site is irrigated and observed until clear. The foramen of Monro is inspected to monitor for obstruction of the flow of spinal fluid from the lateral ventricles into the third ventricle. The neuroendoscope is removed and a ventricular catheter is placed into the lateral ventricle. This catheter is tunneled under the skin and pierces the skin remote from the incision. The neurosurgeon takes a small sample of cerebrospinal fluid and sends it to pathology for analysis. The ventricular catheter is cut to the proper length and secured to a closed extra-ventricular drainage system. The neurosurgeon looks to see that there is spontaneous flow of blood-tinged cerebrospinal fluid throughout the system. The wounds are closed.

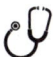

Clinical Example (62163)

A 6-year-old male presents with a history of resolved hydrocephalus and a lost ventricular catheter from a previous shunt attempt. The lost ventricular catheter is found and removed utilizing the neuroendoscope.

Description of Procedure (62163)

The skin is incised and hemostasis achieved with retraction and electrocautery. A power perforator is used to make a burr hole and hemostasis is achieved with bone wax. The dura is coagulated with bipolar coagulation and opened with sharp dissection. The cortex is inspected to make sure that there are no large cortical blood vessels directly in the area where a cortical incision will be made. The cortex is coagulated with bipolar coagulation and opened with sharp dissection. A 5-mm peel-away trocar is introduced through the brain into the ventricle. The inner stylet of the trocar is removed and the flexible neuroendoscope is passed through the trocar into the ventricle. The neurosurgeon orients herself to the intraventricular anatomy and finds the choroid plexus, the foramen of Monro, and the third ventricle. The neuroendoscope is advanced into the occipital horn of the lateral ventricle where the lost ventricular catheter is seen. The catheter is seen to be adherent to the choroid plexus. Using various micro-instruments through the working channel of the neuroendoscope, the catheter is freed from the surrounding scar tissue. Bleeding is controlled with irrigation and bipolar electrocautery. The catheter is grasped with micro-grasping forceps and the neuroendoscope and catheter together are removed from the brain. The neuroendoscope is replaced to inspect the rest of the ventricular system and ensure that there is good communication of spinal fluid throughout the system. The neuroendoscope is then removed. The wounds are closed.

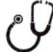

Clinical Example (62164)

A 56-year-old female with a lymphoma in her right caudate nucleus undergoes a neuroendoscopic partial excision of the tumor.

Description of Procedure (62164)

The skin is incised and hemostasis achieved with retraction and electrocautery. A power perforator is used to make a burr hole and hemostasis is achieved with bone wax. The dura is coagulated with bipolar coagulation and opened with sharp dissection. The cortex is inspected to make sure that there are no large cortical blood vessels directly in the area where a cortical incision will be made. The cortex is coagulated with bipolar coagulation and opened with sharp dissection. A 5-mm peel-away trocar is introduced through the brain into the ventricle. The inner stylet of the trocar is removed and the neuroendoscope is passed through the trocar into the ventricle. The neurosurgeon orients herself to the intraventricular anatomy and finds the choroid plexus, the foramen of Monro, and the third ventricle. The neurosurgeon advances the neuroendoscope into the frontal horn of the right lateral ventricle and identifies a discoloration in the ependyma overlying the head of the caudate nucleus, which represents the tumor. In a relatively avascular area, the micro-cup forceps is inserted through the neuroendoscope and into the tumor. A portion of tumor tissue is excised and submitted for later pathological examination. This procedure is repeated several times until approximately 1 cubic centimeter of tumor tissue is removed. Hemostasis is achieved with a bipolar coagulation device introduced into the ventricle through the working channel of the neuroendoscope. Bleeding from the excision site clears after a period of gentle irrigation and observation. The neuroendoscope is removed. The wounds are closed.

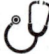

Clinical Example (62165)

A 62-year-old female presents with a six-month history of progressive headaches and blurred vision. Her primary care physician had performed an MRI scan demonstrating a 1-cm pituitary tumor expanding the sella turcica. She undergoes a neuroendoscopic excision of the tumor.

Description of Procedure (62165)

The nasal packs are removed and the endoscope is passed down the left nostril until the sphenoid ostium is visualized. A rongeur is used to open the sphenoid ostium under endoscopic visualization. The sphenoid mucosa is then stripped and electrocautery used for hemostasis. The sinus is irrigated with antibiotic solution. Endoscopic visualization is used to guide a small osteotome into place where the bone of the floor of the sella is removed, exposing the dura. The dura is coagulated by passing bipolar forceps down the right nostril. The dura is opened in a cruciate fashion with a blade and the dural leaflets are coagulated. The tumor capsule is visualized through the endoscope. Biopsy forceps are used to excise several pieces of the tumor which are sent to pathology. The tumor is then removed using a combination of curettage and suction. Once the tumor is removed, the endoscope is released from its clamp and passed through the hole in the dura, into the sella. Using the 30 degree scope, the diaphragma sella is visualized. The endoscope is turned within the cavity to identify any additional tumor remnants. A small dissector is passed through the endoscope and additional tumor remnant(s) are removed with suction. Endoscopic bipolar forceps are used to assist with hemostasis within the sella and endoscopic irrigation is applied. The endoscope is withdrawn into the nasal sinus and clamped there to provide visualization during reconstruction of the sella floor. The dural defect is gently packed with Gelfoam until all bleeding has stopped. The sphenoid sinus is packed with Vaseline-impregnated gauze. The endoscope is withdrawn and the hypopharyngeal pack removed. The Mayfield headholder is removed and the patient awakened and extubated for transport to recovery.

Spine and Spinal Cord

INJECTION, DRAINAGE, OR ASPIRATION

Injection of contrast during fluoroscopic guidance and localization is an inclusive component of codes ▶62263◀, 62270-62273, 62280-62282, 62310-62319, ▶0027T◀. Fluoroscopic guidance and localization is reported by code 76005, unless a formal contrast study (myelography, epidurography, or arthrography) is performed, in which case the use of fluoroscopy is included in the supervision and interpretation codes.

For radiologic supervision and interpretation of epidurography, ...

▶Code 62263 describes a catheter-based treatment involving targeted injection of various substances (eg, hypertonic saline, steroid, anesthetic) via an indwelling epidural catheter. Code 62263 includes percutaneous insertion and removal of an epidural catheter (remaining in place over a several-day period), for the administration of multiple injections of a neurolytic agent(s) performed during serial treatment sessions (ie, spanning two or more treatment days). If required, adhesions or scarring may also be lysed by mechanical means. Code 62263 is NOT reported for each adhesiolysis treatment, but should be reported ONCE to describe the entire series of injections/infusions spanning two or more treatment days. For endoscopic lysis of adhesions, use 0027T.

Code 62264 describes multiple adhesiolysis treatment sessions performed on the same day. Adhesions or scarring may be lysed by injections of neurolytic agent(s). If required, adhesions or scarring may also be lysed mechanically using a percutaneously-deployed catheter.

Codes 62263 and 62264 include the procedure of injection of contrast for epidurography (72275) and fluoroscopic guidance and localization (76005) during initial and/or subsequent sessions.◄

►(For daily hospital management of continuous epidural or subarachnoid drug administration performed in conjunction with codes 62318-62319, see **Evaluation and Management** services)◄

►(For endoscopic lysis of epidural adhesions, use Category III code 0027T)◄

 Rationale

The Spine and Spinal Cord, Injection, Drainage or Aspiration section introductory notes were revised to add instructional intent and delineate differentiation between the procedure described by 62263 and the newly added code, 62264. The first paragraph of the revised introductory notes reflects the addition of the new Category III code 0027T, which describes "endoscopic lysis of epidural adhesions with direct visualization using mechanical means (eg, spinal endoscopic catheter system) or solution injection (eg, normal saline) including radiological localization and epidurography." Additional information in the introductory notes instructs users to report code 0027T when endoscopic lysis of epidural adhesions is performed.

The revised introductory notes now clearly identify inclusive components of the percutaneous lysis of epidural adhesions procedure. For example, insertion and removal of the percutaneous epidural catheter, administration of multiple injections of neurolytic agent(s), or lysis by mechanical means are inclusive components of the overall procedure and should not be separately reported.

▲**62263** Percutaneous lysis of epidural adhesions using solution injection (eg, hypertonic saline, enzyme) or mechanical means (eg, catheter) including radiologic localization (includes contrast when administered), multiple adhesiolysis sessions; 2 or more days

►(62263 includes 72275 and 76005)◄

●**62264** 1 day

►(Do not report 62264 with 62263)◄

►(62264 includes codes 76005 and 72275)◄

 Rationale

Code 62263 was added to *CPT 2000* for the reporting of percutaneous lysis of epidural adhesions using solution injection (eg, hypertonic saline, enzyme) or mechanical means (eg, catheter) including radiologic localization (includes contrast when administered) performed over one or more days. Since the addition of code 62263, this technique has been modified and simplified, resulting in a procedure that may be performed on a one-day basis where the catheter is removed after injecting the drugs or performing mechanical lysis, rather than leaving the catheter in the patient.

Revisions were made to code 62263 for *CPT 2003* to identify this code as a percutaneous epidural adhesiolysis procedure including multiple adhesiolysis sessions performed over two or more days. An additional revision to the descriptor deleted the reference to a "spring wound" type of catheter from the parenthetical note providing examples of mechanical lysis.

New code 62264 was created to specifically address a percutaneous epidural adhesiolysis procedure, including multiple adhesiolysis sessions, performed on a single day. The procedure is essentially the same as described for 62263 but takes place on one day rather than on multiple days.

Both codes, 62263 and 62264, should be reported only one time for the entire series of injections/infusions or mechanical lysis procedures performed, not per adhesiolysis treatment. For code 62263, this treatment series will span two or more treatment days, but the code would still be reported only one time.

Codes 62263 and 62264 are mutually exclusive codes; therefore, they should not be reported together, as indicated in the parenthetical note that follows code 62264.

Explanatory notes were added following codes 62263 and 62264 to direct users that these codes include codes 72275 and 76005.

Clinical Example (62263)

A 35-year-old male has severe pain (rated 8/10) located in the right lower back and radiating down the outside of the right leg to the top of the foot and the big toe after multiple back operations over a 10-year period. Various systemic medications (oral narcotic and non-narcotic) and physical therapy have failed to provide significant long-term pain relief. A catheter is placed percutaneously in the epidural space; an epidurogram is performed to identify the areas of scar, nerve constriction, and possible nerve inflammation and degree of fluid flow (or lack thereof) in the epidural space; and the epidural adhesions are lysed.

[Please note that the catheter is left in place for additional adhesiolysis sessions over the next one or more days. This service encompasses 2 or more days and has a global period of 10 days.]

Description of Procedure (62263)

The skin is locally anesthetized. The introduction needle is directed into the epidural space at the proper vertebral level or the caudal epidural space, under x-ray fluoroscopy. A flexible, directable catheter is introduced through the needle into the epidural space. The catheter tip is carefully maneuvered in the epidural space around bands of scar tissue until it is in the focal scar tissue at the target spinal nerve-nerve root. A contrast injection is performed to confirm needle tip or catheter location and determine degree of free flow liquid in the epidural space (eg, determine areas of scarring in the epidural space). This injection also is used with temporary fluorogram monitor views to evaluate the nerve roots and spinal nerves in the area and any focal constriction or swelling of the nerve. The free flow of dye through the epidural space adjacent to this target spinal nerve-nerve root is also determined. A decision on the number, type, and quantity of injections/infusions is made. For the typical patient described above, an injection is given at this point of hyaluronidase, local anesthetic, and steroid, followed 30 minutes later by an injection of hypertonic (10%) saline. The catheter exit site is dressed for sterility and secured and the patient is admitted to the hospital for two days. At 12-24 hours and at 24-48 hours later, injections are repeated, using local anesthetic, hyaluronidase, steroid, and hypertonic saline. Also, at each series of injections, a repeat epidural contrast injection is performed with temporary fluorogram monitor views to verify correct catheter placement. Also evaluated is the surrounding epidural space, including the gradual opening of constricted scar areas around the target nerves-nerve roots. After the third series of injections, the catheter is removed and a sterile dressing applied.

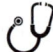

Clinical Example (62264)

A 45-year-old white male has intermittent severe intractable low back pain with radiation into the right lower extremity associated with numbness, tingling, and weakness for over 12 years that started following a work-related injury. Subsequently, he underwent various modalities of treatments, initially conservative management with medication, subsequently physical therapy followed by lumbar laminectomy followed by lumbar fusion with hardware, with intermittent conservative management with physical therapy and continuous medication management, but continued pain problems with significant deterioration of his physical and functional status leading to disability. At this time, he is on significant amounts of narcotics, anxiolytics, as well as other drugs with interrelated depression, generalized anxiety disorder, and significant functional limitations.

Following his presentation to a multidisciplinary pain management program, he was diagnosed to be negative for facet joint-mediated pain. Subsequently, an epidurogram showed significant filling defects. His MRI also showed significant scar tissue on the right side occupying L5 and S1 nerve roots. He failed to respond significantly to transforaminal epidural steroid injections even though diagnosis was confirmed by blocking right L5 and S1 nerve roots and also failed to respond to high-volume caudal epidural steroid injection. The patient is scheduled for a one-day percutaneous lysis of epidural adhesions.

[Please note that this service is a 1-day procedure and has a global period of 10 days.]

Description of Procedure (62264)

After the appropriate preparation and consent, the patient is taken to the operating room or a sterile procedure room where preparation is carried out with povidone-iodine prep. Draping is carried out to cover the patient, extending into the midthoracic or cervical region, even if the procedure is performed in the lumbosacral region. Appropriate monitoring is carried out, with monitoring of BP and pulse and pulse oximetry. Sedation is slowly administered. The fluoroscope is adjusted over the lumbosacral region for AP and lateral views. A physician, scrubbed and in sterile gown and gloves, infiltrates the area for needle insertion with local anesthetic. Following this, an RK needle is introduced into the epidural space under fluoroscopic utilization. Once the needle placement is confirmed to be in the epidural space, a lumbar epidurogram is carried out utilizing approximately 2 to 5 mL of contrast. Finding the filling defects by examining the contrast flow into the nerve roots is the purpose of the epidurogram. Intravascular or subarachnoid placement of the needle or contrast is avoided; if such malpositioning occurs, the needle is repositioned. After appropriate determination of epidurography, a Racz catheter, which is a spring-guided, reinforced catheter, is slowly passed through the RK needle to the area of the filling defect or the site of pathology determined by MRI, CT, or patient symptoms. Following the positioning of the catheter into the appropriate area, adhesiolysis is carried out by mechanical means. After completion of the adhesiolysis, a repeat epidurogram is carried out by additional injection of contrast. If appropriate adhesiolysis is completed, nerve root filling as well as epidural filling will be noted. At this time, variable doses of local anesthetic and steroid are injected. Five to 10 mL of 2% lidocaine hydrochloride or 5 to 10 mL of 0.25% bupivacaine are used for the local anesthetic. Additionally, hyaluronidase may be injected at this time. A steroid is injected in the operating room or recovery room. Following completion of the injection, the catheter is taped utilizing bio-occlusive dressing; and the patient is turned to the supine position and transferred to the recovery room.

62269 Biopsy of spinal cord, percutaneous needle

▶(For fine needle aspiration, see 10021, 10022)◀

▶(For evaluation of fine needle aspirate, see 88172, 88173)◀

Rationale
Parenthetical notes were added to direct users to the fine needle aspiration codes (10021, 10022, 88172, 88173) when fine needle aspiration technique is used to obtain a biopsy of the spinal cord.

⊘▲**62284** Injection procedure for myelography and/or computed tomography, spinal (other than C1-C2 and posterior fossa)

Rationale
For *CPT 2003*, in order to update the language, codes containing the phrases "computerized axial tomography" have been revised to state, "computed tomography." The term "axial" is misleading since computed tomography may be done in any plane (axial, coronal, sagittal, or multiplanar).

62318 Injection, including catheter placement, continuous infusion or intermittent bolus, not including neurolytic substances, with or without contrast (for either localization or epidurography), of diagnostic or therapeutic substance(s) (including anesthetic, antispasmodic, opioid, steroid, other solution), epidural or subarachnoid; cervical or thoracic

62319 lumbar, sacral (caudal)

▶(For daily hospital management of continuous epidural or subarachnoid drug administration performed in conjunction with codes 62318-62319, **see Evaluation and Management** services)◀

Rationale
A cross-reference was added to clarify that an appropriate E/M code should be used to report subsequent day(s) management of an epidural or subarachnoid catheter placed for postoperative pain management rather than to deliver an anesthetic for a surgical procedure.

CATHETER IMPLANTATION

62350   Implantation, revision or repositioning of tunneled intrathecal or epidural catheter, for long-term medication administration via an external pump or implantable reservoir/infusion pump; without laminectomy

62351   with laminectomy

(For refilling and maintenance of an implantable infusion pump ▶for spinal or brain drug therapy, use 95990)◀

RESERVOIR/PUMP IMPLANTATION

62367   Electronic analysis of programmable, implanted pump for intrathecal or epidural drug infusion (includes evaluation of reservoir status, alarm status, drug prescription status); without reprogramming

62368   with reprogramming

▶(For refilling and maintenance of an implantable infusion pump for spinal or brain drug therapy, use 95990)◀

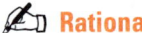

Rationale

A new cross-reference was added following codes 62351, 62368 to instruct that refilling and maintenance of an implantable infusion pump for the spine or brain should be reported with code 95990, Refilling and maintenance of implantable pump or reservoir for drug delivery, spinal (intrathecal, epidural) or brain (intraventricular).

REPAIR

63700   Repair of meningocele; less than 5 cm diameter

63702   larger than 5 cm diameter

▶(Do not report modifier '-63' in conjunction with (63700, 63702)◀

63704   Repair of myelomeningocele; less than 5 cm diameter

63706   larger than 5 cm diameter

▶(Do not report modifier '-63' in conjunction with (63704, 63706)◀

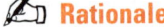

Rationale

For the codes listed above, see page 244, modifier '-63.'

Extracranial Nerves, Peripheral Nerves, and Autonomic Nervous System

INTRODUCTION/INJECTION OF ANESTHETIC AGENT (NERVE BLOCK), DIAGNOSTIC OR THERAPEUTIC

Somatic Nerves

64400*	Injection, anesthetic agent; trigeminal nerve, any division or branch
▲64415*	brachial plexus, single
●64416	brachial plexus, continuous infusion by catheter (including catheter placement) including daily management for anesthetic agent administration

▶(Do not report 01996 in addition to 64416)◀

▲64445*	sciatic nerve, single
●64446	sciatic nerve, continuous infusion by catheter, (including catheter placement) including daily management for anesthetic agent administration

▶(Do not report 01996 in addition to 64446)◀

●64447	femoral nerve, single

▶(Do not report 01996 in addition to 64447)◀

●64448	femoral nerve, continuous infusion by catheter (including catheter placement) including daily management for anesthetic agent administration

▶(Do not report 01996 in addition to 64448)◀

Rationale

The series of codes that describes procedures involving injection of anesthetic agent (nerve block) into the somatic nerves was modified to reflect current clinical practice. Codes 64415 and 64445 were revised to include the word "single" to differentiate a single injection versus continuous administration as described in new codes 64416, 64446, and 64448. New code 64447 was added to describe a single injection of an anesthetic agent at the femoral nerve. Previously, no code adequately described this service. New codes 64416, 64446, 64448 have a 10-day global period and include services provided for daily management of continuous drug administration to the brachial plexus, sciatic nerve and femoral nerve for post operative pain and control and/or chemical sympathectomy.

Cross-references were added following new codes 64416, 64446, 64447 and 64448 to instruct the user not to report code 01996 in addition to these services as daily management of anesthetic agent administration is included in the newly established continuous block codes.

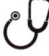

Clinical Example (64415)

A 36-year-old male suffered a crush injury of his thumb and forefinger on the right hand in an auto accident. He has developed marked immobility of these digits and symptoms of reflex sympathetic dystrophy (complex regional pain syndrome). He is to receive a series of axillary blocks to both treat the reflex sympathetic dystrophy and to allow analgesia for physical therapy to his hand.

Description of Procedure (64415)
After obtaining informed consent, the patient's right arm is abducted at the shoulder and flexed at the elbow with his hand positioned above his right shoulder. The axilla is prepped with a betadine solution and a 22-gauge short-bevel needle inserted into the brachial plexus sheath after anesthetizing the skin with a small amount of local anesthetic. The proper location of the needle is ascertained with the use of a nerve stimulator, the elicitation of paresthesias, or the transarterial technique. An axillary block using the injection of 30-40 ml of local anesthetic (usually 1 to 1.5% lidocaine, 0.25 to 0.375% bupivacaine or 1 to 1.5% mepivacaine) is now performed after using a small test dose of the local anesthetic and frequent aspiration during the injection. The density and function of the block is then assessed over the next 30 minutes.

Active physical therapy to the hand and digits is administered while the patient's arm and hand are anesthetized.

The complications of an axillary block include possible infection, injury to the axillary artery with hematoma formation, systemic local anesthetic toxicity and nerve injury. Fortunately these complications are rare.

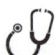

Clinical Example (64416)
A 36-year-old male suffered traumatic amputation of his thumb and forefinger on the right hand in an auto accident. He has had these digits replanted under a general anesthetic and five hours of surgery. The digits are ischemic in appearance and cold with poor capillary filling despite a good surgical repair and anastomoses of the digital arteries. A continuous brachial plexus block using a catheter placed in the brachial plexus at the axilla and the infusion of local anesthetic is planned to provide pain relief and to provide vasodilatation of the arterial supply to the hand and digits in an effort to improve survival of the re-implanted digits.

Description of Procedure (64416)
After obtaining informed consent, the patient is sedated lightly, if necessary, with a small amount of midazolam. His right arm is abducted at the shoulder and flexed at the elbow with his hand positioned above his right shoulder. The axilla is prepped with a betadine solution and an 18 or 20-gauge 2-inch angiocath-type catheter is inserted into the brachial plexus sheath after anesthetizing the skin with a small amount of local anesthetic. The proper location of the needle is ascertained with the use of a nerve stimulator, the elicitation of paresthesias, or the loss of resistance technique. The needle is removed and the plastic sleeve or cannula left in position. Next an epidural-type plastic catheter is inserted through the sleeve into the brachial plexus sheath and fixed in place with tape or suture. An axillary block using the injection of about 30-40 ml of local anesthetic (usually 1 to 1.5% lidocaine, 0.25 to 0.375% bupivacaine or 1 to 1.5% mepivacaine) is now performed after using a small test dose of the local anesthetic and frequent aspiration during the injection. The density and function of the block is then assessed over the next 30 minutes as well as signs and symptoms of

local anesthetic toxicity. A continuous infusion of local anesthetic is now started (0.25% bupivacaine at 5-10 ml/hr).

Clinical Example (64445)

A 55-year-old male sustains a tri-malleolar fracture of his left ankle while rock climbing. He undergoes surgical repair of his left ankle under general anesthesia. To provide post-operative pain control, a sciatic nerve block is performed at the end of surgery. This block will decrease post-op pain, allow earlier ambulation, and lessen the amount of post-op analgesic medication required.

Description of Procedure (64445)

Informed consent is obtained pre-operatively. In the post-anesthesia recovery room or in the operating room after surgery on the foot and ankle is completed, the patient is placed in the right lateral position and the thigh flexed on the hip to 45 degrees. The posterior superior iliac spine (PSIS), the greater femoral trochanter and sacral hiatus are identified and marked. A line is drawn between the superior and posterior aspect of the greater trochanter and the PSIS. The line is bisected and a perpendicular dropped 3-5 cm from the midpoint of the line to the needle insertion site. The point of insertion should lie along a third line drawn between the greater trochanter and the sacral hiatus. The skin is prepped and draped and a 6-inch 22-gauge, short-bevel, insulated nerve stimulator needle advanced perpendicular to the skin. The needle is advanced 6-8 cm with a stimulation intensity of 1.5-2.0 mA and adjusted downwards as evoked motor response increases. Plantar flexion at less than 0.5 mA is the desired goal and indicates placement of the needle near the medial part of the nerve. After a negative aspiration, the needle is held firm and local anesthetic (0.375 to 0.5% bupivacaine with epinephrine 1:200,000, 30 ml) injected incrementally. Attention is paid to the presence of paresthesias, reflex movement and resistance to injection. Efficacy of the block may be improved by depositing the local anesthetic in more than one location, such as laterally (peroneal component) and medially (tibial component). The mean duration of analgesia is 14 hours with 0.5% bupivacaine but can range up to 24 hours.

The complications of a sciatic nerve block include possible infection, injury to the sciatic nerve from intraneural injections, and systemic local anesthetic toxicity. Neural ischemia should be considered in patients with severe peripheral vascular disease who present with nerve injury following sciatic nerve block.

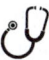

Clinical Example (64446)

A 30-year-old male crushed his left foot in an automobile accident. He undergoes major reconstruction of his left foot and ankle under general anesthesia. To provide post-operative pain control, a continuous sciatic nerve block is performed at the end of surgery. This block will decrease post-op pain, allow earlier ambulation, and lessen the amount of post-op analgesic medication required.

Description of Procedure (64446)

In the post-anesthesia recovery room or in the operating room after surgery on the foot and ankle is completed, the patient is placed in the right lateral position and the thigh flexed on the hip to 45 degrees. The greater femoral trochanter and ischial tuberosity are marked and a line drawn from the popliteal fossa to midway between the two landmarks. A 20-gauge insulated needle is introduced vertically to the skin, just medial to the upper end of the marked line to determine the depth of the sciatic nerve. A brisk motor response in the ankle, foot or toes is noted with less than 0.4 mA stimulation. Next an insulated Tuohy needle is advanced from approximately 5 cm cephalad and angled to intersect the tip of the first needle. Nerve stimulation is again noted, and a catheter then advanced through the Tuohy needle 50 to 100 mm. The electrical connection is then transferred to the catheter and nerve stimulation again noted. The Tuohy needle is removed, the catheter sutured in place, a bacterial filter is attached and 15-20 ml of 0.5% bupivacaine injected through the catheter. Block of the sciatic nerve is then accessed over the next 15-30 minutes and an infusion of 0.375% bupivacaine at 0.1 mL/kg/hr (~7 mL/hr) started. Required infusion rates typically range from 2 to 12 mL/hr. Occasionally bolus injections (10-15 mL) are required. The infusion is usually stopped at about 48 hours post op. The complications of a continuous sciatic nerve block include possible infection, injury to the sciatic nerve with neuralgia, and systemic local anesthetic toxicity.

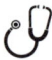

Clinical Example (64447)

A 30-year-old male undergoes a right anterior cruciate ligament repair under general anesthesia. To provide post-operative pain control and increase mobility in his knee, a femoral nerve block is performed. This block will allow earlier discharge from the recovery room, decreased post-op pain and earlier ambulation.

Description of Procedure (64447)

In the post-anesthesia recovery room or in the operating room prior to general anesthesia, the patient's right groin is prepped with a betadine solution and a 22-gauge short-bevel 4 cm needle inserted approximately 1 cm lateral to the femoral artery and 1 cm caudad from the inguinal ligament after anesthetizing the skin with a small amount of local anesthetic. The proper location of the needle is ascertained with the use of a nerve stimulator, the elicitation of paresthesias, the loss of resistance technique, or with a field block technique. Next, between 15 and 30 ml of 0.25% to 0.5% bupivacaine with epinephrine 1:200,000 is injected carefully and with frequent aspiration to avoid the possibility of intravascular injection. The density and function of the block is then assessed. Onset of block may take 30-40 minutes. Postoperative analgesia typically lasts 12 to 24 hours. The complications of a femoral nerve block include possible infection, injury to the femoral artery with hematoma formation, systemic local anesthetic toxicity and nerve injury. Persistent quadriceps weakness suggests neural injury.

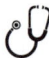

Clinical Example (64448)

A 65-year-old male undergoes a right total knee replacement (CPT code 27447) under general anesthesia. To provide post-operative pain control and increased mobility in his knee, a continuous femoral nerve block is performed. This block will allow earlier discharge from the recovery room, decreased post-op pain, earlier ambulation, improved range of motion of the knee and enhanced rehabilitation.

Description of Procedure (64448)

In the post-anesthesia recovery room or in the operating room prior to general anesthesia, the patient's right groin is prepped with a betadine solution and a 22-gauge short-bevel 10-cm insulated needle is inserted into an 18-gauge long plastic cannula. The femoral nerve is located approximately 1 cm lateral to the femoral artery and 1 cm caudad from the inguinal ligament after anesthetizing the skin with a small amount of local anesthetic. The proper location of the needle is ascertained with the use of a nerve stimulator or with the elicitation of paresthesias, or both. The plastic cannula is then advanced over the needle into the "sheath" of the femoral nerve. Next, between 20 and 30 ml of 0.25% to 0.5% bupivacaine with epinephrine 1:200,000 is injected carefully through the cannula and with frequent aspiration to avoid the possibility of intravascular injection. A 20-gauge epidural catheter is threaded through the cannula and the cannula removed. The catheter is sutured in place and sterilely dressed. Bupivacaine 0.25 to 0.125% at 0.14 mL/kg/hr (~10 mL/hr) is then infused. The complications of a continuous femoral nerve block include possible infection, injury to the femoral artery with hematoma formation, systemic local anesthetic toxicity and nerve injury from direct trauma, intraneural injection or compressive-ischemic injury. Persistent quadriceps weakness suggests neural injury.

Eye and Ocular Adnexa

Anterior Segment

ANTERIOR CHAMBER

Incision

65820 Goniotomy

▶(Do not report modifier '-63' in conjunction with 65820)◀

 Rationale

For the code listed above, see page 244, modifier '-63.'

LENS

OTHER PROCEDURES

+●**66990** Use of ophthalmic endoscope (List separately in addition to code for primary procedure)

▶(66990 may be used only with codes 65820, 65875, 65920, 66985, 66986, 67038, 67039, 67040)◀

66999 Unlisted procedure, anterior segment of eye

67036 Vitrectomy, mechanical, pars plana approach;

67038 with epiretinal membrane stripping

67039   with focal endolaser photocoagulation

67040   with endolaser panretinal photocoagulation

▶(For use of ophthalmic endoscope with 67038, 67039, 67040, use 66990)◀

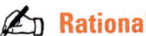

Rationale
An add-on code (66990) has been added to describe ophthalmic procedures using an ophthalmic endoscope to be used only in association with the following codes: 65820 Goniotomy, 65875 Severing adhesions of anterior segment of eye, incisional technique (with or without injection of air or liquid); posterior synechiae, 65920 Removal of implanted material, anterior segment of eye, 66985 Insertion of intraocular lense prosthesis (secondary implant), not associated with concurrent cataract removal, 66986 Exchange of intraocular lens, 67038 Vitrectomy, mechanical, pars plana approach; with epiretinal membrane strpping, 67039 Vitrectomy, mechanical, pars plana approach; with focal endolaser photocoagulation, 67040 Vitrectomy, mechanical, pars plana approach; with endolaser panretinal photocoagulation. The endoscope offers a more extended view of the anatomy not accessible through the operating microscope. This add-on code should not be used in association with removal of cataract code 66982, as endoscopy, when performed, is included in code 66982. Also, this add-on code should not be used in addition to 66710 cyclophotocoagulation. A parenthetic note has also been added to identify how to report use of an ophthalmic endoscope when performed in conjunction with mechanical vitrectomy with 1) epiretinal membrane stripping (66990 with 67038), 2) focal endolaser photocoagulation (66990 with 67039), or 3) endolaser panretinal photocoagulation (66990 with 67040).

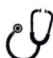

Clinical Example (66990)
A 72-year-old male, 16 months post-op phacoemulsification, who had a posterior chamber lens inserted in the sulcus at the time of surgery due to a broken posterior capsule, presents with glare, poor vision and multiple images due to a "sunset syndrome." A repositioning of the intraocular lens is performed. During the procedure ophthalmic endoscopy is performed to aid in planning and ensuring adequate capsular support.

Description of Procedure (66990)
Two stab incisions are made with a #75 blade at the supero-nasal and temporal surgical limbus. Using a blunt cannula, the anterior segment is filled with viscoelastic material. The viscoelastic material is then gently injected under the iris and in front of the implant to allow visualization of the capsular bag. The sulcus is examined 360 degrees. The zonules are noted to be absent below but intact above. The lower haptic of the intraocular lens is noted to be subluxated into the anterior vitreous. A repositioning is planned based on the anatomy. After the intraocular lens is repositioned and rotated, the endoscope is then reinserted to ensure that there is adequate capsular support for the implant before the completion of the surgical procedure.

Auditory System

Middle Ear

INCISION

▲**69424**   Ventilating tube removal requiring general anesthesia

▶(69424 is a unilateral procedure. To report a bilateral procedure, use 69424 with modifier '-50')◀

▶(Do not report code 69424 in conjunction with codes 69205, 69210, 69420, 69421, 69433-69676, 69710-69745, 69801-69930)◀

 Rationale

Code 69424 was revised to describe the work required for removal of a tympanostomy tube under general anesthesia with an additional cross-reference to exclude use of 69424 when associated with myringoplasty and tympanoplasty procedures. Further, a cross-reference was added to indicate that this is a unilateral procedure. To report a bilateral procedure report 69424 with modifier '-50'.

Code 69424 is used for removal of a tympanostomy tube that has failed or that is causing problems (eg, local infection, granulation, cholesteatoma formation). The work value for placement of a tympanostomy tube does not really reflect the physician work required for its removal under general anesthesia. This work approximates that of placement of a tube. Thus, code 69425 was revised to allow reporting of the tube removal regardless of whether the tube was originally placed by the same surgeon or another surgeon.

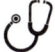 **Clinical Example** (69424)

A five-year-old child had tympanostomy (ventilating) tubes placed at age 2 for recurring acute otitis media with effusion. The left tube extruded 1 year ago and that ear has been free of infection and fluid since then. The right tube has failed to extrude and has granulation tissue around it that has been unresponsive to topical antimicrobial therapy. The surgeon who originally placed the tube has followed the child since placement and feels the remaining indwelling tympanostomy tube should be removed.

Description of Procedure (69424)

The surgeon who originally placed the tympanostomy (ventilating) tubes brings the patient to the outpatient facility. Under general anesthesia and utilizing an operating microscope, the surgeon creates a relaxing incision. The surgeon removes the tube with surrounding granulation tissue, thus creating an optimal situation for closure of the perforation in which the tube was situated. Monitoring of the ear in the office setting revealed the perforation to have closed within several weeks' time.

Radiology

In a return to previous layout conventions for this publication, the codes to be referenced in this section will be found in numerical order by code. The most substantial revision to the Radiology section of the CPT code set is the revision of all of the descriptors within this section for computed tomography imaging procedures. Also, significant revisions have been made to the Obstetrical and Non-obstetrical Ultrasound subsections with the inclusion of guidelines and explanatory notes for this subsection and the addition and revision of several codes.

Radiology Guidelines (Including Nuclear Medicine and Diagnostic Ultrasound)

Administration of Contrast Material(s)

The phrase "with contrast" ▶used in the codes for procedures performed using contrast for imaging enhancement◀ represents contrast material administered intravascularly, intra-articularly, ▶or intrathecally.◀

▶For intra-articular injection, use the appropriate joint injection code. If radiographic arthrography is performed, also use the arthrography supervision and interpretation code for the appropriate joint (which includes fluoroscopy). If CT or MR arthrography are performed without radiographic arthrography, use the appropriate joint injection code, the appropriate CT or MR code ("with contrast" or "without followed by contrast"), and the appropriate imaging guidance code for needle placement for contrast injection.◀

For spine examination using computerized tomography, magnetic resonance imaging, magnetic resonance angiography, "with contrast" includes intrathecal or intravascular injection. For intrathecal injection, use also 61055 or 62284.

Injection of ▶intravascular◀ contrast material is part of the "with contrast" CT, ▶CTA,◀ MRI, and MRA procedure.

Rationale

CPT 2002 and *CPT Changes 2002: An Insider's View* offered revisions related to numerous anatomic sites and related cross-references associated with arthrography procedures. Specifically, revisions included revised cross-references following the arthrography injection codes involving the elbow, wrist, hip, knee, ankle, and temporomandibular joint (21116, 24220, 25246, 27093, 27095, 27370, and 27648), and associated imaging procedures (70332, 73040, 73085, 73115, 73525, 73542, 73580, and 73615). In concert with these revisions, *CPT 2003* has revised the "Administration of Radiologic Contrast" notes in the Radiology section to clarify use of "injection" procedures in addition to CT and MRI filming (other than arthrography).

Radiology

Diagnostic Radiology (Diagnostic Imaging)

Head and Neck

▲ **70450**   Computed tomography, head or brain; without contrast material

▲ **70480** Computed tomography, orbit, sella, or posterior fossa or outer, middle, or inner ear; without contrast material

▲ **70486** Computed tomography, maxillofacial area; without contrast material

▲ **70490** Computed tomography, soft tissue neck; without contrast material

Chest

▲ **71250** Computed tomography, thorax; without contrast material

Spine and Pelvis

▲ **72125** Computed tomography, cervical spine; without contrast material

▲ **72128** Computed tomography, thoracic spine; without contrast material

▲ **72131** Computed tomography, lumbar spine; without contrast material

▲ **72192** Computed tomography, pelvis; without contrast material

 Rationale
For *CPT 2003*, the term "axial" was removed from the descriptor for codes 70450, 70480, 70486, 70490, 71250, 72125, 72128, 72131, and 72192. Typically, direct acquistion images are obtained in the axial plane for computed tomographic studies, but in certain instances direct acquisition may be obtained in other planes (eg, coronal plane for sinus studies). Elimination of the term "axial" will clarify to the user that the CT codes are appropriate for reporting CT direct acquistion imaging performed in any plane (ie, axial, coronal, sagittal or multiplanar).

72275 Epidurography, radiological supervision and interpretation

▶(72275 includes 76005)◀

(For injection procedure, see 62280-62282, 62310-62319, 64479-64484)

 Rationale
A cross-reference was added following code 72275 to instruct that code 76005 is included in 72275 and, therefore, is not separately reportable with code 72275.

Upper Extremities

▲ **73200** Computed tomography, upper extremity; without contrast material

Lower Extremities

▲ **73700** Computed tomography, lower extremity; without contrast material

Rationale

For *CPT 2003*, the term "axial" was removed from the descriptor for codes 73200 and 73700. Typically, direct acquisition of images are obtained in the axial plane for computed tomographic studies, but in certain instances direct acquisition may be obtained in other planes (eg, coronal plane for ankle studies). Elimination of the term "axial" will clarify to the user that the CT codes are appropriate for reporting CT direct acquisition imaging performed in any plane (ie, axial, coronal, sagittal or multiplanar).

Abdomen

74000 Radiologic examination, abdomen; single anteroposterior view

74010 anteroposterior and additional oblique and cone views

74020 complete, including decubitus and/or erect views

▲**74022** complete acute abdomen series, including supine, erect, and/or decubitus views, single view chest

 Rationale

Code 74022 has been revised to delete "upright PA" and include "single view." The designation "upright PA chest" is view specific, thereby limiting the use of code 74022. Broadening the use of this code would provide a mechanism to report any type of single view chest x-ray. This revision is also consistent with the descriptor changes to the knee and spine codes.

▲**74150** Computed tomography, abdomen; without contrast material

 Rationale

For *CPT 2003*, the term "axial" was removed from the code descriptor for 74150. Typically, direct acquisition of images are obtained in the axial plane for computed tomographic studies, but in certain instances direct acquisition may be obtained in other planes (eg, coronal plane for sinus or ankle studies). Elimination of the term "axial" will clarify to the user that the CT codes are appropriate for reporting CT direct acquisition imaging performed in any plane (ie, axial, coronal, sagittal or multiplanar).

Veins and Lymphatics

TRANSCATHETER PROCEDURES

●**75901** Mechanical removal of pericatheter obstructive material (eg, fibrin sheath) from central venous device via separate venous access, radiologic supervision and interpretation

▶(For procedure, use 36536)◀

▶(For venous catheterization, see 36010-36012)◀

●**75902** Mechanical removal of intraluminal (intracatheter) obstructive material from central venous device through device lumen, radiologic supervision and interpretation

▶(For procedure, use 36537)◀

▶(For venous catheterization, see 36010-36012)◀

 Rationale

Codes 75901 and 75902 were added to describe supervision and interpretation services for new codes 36536 and 36537. Cross-references were added to refer the user to the primary procedures. Further, cross-references following codes 75901 and 75902 were added instructing the user to see codes 36010-36012 for venous catheterization services.

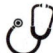 **Clinical Example** (75901 and 75902)

A 68-year-old male with gastric cancer and a subcutaneous port presents with a poorly functioning port. Infusion/injection cannot be aspirated.

▲75953 Placement of proximal or distal extension prosthesis for endovascular repair of infrarenal aortic or iliac artery aneurysm, pseudoaneurysm, or dissection, radiological supervision and interpretation

(For implantation of endovascular extension prostheses, see 34825, 34826)

●75954 Endovascular repair of iliac artery aneurysm, pseudoaneurysm, arteriovenous malformation, or trauma, radiological supervision and interpretation

▶(For implantation of endovascular graft, use 34900)◀

 Rationale

In conjunction with the creation of new codes for endovascular graft placement for repair of iliac artery (34833-34834), code 75953 was 1) editorially revised for terminology to reference "pseudoaneurysm or dissection" and 2) revised to expand the intent of this code to include the correlating radiological supervision and interpretation procedure for placement of a proximal or distal extension prosthesis for endovascular repair of an iliac artery aneurysm.

Code 75954 was created as the correlating radiological supervision and interpretation imaging code for endovascular repair of iliac artery aneurysm with a graft implant procedure, reported with code 34900. As stated in the guidelines preceding 34900, code 75954 includes angiography of the aorta and iliac arteries for diagnostic imaging prior to deployment of the endovascular device (including all routine components), fluoroscopic guidance in the delivery of the endovascular components, and intraprocedural arterial angiography to confirm appropriate position of the graft, detect endoleaks, and evaluate the status of the runoff vessels (eg, evaluation for dissection, stenosis, thrombosis, distal embolization, or iatrogenic injury). A cross-reference has been added following code 75954 to instruct that implantation of endovascular graft is reported with code 34900.

▲75989 Radiological guidance (ie, fluoroscopy, ultrasound, or computed tomography), for percutaneous drainage (eg, abscess, specimen collection), with placement of catheter, radiological supervision and interpretation

Rationale

CPT code 75989 was editorially revised to identify the radiologic guidance procedure for drainage of any type. The previous language limited use of this code to drainage of abscesses or placement of the catheter for specimen collection. The language in this code now reflects provision of this type of imaging for any of a number of percutaneous drainage procedures, citing abscess drainage and specimen collection as examples ("eg"). Further revision of this code descriptor included deletion of the term "axial," as computerized tomographic procedures, typically performed in the axial plane, may be performed in any plane (axial, coronal, sagittal, or multiplanar).

OTHER PROCEDURES

▶(For computed tomography cerebral perfusion analysis, see Category III code 0042T)◀

 Rationale

This cross-reference was added to the Other Procedures subsection to instruct reporting Category III code 0042T for computed tomography cerebral perfusion analysis.

76005 Fluoroscopic guidance and localization of needle or catheter tip for spine or paraspinous diagnostic or therapeutic injection procedures (epidural, transforaminal epidural, subarachnoid, paravertebral facet joint, paravertebral facet joint nerve or sacroiliac joint), including neurolytic agent destruction

(Injection of contrast during fluoroscopic guidance and localization is an inclusive component of codes ▶62263, 62264,◀ 62270-62273, 62280-62282, 62310-62319, ▶0027T◀)

(Fluoroscopic guidance for subarachnoid puncture for diagnostic radiographic myelography is included in supervision and interpretation codes 72240, 72255, 72265, 72270)

(For epidural or subarachnoid needle or catheter placement and injection, see codes 62270-62273, 62280-62282, 62310-62319)

(For sacroiliac joint arthrography, see 27096, 73542. If formal arthrography is not performed, recorded, and a formal radiographic report is not issued, use 76005 for fluoroscopic guidance for sacroiliac joint injections)

(For paravertebral facet joint injection, see 64470-64476. For transforaminal epidural needle placement and injection, see 64479-64484)

(For destruction by neurolytic agent, see 64600-64680)

▶(For percutaneous lysis of epidural adhesions, codes 62263, 62264, 0027T include fluoroscopic guidance and localization.)◀

 Rationale

Several revisions were made to the series of cross-references following code 76005 for fluoroscopic guidance, including the addition of codes 62263, 62264, and 0027T to the "injection of contrast" cross-reference, to indicate that contrast injection for fluoroscopic guidance is an inclusive component of the listed procedures and not separately reported. A cross-reference was added following

76005 to also indicate that, since fluoroscopic guidance is included in codes 62263, 62264, and 0027T, 76005 is not separately reportable when performed in addition to these procedures.

+▲ **76006** Manual application of stress performed by physician for joint radiography, including contralateral joint if indicated

▶(For radiographic interpretation of stressed images, see appropriate anatomic site and number of views)◀

Rationale

CPT code 76006 was editorially revised to clarify the intent of this code. The intent is to identify the manual application of stress during the imaging procedure. This effort is separate from the actual imaging procedure and interpretation. Therefore, this additional effort (ie, the application of the stress) is now separately identified by code 76006. A cross-reference was added instructing users to reference the codes listed by specific anatomic sites for the radiographic interpretation of stressed images.

▲ **76070** Computed tomography, bone mineral density study, one or more sites; axial skeleton (eg, hips, pelvis, spine)

● **76071** appendicular skeleton (peripheral) (eg, radius, wrist, heel)

76075 Dual energy x-ray absorptiometry (DEXA), bone density study, one or more sites; axial skeleton (eg, hips, pelvis, spine)

76076 appendicular skeleton (peripheral) (eg, radius, wrist, heel)

▶(To report dual energy x-ray absorptiometry (DEXA) body composition study, one or more sites, use Category III code 0028T)◀

Rationale

For CPT 2003, the term "axial" was deleted from the descriptor for code 76070. Typically, direct acquisition of images are obtained in the axial plane for computed tomographic studies, but in certain instances direct acquisition may be obtained in other planes (eg, coronal plane for sinus or ankle studies). Elimination of the term "axial" will clarify to the user that the CT codes are appropriate for reporting CT direct acquisition imaging performed in any plane (ie, axial, coronal, sagittal or multiplanar). In addition code 76071 was added to better differentiate this code from code 76070 and to facilitate transition of HCPCS Level III codes into the CPT code set.

A cross-reference following existing codes 76075 and 76076 has been added to direct users to new Category III code 0028T, which allows reporting for body composition studies using DEXA.

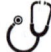
Clinical Example (76071)

A 55-year-old menopausal woman with a family history of osteoporosis is considering estrogen therapy. Lumbar spine hardware prevents obtaining a CT bone mineral density study of the spine.

+▲76085	Digitization of film radiographic images with computer analysis for lesion detection and further physician review for interpretation, mammography (List separately in addition to code for primary procedure)

(Use 76085 in conjunction with ▶76091,◀ 76092)

76090	Mammography; unilateral
76091	bilateral

▶(For computer aided detection applied to a bilateral diagnostic mammogram, use 76085 in conjunction with 76091)◀

76092	Screening mammography, bilateral (two view film study of each breast)

(For computer aided detection applied to a screening mammogram, use 76085 ▶in conjunction with 76092)◀

Rationale
CPT add-on code 76085 was editorially changed to delete "screening" from the code descriptor in order to report computer aided detection (CAD) when used in conjunction with a screening or diagnostic mammography. In addition, correlating cross-references following codes 76085, 76091, and 76092 were revised and added to instruct the user on appropriate reporting use of these codes in conjunction with other services.

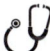
Clinical Example (76085)
A 55-year-old woman is referred to the mammography department complaining of a lump at the two o'clock position of her left breast, corroborated by her referring physician. Her last screening mammogram was taken 22 months ago.

Description of Procedure (76085)
A bilateral diagnostic mammogram is performed with two full-breast views of both the right and left breasts. The film mammograms are loaded into the CAD system, digitized, and analyzed by the software for regions of interest (ROIs). During his review of the films, the physician activates the CAD system display, using the marked ROIs to ensure a thorough review of all breast tissue.

The service includes the time for the clinic staff to load the films into the CAD system and for the physician to activate the CAD display and re-review the mammograms at the location of the marked ROIs.

▲76355	Computed tomography guidance for stereotactic localization
▲76360	Computed tomography guidance for needle placement (eg, biopsy, aspiration, injection, localization device), radiological supervision and interpretation
▲76370	Computed tomography guidance for placement of radiation therapy fields
▲76380	Computed tomography, limited or localized follow-up study

Rationale
For CPT 2003, the term "axial" was removed from the descriptor for codes 76355, 76360, 76370 and 76380. Typically, direct acquisition of images are obtained in

the axial plane for computed tomographic studies, but in certain instances direct acquisition may be obtained in other planes (eg, coronal plane for sinus or ankle studies). Elimination of the term "axial" will clarify to the user that the CT codes are appropriate for reporting CT direct acquisition imaging performed in any plane (ie, axial, coronal, sagittal or multiplanar).

●**76496**   Unlisted fluoroscopic procedure (eg, diagnostic, interventional)

●**76497**   Unlisted computed tomography procedure (eg, diagnostic, interventional)

●**76498**   Unlisted magnetic resonance procedure (eg, diagnostic, interventional)

▲**76499**   Unlisted diagnostic radiographic procedure

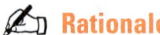 **Rationale**

Continuous advancements in interventional radiology both in terms of new technology and the application of existing techniques in new ways warrant the creation of unlisted interventional radiology codes. In the Radiology section of the CPT code set, unlisted codes currently exist to report unlisted diagnostic procedures, unlisted ultrasound procedures, unlisted radiation oncology procedures, and unlisted nuclear medicine procedures. To promote consistency reflecting modalities utilizing interventional imaging supervision and interpretation, new unlisted codes 76496, 76497, and 76498 have been added and existing code 76499 has been revised in the Radiology section of the CPT code set.

Diagnostic Ultrasound

Pelvis

▶OBSTETRICAL◀

▶Codes 76801and 76802 include determination of the number of gestational sacs and fetuses, gestational sac/fetal measurements appropriate for gestation (<14 weeks 0 days), survey of visible fetal and placental anatomic structure, qualitative assessment of amniotic fluid volume/gestational sac shape and examination of the maternal uterus and adnexa.

Codes 76805 and 76810 include determination of number of fetuses and amniotic/chorionic sacs, measurements appropriate for gestational age (> or = 14 weeks 0 days), survey of intracranial/spinal/abdominal anatomy, four-chambered heart, umbilical cord insertion site, placenta location and amniotic fluid assessment and, when visible, examination of maternal adnexa.

Codes 76811and 76812 include all elements of codes 76805 and 76810 plus detailed anatomic evaluation of the fetal brain/ventricles, face, heart/outflow tracts and chest anatomy, abdominal organ specific anatomy, number/length/ architecture of limbs and detailed evaluation of the umbilical cord and placenta and other fetal anatomy as clinically indicated.

Report should document the results of the evaluation of each element described above or the reason for non-visualization.

Code 76815 represents a focused "quick look" exam limited to the assessment of one or more of the elements listed in code 76815.

Code 76816 describes an examination designed to reassess fetal size and interval growth or re-evaluate one or more anatomic abnormalities of a fetus previously demonstrated on ultrasound, and should be coded once for each fetus requiring re-evaluation using modifier '-59' for each fetus after the first.

Code 76817 describes a transvaginal obstetric ultrasound performed separately or in addition to one of the transabdominal examinations described above. For transvaginal examinations performed for non-obstetrical purposes, use code 76830.◄

- ●76801 Ultrasound, pregnant uterus, real time with image documentation, fetal and maternal evaluation, first trimester (<14 weeks 0 days), transabdominal approach; single or first gestation

- +●76802   each additional gestation ►(List separately in addition to code for primary procedure performed)◄

     ►(Use 76802 in conjunction with 76801)◄

- ▲76805 Ultrasound, pregnant uterus, real time with image documentation, fetal and maternal evaluation, after first trimester (> or =14 weeks 0 days), transabdominal approach; single or first gestation

- +▲76810   each additional gestation (List separately in addition to code for primary procedure performed)

     ►(Use 76810 in conjunction with code 76805)◄

- ●76811 Ultrasound, pregnant uterus, real time with image documentation, fetal and maternal evaluation plus detailed fetal anatomic examination, transabdominal approach; single or first gestation

- +●76812   each additional gestation ►(List separately in addition to code for primary procedure performed)◄

     ►(Use 76812 in conjunction with code 76811)◄

- ▲76815 Ultrasound, pregnant uterus, real time with image documentation, limited (eg, fetal heart beat, placental location, fetal position and/or qualitative amniotic fluid volume), one or more fetuses

     ►(Use 76815 only once per exam and not per element)◄

- ▲76816 Ultrasound, pregnant uterus, real time with image documentation, follow-up (eg, re-evaluation of fetal size by measuring standard growth parameters and amniotic fluid volume, re-evaluation of organ system(s) suspected or confirmed to be abnormal on a previous scan), transabdominal approach, per fetus

     ►(Report 76816 with modifier '-59' for each additional fetus examined in a multiple pregnancy)◄

- ●76817 Ultrasound, pregnant uterus, real time with image documentation, transvaginal

     ►(For non-obstetrical transvaginal ultrasound, use 76830)◄

     ►(If transvaginal examination is done in addition to transabdominal obstetrical ultrasound exam, use 76817 in addition to appropriate transabdominal exam code)◄

76818 Fetal biophysical profile; with non-stress testing

76819 without non-stress testing

(Fetal biophysical profile assessments for the second and any additional fetuses, should be reported separately by code 76818 or 76819 with modifier ▶'-59'◀ appended)

▶NON-OBSTETRICAL◀

76830 Ultrasound, transvaginal

▶(For obstetrical transvaginal ultrasound, see 76817)◀

▶(If transvaginal examination is done in addition to transabdominal non-obstetrical ultrasound exam, use 76830 in addition to appropriate transabdominal exam code)◀

76831 Hysterosonography, with or without color flow Doppler

(For introduction of saline or contrast for hysterosonography, use 58340)

(76855 has been deleted. To report, see 93975-93979)

76856 Ultrasound, pelvic (non-obstetric), B-scan and/or real time with image documentation; complete

76857 limited or follow-up (eg, for follicles)

Rationale

The practice of obstetrical ultrasound has changed significantly since the ultrasound codes for these services were originally developed. Advances in ultrasound technology enable evaluations and measurement of fetal characteristics and organ systems in much greater detail.

A new heading and instructional notes to define the services included in the obstetric ultrasound series of codes 76801-76817 were added. Codes 76805 and 76810 continue to represent ultrasonic examinations after the first trimester. However, the term "complete" has been omitted and replaced with a definition included in the instructional notes that identifies the specific components included in codes 76805 and 76810. Code 76810 continues to describe services pertinent to examinations of multiple fetuses; however, it now is consistent with other "add-on" codes in the CPT code set. Two new codes, 76801 and 76802, have been added for obstetric ultrasound examinations performed during the first trimester. The add-on code structure applies to codes 76801 and 76802 for reporting multiple gestations. Codes 76801 and 76802 are also further defined in the instructional notes.

Code 76811 was added to describe an extensive evaluation and detailed anatomic survey for pregnancies at elevated risk of congenital abnormalities of fetal development (birth defects). New codes 76811, 76812 for extensive obstetric evaluations include all elements described in code 76805, plus an extensive evaluation of fetal anatomy, such as "cardiac outflow tracks," "lip formation," "measurement of feet and hands," "head and brain." Code 76812 is an add-on code to report examination of multiple births and should be reported separately in addition to the code for the primary procedure performed on the same day. If the same fetus is examined at a separate session on the same date of service, use 76811-59. If the same fetus is examined on a different date, then code 76811 should be reported with use of the '-59' modifier. If a separate fetus of a multiple birth is examined on a separate date, then code 76811 should be reported without modifier '-59.'

The intent of 76815 remains the same. However, the descriptor has been revised for better specificity. The term applied to 76815, "or emergency in the delivery room," was omitted due to its restrictiveness, since these examinations are not limited to the delivery room. Language identifying the measurement of "amniotic fluid volume" was added to 76815, as was language identifying examination of one or more fetuses. It has also been clarified that code 76815 should not be reported separately for each element examined. Instead code 76815 includes the assessment of one or more elements examined.

The intent of code 76816 also remains the same, but it is now better defined to describe a re-assessment or re-evaluation of a fetus previously examined. An example of the types of re-evaluations that may be done are included in 76816. Instructions to report modifier '-59' for examination of additional fetuses have been added.

The last change of this revised section is the addition of a separate code (76817) to distinguish between obstetrical and non-obstetrical transvaginal ultrasonic examinations. New code 76817 represents an obstetrical transvaginal ultrasound and 76830 is now included under a new subsection heading "Non-Obstetrical," which designates it as a non-obstetrical transvaginal ultrasound.

Also related to this series of code revisions was a modification of the instructional notes applicable to codes 76818 or 76819 to instruct the use of modifier '-59' for consistency with the instructional notes for code 76816.

OTHER PROCEDURES

▲ **76999** Unlisted ultrasound procedure (eg, diagnostic, interventional)

Rationale
Unlisted code 76999 has been added to promote consistency reflecting modalities utilizing interventional imaging supervision and interpretation.

Radiation Oncology

Medical Radiation Physics, Dosimetry, Treatment Devices, and Special Services

▲ **77326** Brachytherapy isodose plan; simple (calculation made from single plane, one to four sources/ribbon application, remote afterloading brachytherapy, 1 to 8 sources)

77327 intermediate (multiplane dosage calculations, application involving 5 to 10 sources/ribbons, remote afterloading brachytherapy, 9 to 12 sources)

77328 complex (multiplane isodose plan, volume implant calculations, over 10 sources/ribbons used, special spatial reconstruction, remote afterloading brachytherapy, over 12 sources)

Rationale

Codes 77326, 77327, and 77328 have been revised to replace the word "calculation" with the word "plan." The word "calculation" indicates a lesser service than what is being performed. The word "plan" more accurately describes the process being performed.

Pathology and Laboratory

The revisions of the Pathology and Laboratory section begin again with the deletion of a panel code. Substantial revisions include addition, revision, and deletion of many codes in the hematology subsection. Two new antibody detection codes and a virus isolation code have been added to the microbiology subsection, a new fecal leukocyte count code and two codes added to report cervical smears, with correlating code deletions for outdated testing methodologies.

Disclaimer
The clinical examples included with the Laboratory series of codes in some circumstances describe the methodology of the test performed. In other cases, a scenario is described to illustrate for the user the circumstances under which this test might be performed. These clinical examples are not intended to describe only or completely the service performed, but are for illustrative purposes only.

Pathology and Laboratory

Organ or Disease Oriented Panels

▶(80090 has been deleted. To report, see codes for specific tests)◀

 Rationale

CPT code 80090, toxoplasmosis, other infections, rubellla, cytomegalovirus, herpes simplex virus (TORCH) antibody panel has been deleted. A cross-reference directing the user to the specific tests to report has been added.

When the TORCH panel became part of the CPT code set, tests were only available for total antibody levels (IgG and IgM). In recent years, IgM-specific tests have become available for some of the included assays. Since a universally common panel of analytes no longer exists, the TORCH antibody panel (80090) has been deleted.

The TORCH panel was used to screen for serologic response to toxoplasmosis, rubella, cytomegalovirus, and herpes virus infection. It was also used to evaluate newborn infants for possible congenital infection.

Urinalysis

▶(For urinalysis, infectious agent detection, semi-quantitative analysis of volatile compounds, use Category III code 0041T)◀

81000 Urinalysis, by dip stick or tablet reagent for bilirubin, glucose, hemoglobin, ketones, leukocytes, nitrite, pH, protein, specific gravity, urobilinogen, any number of these constituents; non-automated, with microscopy

81007 bacteriuria screen, except by culture or dipstick

 Rationale

A cross-reference has been added to direct the user to the new Category III code 0041T.

Chemistry

82205 Barbiturates, not elsewhere specified

(For qualitative analysis, see 80100-80103)

▶(For B-Natriuretic peptide, use 83880)◀

82375 Carbon monoxide, (carboxyhemoglobin); quantitative

82376 qualitative

▶(To report end-tidal carbon monoxide, use Category III code 0043T)◀

● **83880** Natriuretic peptide

Note: Code 83880 has been reassigned. Previously, code 83880 described a test for the measurement of Nalorphine and is currently included in code 83925. The reference to the deletion of 83880 will be revised in 2004. The original code 83880 was deleted in 1993.

Rationale

A cross-reference has been added to direct the user to the new Category III code 0043T.

Rationale

New code 83880 describes natriuretic peptide testing. This test measures a specific analyte to provide diagnostic information for patients with heart failure and to assist with the differentiation of heart failure from other disorders. A cross-reference following code 82205 has been added directing users to this newly established code because many recognize this test as "BNP" or b natriuretic peptide.

Heart failure may be difficult to diagnose, especially in the emergency department or other urgent care setting. Symptoms and some standard diagnostic tests may not be sensitive to diagnose heart failure in all populations. It is essential to diagnose heart failure early to provide patients with treatments proven to decrease morbidity and mortality.

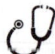

Clinical Example (83880)

A 64-year-old man with a history of chronic obstructive pulmonary disease and prior myocardial infarction presents to the emergency department with a complaint of shortness of breath worsening over the past few months. He is now unable to walk more than 10 steps and is coughing with production of tenacious brownish sputum. The patient used a bronchodilator inhaler with partial relief but was unable to sleep due to continued shortness of breath. The patient is 2 years post-myocardial infarction. The patient has been poorly compliant with his medications for the past 3 months. The natriuretic peptide test is performed to assist with the differentiation of pulmonary disease from heart failure and to aid in the guidance of further diagnostic testing (eg, chest x-ray, echocardiogram) and to help guide treatment.

In this patient, the results of natriuretic peptide testing showed elevated levels consistent with moderate heart failure and helped to distinguish between decompensated heart failure and exacerbation of pulmonary disease as the basis for the symptoms. The patient was treated with angiotensin converting enzyme inhibitors and diuretics. Symptoms improved. Follow-up natriuretic peptide testing showed reduced levels consistent with compensated heart failure.

Description of Procedure (83880)

Specimen of whole blood or plasma is collected (eg, by venipuncture) using EDTA as the anticoagulant. Natriuretic peptide testing can be performed on an automated platform or using an immunoassay test. An immunoassay may be performed using murine monoclonal and polyclonal antibodies against natriuretic peptide, labeled with a fluorescent dye and immobilized on the solid phase. The EDTA whole blood or plasma specimen is added to the sample chamber and the analysis is run. The results are provided to the treating physician to assist with diagnosis and treatment decision making.

▲ **83015** Heavy metal (eg, arsenic, barium, beryllium, bismuth, antimony, and mercury); screen

83018 quantitative, each

Rationale
Code 83015 was editorially revised to include an "eg" to avoid restricting this code to the metals listed.

84295 Sodium; serum

84300 urine

● **84302** other source

Rationale
New code 84302 was added to allow a reporting mechanism for sodium analyses other than serum and urine.

In addition, the cross-reference following code 89360 was revised to clarify the codes used to measure chloride and sodium on a sweat specimen. The cross-reference instructs the user to report new code 84302 for sodium analyses on a sweat specimen.

Hematology and Coagulation

● **85004** Blood count; automated differential WBC count

▲ **85007** blood smear, microscopic examination with manual differential WBC count

▲ **85008** blood smear, microscopic examination without manual differential WBC count

▲ **85009** manual differential WBC count, buffy coat

85013 spun microhematocrit

▲ **85014** hematocrit (Hct)

▲ **85018** hemoglobin (Hgb)

▶(85021 has been deleted)◀

▶(85022 has been deleted)◀

▶(85023 has been deleted. To report, use 85007 and 85027)◀

▶(85024 has been deleted. To report, use 85025)◀

▲ **85025** complete (CBC), automated (Hgb, Hct, RBC, WBC and platelet count) and automated differential WBC count

▲ **85027** complete (CBC), automated (Hgb, Hct, RBC, WBC and platelet count)

▶(85031 has been deleted. To report, use 85014, 85018 and 85032)◀

●85032		manual cell count (erythrocyte, leukocyte, or platelet) each
▲85041		red blood cell (RBC), automated
	▶(Do not report code 85041 in conjunction with 85025 or 85027)◀	
▲85044		reticulocyte, manual
▲85045		reticulocyte, automated
85046		reticulocyte, hemoglobin concentration
▲85048		leukocyte (WBC), automated
●85049		platelet, automated
85576		Platelet, aggregation (in vitro), each agent

▶(85585 has been deleted. To report, use 85008)◀

▶(85590 has been deleted. To report, use 85032)◀

▶(85595 has been deleted. To report, use 85049)◀

 Rationale

To better organize and update the codes in the Hematology section, some of the code descriptors have been revised, new codes have been added, and some codes have been deleted.

Current hematology laboratory practice performs non-physician manual microscopic review of peripheral blood in three basic categories: the traditional manual leukocyte (WBC) differential, a non-leukocyte differential smear review when the automated complete blood count (CBC) data suggest other abnormalities of clinical significance necessitating evaluation (eg, abnormal RDW, thrombocytopenia), and a buffy coat preparation when the leukocyte count is insufficient to allow adequate examination by the traditional differential. For this reason, three microscopic evaluation codes have been updated in the *CPT 2003* edition (85007, 85008, and 85009).

In addition, the word "manual" was added to code 85009 for clarity. It should be used as it was previously, to report a manual differential WBC count buffy coat smear study.

Code 85013 has remained unchanged and should continue to be used to report spun hematocrit. Likewise, code 85014 should be used to report hematocrit, other than spun hematocrit.

An editorial revision to code 85018 was made to add the abbreviation for hemoglobin (Hgb) to the code descriptor.

Codes 85021-85024 have been deleted. Differentiation between partial and complete automated WBC differential counts are no longer necessary as the difference in work or cost do not warrant separation and have been eliminated. For practices that reflect the appropriate WBC differential counting technique, depending on the results of the automated CBC, the revised code 85027 may serve as the base code for the CBC, on which the most appropriate WBC differential code (85007, 85008, or 85009) may be added. Conversely for labs that routinely perform only the automated differentials (eg, large reference laboratories) the revised 85025 code can also be used to report an automated complete CBC (ie, Hgb, Hct, RBC, WBC, and platelet count) with automated differential WBC count.

It is recognized that complete manual CBC has become virtually non-existent; therefore, code 85031 has been deleted. Individual parts of this evaluation (eg, manual WBC and platelet counts) continue to occasionally be necessary. Report code 85032 for each manual erythrocyte, leukocyte, or platelet count. To report a manual complete CBC (ie, RBC, WBC, Hgb, Hct, differential, and indices), use codes 85014, 85018, and code 85032 times two.

A new code (85032) has been added for a manual cell count. Previously, this code was reported using code 85595 for the manual platelet count. However, it has been replaced by code 85032 for consistency to keep related codes in the same family.

Code 85041 has been revised. It should be used to report automated red blood cell counts only. This code should not be reported in conjunction with codes 85025 or 85027.

Code 85044 was editorially revised with removal of the word "count" from the descriptor.

Code 85045 has been revised. It should be used to report automated reticulocyte count.

Code 85048 has been revised to reflect current terminology. It should continue to be used to report automated leukocyte count.

Additionally, the platelet count codes were moved from the coagulation section and revised. Code 85595 was deleted and replaced with 85049 (platelet, automated). The manual platelet count that was previously reported with 85590 should now be reported with 85032, as noted above. The platelet estimation code previously reported with 85585 should now be reported using the new code, 85008 (blood smear microscopic examination without manual differential WBC count).

▲85378 Fibrin degradation products, D-dimer; qualitative or semiquantitative

85379 quantitative

●85380 ultrasensitive (eg, for evaluation for venous thromboembolism), qualitative or semiquantitative

 Rationale

CPT code 85378 was revised to differentiate specific methodologies for measuring D-dimer, based on the sensitivity of the analysis. The indented new code 85380 was added to describe a new test to help aid in the diagnosis of venous thromboembolic disease.

The diagnosis of deep vein thrombosis (DVT) of the lower extremity and pulmonary embolism (PE) requires objective diagnostic testing. The primary screening test for proximal DVT is compression ultrasound (US), which has a reported sensitivity of greater than 95%. However, ultrasound is insensitive to calf deep-vein thromboses, 20%-30% of which may progress to primal DVT, posing a risk of pulmonary embolism. Therefore, patients with suggestive symptoms and a negative ultrasound require serial ultrasounds for 7-10 days to rule out extension.

For the initial evaluation of PE, ultrasound can identify a minority of patients with proximal DVT, obviating further workup. For the remaining patients, ventilation-perfusion lung scanning has been the standard initial test. Unfortunately, over one half of patients will have a non-diagnostic exam and less than half of these will have angiographically demonstrable PE.

To improve the diagnostic yield of standard testing and to provide rapid availability of an accurate diagnostic test, ultrasensitive D-dimer assays with high negative predictive value have been developed. The high sensitivity and negative predictive value of this method allow it to be used for the exclusion of venous thromboembolic disease.

This test is intended for use as one component for determining the likelihood that an outpatient has venous thromboembolic disease. The clinical use of this assay has been shown to decrease the number of invasive and expensive diagnostic tests, thereby reducing costs.

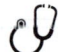

Clinical Example (85380)

A 55-year-old female on hormone replacement therapy who has just traveled for 5 hours by automobile to visit her daughter is admitted to the emergency room with severe leg pain. Physical examination reveals a swollen, erythematous left calf. During examination, patient becomes acutely short of breath.

The sensitive D-dimer test is performed using an immunoassay analyzer. D-dimer is measured using an ELISA method with a fluorescent endpoint. The high sensitivity and negative predictive value of the method allow it to be used for exclusion of venous thromboembolic disease.

Immunology

86148   Anti-phosphatidylserine (phospholipid) antibody

▶(To report antiprothrombin (phospholipid cofactor) antibody, use Category III code 0030T)◀

Rationale

A cross-reference has been added to direct the user to the newly established Category III code 0030T.

Transfusion Medicine

▶(86915 has been deleted. To report, use 38210- 38213)◀

▲**86930** Frozen blood, each unit; freezing (includes preparation)

▲**86931** thawing

▲**86932** freezing (includes preparation) and thawing

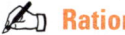
Rationale

In *CPT 2003* the transfusion medicine codes 86930, 86931, and 86932 have been revised to eliminate confusion and misinterpretation of the services.

Situations occur when an institution only thaws the frozen unit prior to transfusion. These instances are not covered by the existing family 86930, 86931, and 86932. Although code 86931 might appear to be the appropriate code, because of the placement of the semicolon and the order of the wording, it is not the correct choice. Code 86930 is also incorrect because it includes preparation for freezing. Revised CPT codes 86930, 86931, and 86932 now offer institutions a reporting mechanism for thawing prior to transfusion into the patient. The revision also provides a reporting mechanism for institutions that process and freeze units.

Finally, code 86915 was moved to the Surgery section of the CPT book. For a complete explanation regarding relocation of this code, see the information included in the Surgery section (codes 38210-38213).

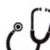
Clinical Example

A patient presents with anemia and has multiple red cell antibodies. No compatible fresh units are identified at the institution where the patient is located. For this reason, a search of rare units is undertaken and archived frozen units are identified at another institution. These units are processed and frozen at a facility other than where the units are being given. Therefore, the units are sent to the institution currently treating the patient where they are thawed and transfused into the patient.

Microbiology

87177 Ova and parasites, direct smears, concentration and identification

(Do not report 87177 in conjunction with 87015)

▶(For direct smears from a primary source, use 87207)◀

▲**87207** Smear, primary source with interpretation; special stain for inclusion bodies or parasites (eg, malaria, coccidia, microsporidia, trypanosomes, herpes viruses)

▶(For direct smears with concentration and identification, use 87177)◀

(For thick smear preparation, use 87015)

(For complex special stains, see 88312, 88313)

(For fat, meat, fibers, nasal eosinophils, and starch, see miscellaneous section)

(87208 has been deleted)

Rationale

The "eg" statement in code 87207 has been revised and two cross-references added following codes 87177 and 87207 directing users to the appropriate smear techniques procedures.

87250	Virus isolation; inoculation of embryonated eggs, or small animal, includes observation and dissection
87252	tissue culture inoculation, observation, and presumptive identification by cytopathic effect
87253	tissue culture, additional studies or definitive identification (eg, hemabsorption, neutralization, immunofluorescence stain), each isolate
▲87254	centrifuge enhanced (shell vial) technique, includes identification with immunofluorescence stain, each virus
●87255	including identification by non-immunologic method, other than by cytopathic effect (eg, virus specific enzymatic activity)

Rationale

Code 87254 was editorially revised to clarify the use of the centrifuge with the shell vial technique of virus identification. In addition, a new virus isolation and identification code 87255 has been added to reflect newer technologies such as virus specific enzymatic activity.

87260	Infectious agent antigen detection by immunofluourescent technique; adenovirus
●87267	Enterovirus, direct fluorescent antibody (DFA)
●87271	Cytomegalovirus, direct fluorescent antibody (DFA)

Rationale

Previously, codes for enterovirus (87199) and cytomegalovirus (87198) by direct fluorescent antibody were included under the Microbiology section with bacterial testing procedures. In *CPT 2003*, these codes have been appropriately relocated under the infectious agent antigen detection listing in the Microbiology section as new codes 87267 (Enterovirus, direct fluorescent antibody [DFA]) and 87271 (Cytomegalovirus, direct fluorescent antibody [DFA]). Codes 87198 and 87199 have been deleted with cross-references added to direct the user to these newly established codes.

Cytopathology

88142 Cytopathology, cervical or vaginal (any reporting system), collected in preservative fluid, automated thin layer preparation; manual screening under physician supervision

88143 with manual screening and rescreening under physician supervision

▶(88144 has been deleted)◀

▶(88145 has been deleted)◀

▶(For automated screening of automated thin layer preparation, see 88174 and 88175)◀

88164 Cytopathology, slides, cervical or vaginal (the Bethesda system); manual screening under physician supervision

88167 with manual screening and computer-assisted rescreening using cell selection and review under physician supervision

(88170 has been deleted. To report, ▶see◀ 10021, ▶10022◀)

(88171 has been deleted. To report, ▶see 10021,◀ 10022)

●**88174** Cytopathology, cervical or vaginal (any reporting system), collected in preservative fluid, automated thin layer preparation; screening by automated system, under physician supervision

●**88175** with screening by automated system and manual rescreening, under physician supervision

▶(For manual screening, see 88142 and 88143)◀

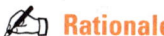

Rationale

The Cytopathology series of codes has been modified and appropriate cross-references have been added to more accurately reflect current screening and re-screening of cytopathology procedures resulting from automation in the field. In addressing changes in clinical practice, two new codes, 88174 and 88175, have been added, codes 88144 and 88145 have been deleted, and cross-references have been added directing the user to the automated screening and manual re-screening of automated thin layer preparation codes.

The cross-references following deleted codes 88170-88171 have been revised to include both fine needle aspiration procedures 10021-10022 to clarify that these procedures are no longer distinguished by the terms "deep" and "superficial" to describe the anatomy, but rather by whether imaging was or was not necessary to perform the procedure.

Cytogenetic Studies

88240 Cryopreservation, freezing and storage of cells, each cell line

▶(For therapeutic cryopreservation and storage, see 38207)◀

88241 Thawing and expansion of frozen cells, each aliquot

▶(For therapeutic thawing of previous harvest, see 38208)◀

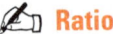 **Rationale**

Cross-references have been added to codes 88240 and 88241 to indicate that codes 38207 and 38208 should be reported for performance of therapeutic cryopreservation and storage and therapeutic thawing of frozen cells procedures, where "therapeutic" indicates the planned use of this material for transplantation.

Other Procedures

●**89055** Leukocyte count, fecal

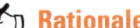 **Rationale**

A new code has been added to describe laboratory testing for fecal leukocytes. New code 89055 correlates with HCPCS Level II G code: G0026 Fecal leukocyte examination.

89300 Semen analysis; presence and/or motility of sperm including Huhner test (post coital)

▲**89310** motility and count (not including Huhner test)

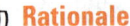 **Rationale**

Code 89310 was revised to describe laboratory analysis of semen that excludes Huhner testing. Revised code 89310 correlates with the HCPCS Level II G code: G0027 Semen analysis presence and/or motility of sperm excluding Huhner test.

89360 Sweat collection by iontophoresis

(For chloride ▶analysis, use 82438,◀ and sodium analysis, use ▶84302◀)

Rationale

The cross-reference following code 89360 has been revised to direct the user to report 82438 for chloride analysis and 84302 for sodium analyses.

Medicine

Most notable of the changes to the Medicine section is the addition of subheadings to the Neurology and Neuromuscular Procedures subsection for greater clarity of the organization of this section. Significant changes also include the addition of a new section and many codes to report evaluation of swallowing function, and the services for patients with cochlear implants and communication devices. Two new codes have been added to the Cardiac Catheterization section to report transcatheter closure of congenital interatrial and ventricular septal defects with an implant. Also revised are the Home Infusion codes with the addition of these codes to the same subsection as the Home Visit codes, and revision to indicate the appropriate reporting timeframe for these procedures.

Medicine

Vaccines, Toxoids

▶(90709 has been deleted)◀

 Rationale

Code 90709 was deleted, as this product is no longer available.

Therapeutic, Prophylactic or Diagnostic Injections

90788   Intramuscular injection of antibiotic (specify)

(90790-90796 has been deleted. To report, see ▶95990◀, 96408-96414, 96420-96425, 96440, 96450, 96530, 96545, 96549)

 Rationale

The cross-reference following code 90788 was revised to include new code 95990 for refilling and maintenance of implantable pump or reservoir for drug delivery, spinal (intrathecal, epidural) or brain (intraventricular).

Biofeedback

90911   Biofeedback training, perineal muscles, anorectal or urethral sphincter, including EMG and/or manometry

▶(For incontinence treatment by pulsed magnetic neuromodulation, use Category III code 0029T)◀

 Rationale

A Category III code 0029T was added to the Category III subsection of the CPT code set to report incontinence treatment by pulsed magnetic neuromodulation. In support of this action, a cross-reference was added following 90911 to instruct that incontinence treatment by pulsed magnetic neuromodulation is reported with codes 90911.

Special Otorhinolaryngologic Services

▶(92525 has been deleted. To report, see 92610-92611 for specific evaluation)◀

Audiologic Function Tests With Medical Diagnostic Evaluation

▲**92597** Evaluation for use and/or fitting of voice prosthetic device to supplement oral speech

▶(To report augmentative and alternative communication device services, see 92605, 92607, 92608)◀

▶(92598 has been deleted)◀

▶(92599 has been deleted. To report use 92700)◀

▶Evaluative and Therapeutic Services◀

▶Codes 92601 and 92603 describe post-operative analysis and fitting of previously placed external devices, connection to the cochlear implant, and programming of the stimulator. Codes 92602 and 92604 describe subsequent sessions for measurements and adjustment of the external transmitter and re-programming of the internal stimulator.◀

▶(For placement of cochlear implant, use 69930)◀

●**92601** Diagnostic analysis of cochlear implant, patient under 7 years of age; with programming

●**92602**   subsequent reprogramming

▶(Do not report 92602 in addition to 92601)◀

▶(For aural rehabilitation services following cochlear implant, including evaluation of rehabilitation status, use 92507)◀

●**92603** Diagnostic analysis of cochlear implant, age 7 years or older; with programming

●**92604**   subsequent reprogramming

▶(Do not report 92604 in addition to 92603)◀

●**92605** Evaluation for prescription of non-speech-generating augmentative and alternative communication device

●**92606** Therapeutic service(s) for the use of non-speech-generating device, including programming and modification

●**92607** Evaluation for prescription for speech-generating augmentative and alternative communication device, face-to-face with the patient; first hour

▶(For evaluation for prescription of a non-speech-generating device, use 92605)◀

+●**92608**   each additional 30 minutes (List separately in addition to code for primary procedure)

▶(Use 92608 in conjunction with 92607)◀

●**92609** Therapeutic services for the use of speech-generating device, including programming and modification

▶(For therapeutic service(s) for the use of a non-speech-generating device, use 92606)◀

●**92610** Evaluation of oral and pharyngeal swallowing function

▶(For motion fluoroscopic evaluation of swallowing function, use 92611)◀

▶(For flexible endoscopic examination, use 92612-92617)◀

●**92611** Motion fluoroscopic evaluation of swallowing function by cine or video recording

▶(For radiological supervision and interpretation, use 74230)◀

▶(For evaluation of oral and pharyngeal swallowing function, use 92610)◀

●**92612** Flexible fiberoptic endoscopic evaluation of swallowing by cine or video recording;

▶(If flexible fiberoptic or endoscopic evaluation of swallowing is performed without cine or video recording, use 92700)◀

●**92613** physician interpretation and report only

▶(To report an evaluation of oral and pharyngeal swallowing function, use 92610)◀

▶(To report motion fluoroscopic evaluation of swallowing function, use 92611)◀

●**92614** Flexible fiberoptic endoscopic evaluation, laryngeal sensory testing by cine or video recording;

●**92615** physician interpretation and report only

●**92616** Flexible fiberoptic endoscopic evaluation of swallowing and laryngeal sensory testing by cine or video recording;

●**92617** physician interpretation and report only

▶Other Procedures◀

●**92700** Unlisted otorhinolaryngological service or procedure

Rationale

Eighteen new codes were added, three were deleted and one code was revised in the Special Otorhinolaryngologic Services subsection of the *CPT 2003* book. Cross-references were also provided to direct the users to the appropriate codes and instruct them in the appropriate use of the new codes for the services provided. The "Other Procedures" subsection was relocated to accommodate the revisions to this section.

Codes 92525 and 92598 have been deleted to avoid duplicate codes described by the newly established codes, and a cross-reference was added to code 92525 to instruct that evaluation for feeding is reported with codes 92610 and 92611. The two new codes, 92610 and 92611, were added to describe different swallowing function evaluations.

Code 92597 has been revised by deleting "or augmentative/alternative communication" from the code descriptor to reflect the establishment of five new codes, 92605-92609, for reporting speech-generating and non-speech-generating, augmentative, and alternative communication device-related services. It is important to note that the low technology non-speech-generating devices described by codes 92605 and 92606 include Plexiglas devices, touch screen monitors, and communication boards. A cross-reference was added following code 92597 to direct the users to the new codes.

A new subheading, "Evaluative and Therapeutic Services," has been added with introductory language to indicate that codes 92601 and 92603 describe post-operative analysis and fitting of previously placed external devices, connection to the cochlear implant, and programming of the stimulator. The introductory language also indicates that codes 92602 and 92604 are intended to report subsequent sessions for measurement and adjustment of the external transmitter and re-programming of the internal stimulator. It is important to note that the cochlear implant periodic reprogramming, described by codes 92602 and 92604, includes any services performed after the first day. A cross-reference has also been added after the introductory note directing the user to report code 69930 for placement of cochlear implant.

Codes 92610 and 92611 were added to report swallowing function evaluation. Cross-references were added to direct the user to the appropriate code for reporting motion fluoroscopic evaluation of swallowing and evaluation of oral and pharyngeal swallowing. A cross-reference was also added following code 92611 directing the user to the appropriate radiological supervision and interpretation code.

Six new codes, 92612-92617, were added for reporting flexible, fiberoptic endoscopic laryngeal/swallowing evaluations. The swallowing evaluation reported by code 92612 is intended to describe an evaluation of the digestive system as opposed to the laryngeal sensory testing reported by code 92614, which is intended to describe diagnostic evaluation of the respiratory system. Laryngeal evaluations are based upon videotaping of vocal cord movement performed by a speech pathologist or other qualified provider. Therefore, the service of the physician review, report, and rendering of a medical diagnosis is performed with the aid of videotape review.

The unlisted otorhinolaryngological service or procedure code 92599 was deleted for the purpose of relocation and was renumbered to 92700 to allow expansion of this section.

New codes 92612-92617 were developed to fully capture the endoscopic work involved with swallowing and laryngeal sensory testing. In the laryngeal sensory testing evaluation, reported with codes 92615-92616, positive findings of paresis and paralysis can unmask subtle vocal fold movement disorders not generally seen during a cursory examination of the larynx. Similarly for this evaluation, distinct differences found in the examination of the right and left sides of the laryngopharynx during the symmetry evaluation of sensory testing can indicate site of lesion findings in the brain or skull base.

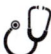 **Clinical Example (92612)**

A 60-year-old man diagnosed with aortic root aneurysm undergoes coronary artery bypass grafting times one. The postoperative course is difficult, with prolonged ventilation via endotracheal tube. The patient's nutrition and hydration are maintained via total parenteral nutrition. On postoperative day seven the process of weaning from the ventilator is initiated and the endotracheal tube removed. An oral diet is ordered and initiated. The patient is noted to cough and choke during feeding, indicating that food and/or liquid are entering the airway (aspiration). The findings of the bedside examination do not allow for complete and confident management of the patient's oral intake, so a flexible fiberoptic endoscopic evaluation of swallowing (FEES) is scheduled to directly assess pharyngeal swallowing function.

Description of Procedure (92612)

The physician passes a flexible endoscope via the nasal cavity into the widest portion of the oropharynx, noting anatomic and vocal fold movement abnormalities. Abnormalities are noted, as they may immediately affect how the food administration trials are delivered. During the examination, the endoscope is positioned in order that the epiglottis is at the inferior aspect of the monitor displaying a real-time image of the laryngopharynx to insure proper visual orientation and recognition of the effects of the various swallowing safety maneuvers. The tip of the endoscope lens is kept unobstructed and free of debris to permit detection of laryngeal penetration and aspiration. The endoscope tip is adjusted at various times during swallowing maneuvers to avoid entering the trachea during laryngeal elevation, to evaluate for instances of aspiration, and to obtain key information regarding reflux of administered food and function of the cricopharyngeal muscle.

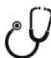 **Clinical Example (92613)**

A 60-year-old man diagnosed with aortic root aneurysm undergoes coronary artery bypass grafting times one. The postoperative course is difficult, with prolonged ventilation via endotracheal tube. The patient's nutrition and hydration are maintained via total parenteral nutrition. On postoperative day seven the process of weaning from the ventilator is initiated and the endotracheal tube removed. An oral diet is ordered and initiated. The patient is noted to cough and choke during feeding, indicating that food and/or liquid are entering the airway (aspiration). The findings of the bedside examination do not allow for complete and confident management of the patient's oral intake, so a flexible fiberoptic endoscopic evaluation of swallowing (FEES) is scheduled to directly assess pharyngeal swallowing function.

Description of Procedure (92613)

The physician reviews the videotape containing the endoscopic swallowing evaluation at the appropriate junctures to assess for evidence of: 1) anatomic abnormalities of the laryngopharyngeal structures such as tumors (solid, cystic, vascular), areas of edema, exudate and mucosal irregularity appearing in the nasopharyngeal and superior oropharyngeal regions; 2) vocal fold paresis or paralysis during the swallowing evaluation located on the tape at the pre-food administration sector; 3) laryngeal evaluation from the taped evaluation; 4) laryngeal penetration and aspiration, which would be captured in the food administration portion of the examination; and 5) cricopharyngeal function demonstrated by contraction and relaxation of the structure during swallowing.

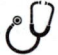

Clinical Example (92614)

A 64-year-old man develops a stroke and is hospitalized immediately. The patient cannot move the left side of his body, and is choking, hoarse, and unable to swallow. Full workup, including MRI of the brain, reveals the patient to have sustained a stroke. The patient is unable to eat and swallow without choking and coughing uncontrollably. The patient requires a diagnostic test of his ability to protect his airway both from ingestants and secretions so that he will sustain his nutrition and not have a respiratory arrest or develop aspiration pneumonia.

Description of Procedure (92614)

Endoscopic sensory testing takes place by passing the sensory endoscope via the nasal cavity into the hypopharynx and bringing the tip of the endoscope to within 3 mm of the tissue surface. Both the right side and the left side are always tested. Air pulses of varying strengths (mm Hg) and pulse durations (msec) are then administered to the arytenoid mucosa innervated by the internal branch of the superior laryngeal nerve to elicit the laryngeal adductor reflex. The foot pedal is depressed at least one time at suprathreshold values to clear debris from the endoscope tip prior to each air pulse delivery sequence. Once a clear image is seen, the endoscope is then directed towards the mucosa of the arytenoids and sensory testing generally begins by administering an air pulse to the tissues, to elicit the laryngeal adductor reflex. Depending on the response of the patient to this initial pulse, one of two things must then be carried out by the physician:

If the adductor reflex is not elicited, a continuous air pulse mode is then administered to the tissues. The endoscope is brought toward the tissue target. At the instant the continuous pulse is emanating from the endoscope tip, it must be at the precise location on the arytenoid mucosa. Subsequently, the physician immediately withdraws the tip of the endoscope from the arytenoid mucosa, because elicitation of the airway protective reflex typically results in elicitation of the swallow reflex, which in turn causes the larynx to begin elevating upward toward the tongue base. Whether or not the airway protective reflex is then elicited, the testing of the contralateral side is then performed. If the reflex is not elicited on both sides, the patient does not have intact airway protective reflexes and all testing then stops. In general, if bilateral absent laryngeal adductor reflexes are noted, no food administration trials are then given.

If the adductor reflex is elicited, the air pulse strength is then reduced and a pulse given. If the adductor reflex is elicited, then the patient is noted to have a normal airway protective reflex and the contralateral side is then tested. If the reflex is not elicited, the pulse strength is then increased. If the reflex occurs at this higher pulse strength, the dial is then reduced in increments and another pulse given. The point where the pulse strength switches from positive (reflex intact) to negative (reflex absent) is noted.

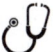
Clinical Example (92615)

A 64-year-old man develops a stroke and is hospitalized immediately. The patient cannot move the left side of his body, and is choking, hoarse, and unable to swallow. Full workup, including MRI of the brain, reveals the patient to have sustained a stroke. The patient is unable to eat and swallow without choking and coughing uncontrollably. The patient requires a diagnostic test of his ability to protect his airway both from ingestants and secretions so that he will sustain his nutrition and not have a respiratory arrest nor develop aspiration pneumonia.

Description of Procedure (92615)

The elements assessed during the physician review of the videotape containing the sensory testing findings are: 1) anatomic abnormalities of the laryngopharyngeal structures such as tumors (solid, cystic, vascular), areas of edema, exudate, and mucosal irregularity found in the visualization of the nasopharyngeal and superior oropharyngeal regions; 2) evidence of vocal fold paresis or paralysis during the sensory testing; 3) symmetry of the sensory testing results including visualization of sequences of both the right and left sides; and 4) determination of presence or absence of the laryngeal adductor reflex, located at the threshold evaluation juncture of the videotape examination. The threshold point is defined as the lowest air pulse pressures where the reflex is elicited for both the right and left sides of the laryngopharynx.

As sensory testing depends on intact vocal fold movements (opening and closing), sensory testing often unmasks subtle vocal fold movement disorders not generally seen during a cursory examination of the larynx. Generally, a frame-by-frame, or at least a slow-motion analysis of the sensory findings must be observed on the videotape machine in order to clearly make these diagnoses.

The review of the videotape must include sequences of both the right and left sides that were tested. Distinct differences between the right and left sides of the laryngopharynx can herald site of lesion findings in the brain or skull base.

In order to make this assessment the tape must be forwarded to the threshold points-the lowest air pulse pressures where the reflex is elicited for both the right and left sides of the laryngopharynx.

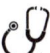
Clinical Example (92616)

A 59-year-old woman develops a stroke and is hospitalized immediately. The patient cannot move the left side of her body, and is choking, hoarse, and unable to swallow. Full workup, including MRI of the brain, reveals the patient to have sustained a stroke. The patient is unable to eat and swallow without choking and coughing uncontrollably. The patient requires a diagnostic test of her ability to protect her airway both from ingestants and secretions so that she will sustain her nutrition and not have a respiratory arrest or develop aspiration pneumonia. The patient also requires endoscopic evaluation of pharyngeal swallowing function to determine appropriate nutritional intake.

Description of Procedure (92616)

During scope passage via the nasal cavity, the physician must first note anatomic abnormalities and vocal fold movement abnormalities. Abnormalities are noted as they may immediately affect how the food administration trials are delivered.

Endoscopic sensory testing is performed, passing the sensory endoscope via the nasal cavity into the hypopharynx and bringing the tip of the endoscope to within 3 mm of the tissue surface. Both the right side and the left side are tested. Air pulses of varying strengths (mm Hg) and pulse durations (msec) are administered to the arytenoid mucosa innervated by the internal branch of the superior laryngeal nerve to elicit the laryngeal adductor reflex. The foot pedal is depressed at least one time at a suprathreshold value to clear debris from the endoscope tip prior to each air pulse delivery sequence. Once a clear image is seen, the endoscope is then directed towards the mucosa of the arytenoids and sensory testing generally begins by administering an air pulse to the tissues, to elicit the laryngeal adductor reflex.

If the adductor reflex is not elicited, a continuous air pulse is administered to the tissues. The endoscope is brought towards the tissue target. At the instant the continuous pulse is emanating from the endoscope tip, the tip must be at the precise location on the arytenoid mucosa. Subsequently, the physician immediately withdraws the tip of the endoscope from the arytenoid mucosa, because elicitation of the airway protective reflex typically results in elicitation of the swallow reflex, which in turn causes the larynx to begin elevating upward toward the tongue base. Testing of the contralateral side is then performed. If the reflex is not elicited on both sides, the patient does not have intact airway protective reflexes and all testing then stops. If bilateral laryngeal adductor reflexes are absent, no food administration trials are then given.

If the adductor reflex is elicited, the air pulse strength is then reduced and a pulse given. If the adductor reflex is elicited, the patient is noted to have a normal airway protective reflex and the contralateral side is then tested. If the reflex is not elicited, the pulse strength is then increased. If the reflex occurs at this pressure, the dial is then reduced in small increments and another pulse given. Where the pulse strength switches from positive (reflex intact) to negative (reflex absent) is noted.

If it is determined from the sensory test that the patient has intact airway protective reflexes then the food administration trials commence. During the examination, the endoscope is positioned with the epiglottis at the inferior aspect of the monitor displaying a real-time image of the laryngopharynx to ensure proper visual orientation and recognition of the effects of the various swallowing safety maneuvers. It is necessary to keep the tip of the endoscope lens unobstructed and free of debris to permit detection of laryngeal penetration and aspiration, and to slightly withdraw the tip during the actual swallow to avoid entering the trachea during elevation of the larynx. Visualization of various swallowing maneuvers also requires adjustment of the position of the endoscope tip. This helps to visualize all instances of aspiration with periodic movement of the tip of the endoscope into the most posterior and inferior aspects of the hypopharynx to obtain key information regarding reflux of administered food and function of the cricopharyngeus muscle.

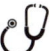 **Clinical Example (92617)**

A 59-year-old woman develops a stroke and was hospitalized immediately. The patient cannot move the left side of her body, and is choking, hoarse, and unable to swallow. Full workup, including MRI of the brain, reveals the patient to have sustained a stroke. The patient is unable to eat and swallow without choking and coughing uncontrollably. The patient requires a diagnostic test of her ability to protect her airway both from ingestants and secretions so that she will sustain her nutrition and not have a respiratory arrest or develop aspiration pneumonia. The patient also requires endoscopic evaluation of pharyngeal swallowing function to determine appropriate nutritional intake.

Description of Procedure (92617)

The elements assessed during the physician review of the videotape containing the sensory testing findings are: 1) anatomic abnormalities of the laryngopharyngeal structures such as tumors (solid, cystic, vascular), areas of edema, exudate and mucosal irregularity found in the visualization of the nasopharyngeal and superior oropharyngeal regions; 2) evidence of vocal fold paresis or paralysis during the sensory testing; 3) symmetry of the sensory testing results including visualization of sequences of both the right and left sides; and 4) determination of presence or absence of the laryngeal adductor reflex, located at the threshold evaluation juncture of the videotape examination. The threshold point is defined as the lowest air pulse pressures where the reflex is elicited for both the right and left sides of the laryngopharynx.

As sensory testing depends on intact vocal fold movements (opening and closing), sensory testing often unmasks subtle vocal fold movement disorders not generally seen during a cursory examination of the larynx. Generally, a frame-by-frame, or at least a slow-motion analysis of the sensory findings must be observed on the videotape machine in order to clearly make these diagnoses.

The review of the videotape must include sequences of both the right and left sides that were tested. Distinct differences between the right and left sides of the laryngopharynx can herald site of lesion findings in the brain or skull base.

In order to make this assessment the tape must be forwarded to the threshold points—the lowest air pulse pressures where the reflex was elicited for both the right and left sides of the laryngopharynx.

Cardiovascular

Cardiography

▲93012   Telephonic transmission of post-symptom electrocardiogram rhythm strip(s), 24-hour attended monitoring, per 30 day period of time; tracing only

93014   physician review and interpretation only

▲**93268**   Patient demand single or multiple event recording with presymptom memory loop, 24-hour attended monitoring, per 30 day period of time; includes transmission, physician review and interpretation

93270   recording (includes hook-up, recording, and disconnection)

93271   monitoring, receipt of transmissions, and analysis

93272   physician review and interpretation only

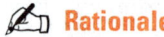
Rationale

CPT codes 93012 and 93014 were editorially revised to correlate with the HCPCS Level II G codes G0015-G0016 specifying the requirement of 24-hour attended monitoring.

Code 93268 was editorially revised to correlate with the HCPCS level II G codes G0004-G0007 specifying the requirement of 24-hour attended monitoring.

Cardiac Catheterization

▶REPAIR OF SEPTAL DEFECT◀

●**93580**   Percutaneous transcatheter closure of congenital interatrial communication (ie, fontan fenestration, atrial septal defect) with implant

▶(Percutaneous transcatheter closure of atrial septal defect includes a right heart catheterization procedure. Code 93580 includes injection of contrast for atrial and ventricular angiograms. Codes 93501, 93529-93533, 93539, 93543, 93555 should not be reported separately in addition to code 93580)◀

●**93581**   Percutaneous transcatheter closure of a congenital ventricular septal defect with implant

▶(Percutaneous transcatheter closure of ventricular septal defect (ie, fontan fenestration) includes a right heart catheterization procedure. Code 93581 includes injection of contrast for atrial and ventricular angiograms. Codes 93501, 93529-93533, 93539, 93543, 93555 should not be reported separately in addition to code 93581)◀

▶(For echocardiographic services performed in addition to 93580, 93581, see 93303-93317 as appropriate)◀

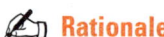
Rationale

Two new codes (93580, 93581) were created to identify transcatheter repair of congenital heart defects. Code 93580 describes percutaneous transcatheter closure of a congenital interatrial communication (ie, fontan fenestration, atrial septal defect) and code 93581 describes percutaneous transcatheter closure of congenital ventricular septal defects. These codes are not intended for post-myocardial infarction septal defects, but are intended for reporting the repair of congenital defects. Patients range from infants to adults. The physician work is comparable whether the patient is an infant or an adult.

Explanatory notes were added to identify the inclusive elements within these procedures, such as right heart catheterizations and contrast injection for atrial and ventricular angiograms. A cross-reference was added to direct users not to report codes 93501, 93529-93533, 93539, 93543, and 93555 separately. An additional parenthetical cross-reference is included to direct users to codes 93303-93317 to report echocardiographic services performed in addition to codes 93580 and 93581.

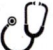

Clinical Example (93580)

The typical patient has atrial defects amenable to device closure including congenital atrial septal defects (ASDs), surgically created fenestrations in atrial baffles (eg, fenestrated fontan or in patches to partially close ASDs in selected circumstances) and leaks in surgically created baffles or patches. Patients range from infants to adults with similar time and effort required regardless of age.

Description of Procedure (93580)

Trans-esophageal echocardiography (TEE) or intracardiac echocardiography (ICE) may be required (separately reported). General anesthesia (separately reported) is commonly used when TEE is required; otherwise conscious sedation is usually employed. The patient is heparinized and the ACT is maintained throughout the case. Prophylactic antibiotics are given. A combined right heart catheterization and left heart catheterization through existing septal opening including angiography (93529 or 93533, 93542 or 93543 and 93555) is performed to delineate the anatomy and physiology.

Using an end-hole catheter, wedge or preformed catheter such as a multipurpose catheter, the atrial defect is crossed from right to left atrium. The catheter is then advanced into the left upper pulmonary vein. This catheter is exchanged for a sizing balloon over a guidewire. The balloon is positioned across the defect and inflated at low pressure to measure the "stretched" diameter. The device size is based on this measurement. In patients with fenestrated fontans, and in some with right-to-left shunts through the atrial defect, right-sided pressures and saturations are re-measured while temporarily balloon occluding the defect to ensure that device closure will be hemodynamically tolerated.

A long sheath and dilator are then advanced over the wire and positioned in the left atrium. The device is then deployed across the atrial opening. The position of the device must be evaluated by echocardiography and fluoroscopy prior to release. If the device is in good position, the release mechanism is activated and the device position checked again. Abnormal placement or an inappropriate-sized device may have to be removed if there is a large leak, potential encroachment on cardiac structures, or risk of embolization, and a second device is placed.

After device position is confirmed using TEE or angiography, the catheters and sheaths are removed and hemostasis is achieved.

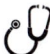

Clinical Example (93581)

The patient has a ventricular septal defect appropriate for device closure. The defect is congenital and unoperated or residual following attempted surgical closure.

Description of Procedure (93581)

The ventricular septal defect (VSD) closure is performed using general anesthesia (separately reported). Trans-esophageal or intracardiac echocardiography may be performed. The patient is prepped and draped.

Percutaneous access is obtained in the femoral vein and artery and sheaths are placed. The patient is heparinized and the ACT is maintained throughout the case. Prophylactic antibiotics are given.

Depending on the location of the VSD, additional venous access will be required in the other femoral vein or the internal jugular vein. A right and left heart catheterization, including angiography, is performed to define the anatomy and physiology of the defect(s).

Device closure of VSDs involves crossing the VSD, sizing the defect, and then delivering the device. Multiple options to cross the defect are available and depend on the anatomy and location of the defect. Usually the VSD is crossed from left to right ventricle rather than right to left from the trabeculated right ventricle. From the left ventricle, the VSD can be crossed using a retrograde approach from the femoral artery or antegrade using the catheter in the femoral vein. The latter is accomplished by performing a transseptal (atrial septum) puncture (Brockenbrough) to enter the left atrium. The catheter is then passed from the left atrium to the left ventricle. The VSD can be crossed using a flow-directed, balloon-tipped wedge catheter or more commonly, preformed catheters are used to aim a guidewire, which is then advanced through the defect into the right ventricle and then into a pulmonary artery or retrograde through the tricuspid valve in the right atrium. This wire is then snared from the venous side. The venous site from which the wire is snared will depend on how one intends to deliver the device. Devices are occasionally delivered retrograde from an artery. Mid- and apical muscular defects are most easily closed using the internal jugular vein. Anterior muscular defects and residual membranous and cono-ventricular defects are most easily closed from the femoral vein. At the completion of this stage, there is an exchange-length guidewire entering the body at one site, passing through the VSD and exiting the body at another site.

An angiographic catheter is passed over the wire for selective contrast injections in the defect to define the commonly complex anatomy. Following this, a balloon-tipped catheter (over the wire) is pulled through or inflated in the defect to determine the "stretched" diameter. With this information, the appropriate device can be chosen. A long sheath and dilator are advanced over the guidewire and positioned across the VSD. The guidewire and dilator are removed and the device is delivered. Angiography, using a retrograde left ventricular catheter, is performed during delivery to ensure correct positioning of the device. Following delivery, angiography is performed to confirm device position and hemodynamics are repeated to determine residual shunting.

If there is a large leak, potential encroachment on cardiac structures, or risk of embolization, the device may have to be removed and a second device placed. Occasionally (10% to 15% of the time), multiple devices must be placed to close separate muscular defects that cannot be covered with a single device.

Intracardiac Electrophysiological Procedures/Studies

Intracardiac electrophysiologic studies ...

Definitions

Arrhythmia Induction: In most electrophysiologic ...

Mapping: Mapping is a distinct procedure performed in addition to a diagnostic electrophysiologic procedure and should be separately reported using code 93609 or 93613. ▶Do not report standard mapping (93609) in addition to 3-D mapping (93613).◀ When a tachycardia is induced, the site of tachycardia origination ...

Ablation: Once the part of the heart involved in the tachycardia is localized ...

+ **93609** Intraventricular and/or intra-atrial mapping of tachycardia site(s) with catheter manipulation to record from multiple sites to identify origin of tachycardia (List separately in addition to code for primary procedure)

(Use 93609 in conjunction with codes 93620, 93651, 93652)

▶(Do not report 93609 in addition to 93613)◀

+ **93613** Intracardiac electrophysiologic 3-dimensional mapping (List separately in addition to code for primary procedures)

(Use 93613 in conjunction with codes 93620, 93651, 93652)

▶(Do not report 93613 in addition to 93609)◀

⊘▲ **93620** Comprehensive electrophysiologic evaluation including insertion and repositioning of multiple electrode catheters with induction or attempted induction of arrhythmia; with right atrial pacing and recording, right ventricular pacing and recording, His bundle recording

 Rationale

In the electrophysiological procedures guidelines, a cross-reference was added within the definition of mapping to direct users not to report code 93609 in addition to code 93613. Code 93609 describes intraventricular and/or intra-arterial mapping of tachycardia site(s) with catheter manipulation to record from multiple sites to identify the origin of tachycardia. Code 93613 describes a mapping technique that allows simultaneous recording from many electrodes on the same catheter and computer-assisted three-dimensional reconstruction of the tachycardia activation sequence. Parenthetical cross-references were also added after codes 93609 and 93613 to indicate that these two codes are not reported together.

Code 93620 within the Intracardiac Electrophysiological Procedures/Studies section was revised to accurately depict the procedures performed and allay confusion resulting from placement of the semicolon. Code 93620 was restructured so that the type of pacing and recording performed (eg, right atrial, right ventricular) is described in the descriptor after the semicolon.

Clinical Example (93620)

A 70-year-old man with prior myocardial infarction presents with syncope. Following injection of local anesthetic, multiple electrode catheters are positioned in the heart from the venous site. Right atrial pacing and recording and ventricular pacing and recording are performed with induction of ventricular tachycardia.

Non-Invasive Vascular Diagnostic Studies

Vascular studies include patient care required to perform the studies, supervision of the studies and interpretation of study results with copies for patient records of hard copy output with analysis of all data, including bi-directional vascular flow or imaging when provided.

The use of a simple hand-held or other Doppler device that does not produce hard copy output, or that produces a record that does not permit analysis of bi-directional vascular flow, is considered to be part of the physical examination of the vascular system and is not separately reported.

Duplex scan ▶(eg, 93880, 93882)◀ describes an ultrasonic scanning procedure ▶for characterizing the pattern and direction of blood flow in arteries or veins with the production of real time images integrating B-mode two-dimensional vascular structure with spectral and/or color flow Doppler mapping or imaging.◀

▶Non-invasive physiologic studies are performed using equipment separate and distinct from the duplex scanner. Codes 93875, 93965, 93922, 93923, and 93924 describe the evaluation of non-imaging physiologic recordings of pressures, Doppler analysis of bi-directional blood flow, plethysmography, and/or oxygen tension measurements appropriate for the anatomic area studied.◀

 Rationale

The introductory language in the Non-Invasive Vascular Studies section was revised to provide distinction between duplex scanning and non-invasive physiologic studies. The third paragraph was revised to include language indicating that a duplex scan describes an ultrasonic scan procedure for characterizing the pattern and direction of blood flow in arteries or veins with the production of real time images integrating B-mode two-dimensional vascular structure with spectral and/or color flow Doppler mapping or imaging.

A fourth paragraph was added to the introductory notes to describe physiologic studies. Code 93875 typically involves the analysis of hard copy bi-directional Doppler ultrasonic recordings of blood flow about the eye or analysis of ocular blood pressure using oculoplethysmography. CPT code 93965 is an analysis of extremity venous blood flow using impedance plethysmography or air plethysmography. Codes 93922-93924 provide analysis of upper or lower extremity arterial blood flow using methods such as Doppler waveform analysis, Doppler-derived ankle/brachial indices, volume plethysmography, or transcutaneous oxygen tension measurements.

Pulmonary

▲ **94640** Pressurized or nonpressurized inhalation treatment for acute airways obstruction or for sputum induction for diagnostic purposes (eg, with an aerosol generator, nebulizer, metered dose inhaler or intermittent positive pressure breathing (IPPB) device)

▶(For more than one inhalation treatment performed on the same date, append modifier '-76')◀

▶(94650-94652 have been deleted)◀

▲ **94664** Demonstration and/or evaluation of patient utilization of an aerosol generator, nebulizer, metered dose inhaler or IPPB device

▶(94664 can be reported one time only per day of service)◀

▶(94665 has been deleted)◀

 Rationale

To both simplify and clarify the use of aerosols and bronchodilators in accord with current medical practice, existing CPT codes were revised while others were deleted. Code 94640 was revised to report pressurized and nonpressurized inhalation treatment for acute airway obstruction or for sputum induction for diagnostic services. The code descriptor includes different modes of treatment such as aerosol generator, nebulizer, metered dose inhaler or intermittent positive pressure breathing (IPPB) device. Codes 94650-94652, previously used to report intermittent positive pressure breathing (IPPB) treatment, have been deleted and are included in code 94640. A parenthetical cross-reference was added to direct users to append modifier '-76' if more than one treatment is performed on the same date.

Code 94664 was revised to report the demonstration and/or evaluation of patient utilization of an aerosol generator, nebulizer, metered dose inhaler, or IPPB device. The term "initial" was deleted from the code descriptor since the code will no longer distinguish between initial and subsequent demonstrations and or/evaluations. This code is intended to be reported only once per day of service. Therefore, code 94665 was deleted since it was no longer relevant. An explanatory note was added to direct users that 94664 can be reported one time only per day of service.

Allergy and Clinical Immunology Allergy Testing

▲ **95027** Intracutaneous (intradermal) tests, sequential and incremental, with allergenic extracts for airborne allergens, immediate type reaction, specify number of tests

 Rationale

Code 95027 was revised to clarify the intent and use of this code to describe testing of airborne allergen(s) using various dilutional strengths. Previously, this was described in code 95027 using the term "skin end-point titration." End-point titration analyzes the highest dilution (or lowest level of concentration) of a substance that produces a significant positive reaction with a given concentration of another substance. This defines the endpoint of testing, and is used to determine the starting dose(s) of allergen immunotherapy (ie, it is used to determine the safe starting dose for immunotherapy). The language in the descriptor of this code was revised in order to make it more consistent with other allergy intradermal diagnostic testing codes, and at the same time, distinguish it from codes 95015, 95024, and 95028.

Neurology and Neuromuscular Procedures

▶Routine Electroencephalography (EEG)◀

▶EEG codes 95812-95822 include hyperventilation and/or photic stimulation when appropriate. Routine EEG codes 95816-95822 include 20 to 40 minutes of recording. Extended EEG codes 95812-95813 include reporting times longer than 40 minutes.◀

▲ 95812　Electroencephalogram (EEG) extended monitoring; 41-60 minutes

95813　　　greater than one hour

▲ 95816　Electroencephalogram (EEG); including recording awake and drowsy

▲ 95819　　　including recording awake and asleep

▲ 95822　　　recording in coma or sleep only

95824　　　cerebral death evaluation only

▲ 95827　　　all night recording

(For 24-hour EEG monitoring, ▶see 95950-95953 or 95956◀)

(For EEG during nonintracranial surgery, use 95955)

(For Wada ▶test◀, use 95958)

▶(For digital analysis of EEG, use 95957)◀

95829　Electrocorticogram at surgery (separate procedure)

95830　Insertion by physician of electrodes for electroencephalographic (EEG) recording

▶Muscle and Range of Motion Testing◀

95831　Muscle testing, manual (separate procedure) with report; extremity (excluding hand) or trunk

▶Electromyography and Nerve Conduction Tests◀

95860	Needle electromyography; one extremity with or without related paraspinal areas
95861	two extremities with or without related paraspinal areas
95863	three extremities with or without related paraspinal areas
95864	four extremities with or without related paraspinal areas
▲95867	cranial nerve supplied muscle(s), unilateral
95868	cranial nerve supplied muscles, bilateral
▲95869	thoracic paraspinal muscles (excluding T1 or T12)
95870	limited study of muscles in one extremity or non-limb (axial) muscles (unilateral or bilateral), other than thoracic paraspinal, cranial nerve supplied muscles, or sphincters
95872	Needle electromyography using single fiber electrode, with quantitative measurement of jitter, blocking and/or fiber density, any/all sites of each muscle studied
▲95875	Ischemic limb exercise test with serial specimen(s) acquisition for muscle(s) metabolite(s)
⊘95900	Nerve conduction, amplitude and latency/velocity study, each nerve; motor, without F-wave study
⊘95903	motor, with F-wave study
⊘95904	sensory

▶Intraoperative Neurophysiology◀

+95920 Intraoperative neurophysiology testing, per hour (List separately in addition to code for primary procedure)

(Use code 95920 in conjunction with the study performed, 92585, 95822, 95860, 95861, 95867, 95868, 95900, 95904, 95925, 95926, 95927, 95930, 95933, 95934, 95936, 95937)

(Code 95920 describes ongoing electrophysiologic testing and monitoring performed during surgical procedures. Code 95920 is reported per hour of service, and includes only the ongoing electrophysiologic monitoring time distinct from performance of specific type(s) of baseline electrohysiologic study(ies) (95860, 95861, 95867, 95868, 95900, 95904, 95933, 95934, 95936, 95937) or interpretation of specific type(s) of electrophysiologic study(ies) (92585, 95922, 95925, 95926, 95927, 95930). The time spent performing or interpreting the baseline electrophysiologic study(ies) should not be counted as intraoperative monitoring, but represent separately reportable procedures. Code 95920 should be used once per hour even if multiple electrophysiologic studies are performed. The baseline electrophysiologic study(ies) should be used once per operative session.)

▶(For electrocorticography, use 95829)◀

▶(For intraoperative EEG during nonintracranial surgery, use 95955)◀

▶(For intraoperative functional cortical or subcortical mapping, see 95961-95962)◀

▶(For intraoperative neurostimulator programming and analysis, see 95970-95975)◀

▶Autonomic Function Tests◀

95921 Testing of autonomic nervous system function; cardiovagal innervation (parasympathetic function), including two or more of the following: heart rate response to deep breathing with recorded R-R interval, Valsalva ratio, and 30:15 ratio

95922 vasomotor adrenergic innervation (sympathetic adrenergic function), including beat-to-beat blood pressure and R-R interval changes during Valsalva maneuver and at least five minutes of passive tilt

95923 sudomotor, including one or more of the following: quantitative sudomotor axon reflex test (QSART), silastic sweat imprint, thermoregulatory sweat test, and changes in sympathetic skin potential

▶Evoked Potentials and Reflex Tests◀

95925 Short-latency somatosensory evoked potential study, stimulation of any/all peripheral nerves or skin sites, recording from the central nervous system; in upper limbs

95926 in lower limbs

95927 in the trunk or head

(To report a unilateral study, use modifier '-52')

(For auditory evoked potentials, use 92585)

▶Special EEG Tests◀

95950 Monitoring for identification and lateralization of cerebral seizure focus, electroencephalographic (eg, 8 channel EEG) recording and interpretation, each 24 hours

95951 Monitoring for localization of cerebral seizure focus by cable or radio, 16 or more channel telemetry, combined electroencephalographic (EEG) and video recording and interpretation (eg, for presurgical localization), each 24 hours

95953 Monitoring for localization of cerebral seizure focus by computerized portable 16 or more channel EEG, electroencephalographic (EEG) recording and interpretation, each 24 hours

Rationale

Following the identification of inaccuracies in the headings and the organization of the codes in the Neurology and Neuromuscular Procedures subsection of the Medicine section of the CPT book, for *CPT 2003* appropriate subheadings were created and revised, redundancies eliminated, and codes reformatted to appear as subset codes (95816-95827). In addition, unnecessary cross-references were omitted, and instructional references, notes, and explanatory cross-references added (eg, modifier '-51' is not appropriate when reporting nerve conduction studies [95900-95904] performed on multiple nerves). These revisions are strictly editorial in nature.

Other Procedures

● **95990** Refilling and maintenance of implantable pump or reservoir for drug delivery, spinal (intrathecal, epidural) or brain (intraventricular)

▶(For analysis and/or reprogramming of implantable infusion pump, see 62367-62368)◀

▶(For refill and maintenance of implanted infusion pump or reservoir for systemic drug therapy (eg, chemotherapy or insulin), use 96530)◀

 Rationale

Code 95990 was established to report refilling and maintenance of implantable pumps or reservoirs for spinal and brain drug delivery to specifically identify drug delivery systems that include intrathecal, intraventricular, and epidural drug delivery. The refill and maintenance of the different pumps is very different in terms of risks, knowledge required, skill required, and severity of potential complications. The addition of code 95990 provides a more granular system of codes that reflect the work, time, and intensity for the refill and maintenance of pumps providing spinal or brain infusion (epidural, intrathecal, intraventricular) versus systemic infusion.

A cross-reference was added to direct users to codes 62367-62368 for analysis and/or reprogramming of an implantable infusion pump. An additional cross-reference was added to direct users to report code 96530 for refill and maintenance of implanted infusion pump or reservoir for systemic drug delivery (eg, chemotherapy or insulin).

Health and Behavior Assessment/Intervention

Health and behavior assessment procedures are used to identify the psychological, behavioral, emotional, cognitive, and social factors important to the prevention, treatment or management of physical health problems. The focus of the assessment is not on mental health, but on the biopsychosocial factors important to physical health problems and treatments.

The focus of the intervention is to improve the patient's health and well-being utilizing cognitive, behavioral, social, and/or psychophysiological procedures designed to ameliorate specific disease-related problems.

Codes 96150-96155 describe services ▶offered to patients who present with established illnesses or symptoms, who are not diagnosed with mental illness, and may benefit from evaluations that focus on the biopsychosocial factors related to the patient's physical health status. These services do not represent preventive medicine counseling and risk factor reduction interventions.◀

For patients that require psychiatric ...

Evaluation and Management services codes ▶(including **Preventive Medicine, Individual Counseling** codes 99401-99404, and **Preventive Medicine, Group Counseling** codes 99411-99412),◀ should not be reported on the same day.

▶(For health and behavior assessment and/or intervention performed by a physician, see **Evaluation and Management** or **Preventive Medicine** services codes)◀

96150 Health and behavior assessment (eg, health-focused clinical interview, behavioral observations, psychophysiological monitoring, health-oriented questionnaires), each 15 minutes face-to-face with the patient; initial assessment

96151   re-assessment

96152 Health and behavior intervention, each 15 minutes, face-to-face; individual

96153   group (2 or more patients)

96154   family (with the patient present)

96155   family (without the patient present)

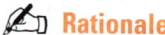

Rationale

The Health and Behavior Assessment Intervention introductory language was revised to specifically state that these services do not represent "preventive medicine" services. The *CPT 2002* introductory language for this subsection included the term "preventive," creating the impression that these services would be interpreted to represent the preventive medicine counseling/education. References to preventive medicine were therefore omitted in the introductory notes to allay confusion and misinterpretation among payers.

A parenthetical note referencing specific preventive medicine evaluation and management codes, 99401-99404, and 99411-99412, was added to further emphasize that these are not to be reported on the same day. For ease of reference, a parenthetical note that was previously listed at the end of the section after the code listings was relocated to the end of the introductory notes.

Chemotherapy Administration

96408 Chemotherapy administration, intravenous; push technique

96410   infusion technique, up to one hour

+96412   infusion technique, one to 8 hours, each additional hour (List separately in addition to code for primary procedure)

(Use 96412 in conjunction with code 96410)

96414   infusion technique, initiation of prolonged infusion (more than 8 hours), requiring the use of a portable or implantable pump

▶(For refilling and maintenance of a portable pump or an implantable infusion pump or reservoir for drug delivery,◀ see 96520, 96530)

96420   Chemotherapy administration, intra-arterial; push technique

96425   infusion technique, initiation or prolonged infusion (more than 8 hours), requiring the use of a portable or implantable pump

(For refilling ▶and maintenance of a portable pump or an implantable infusion pump or reservoir for drug delivery,◀ see 96520, 96530)

▲**96530**   Refilling and maintenance of an implantable pump or reservoir for drug delivery, systemic (eg, intravenous, intra-arterial)

▶(For refilling and maintenance of an implantable infusion pump for spinal or brain drug infusion, use 95990)◀

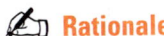
Rationale
Code 96530 was revised to report refilling and maintenance of implantable pumps or reservoirs for systemic drug delivery, to specifically identify drug delivery systems that include intravenous, intra-arterial drug delivery.

Previously, code 96530 was reported to encompass the refill and maintenance of all implanted infusion pumps or reservoirs. Medical practice has changed to allow new routes of drug delivery via an implant. To accommodate the advances in medical practice, and to uniquely identify these services, some revisions and additions to the CPT code set were necessary. In support of these revisions, 95990 was established to report refilling and maintenance of implantable pumps or reservoirs for spinal and brain drug delivery to specifically identify drug delivery systems that include intrathecal, intraventricular, epidural drug delivery.

Appropriate cross-references were added and existing cross-references were revised to direct users to the correct refilling/maintenance procedures for the technology/anatomy involved. A cross-reference following code 96530 was added to direct users to report code 95990 for refilling and maintenance of an implantable infusion pump for spinal or brain drug infusion. Also, cross-references following codes 96414 and 96425 were revised to direct users to use codes 96520 or 96530 for refilling and maintenance of a portable pump or an implantable infusion pump or reservoir for drug delivery.

Special Dermatological Procedures

▶(For whole body photography, see Category III code 0044T)◀

●**96920**   Laser treatment for inflammatory skin disease (psoriasis); total area less than 250 sq cm

●**96921**   250 sq cm to 500 sq cm

●**96922**   over 500 sq cm

Rationale

A new series of laser codes (96920, 96921, and 96922) for treatment of psoriasis has been added to *CPT 2003*. These codes were added to the Medicine section, as they differ from the existing 17000 series of laser destruction codes. The laser treatment described by the codes in the 17000 series are intended for the destruction of skin lesions as opposed to the laser treatment described in new codes 96920, 96921, and 96922, which are intended to report laser treatment of inflammatory skin diseases.

Clinical Example (96920)

The patient is a 35-year-old Caucasian male with a 10-year history of stable moderate plaque psoriasis, which worsens during the winter months. There is a family history of psoriasis. Physical findings include inflamed, scaly, somewhat tender lesions present on the extensor surfaces of elbows and knees, hips, sacrum, and scalp involving 10% of the body surface area, or about 1500 square centimeters.

Currently the patient's therapy includes daily use of both moderate-potency topical corticosteroid ointment and calcipotriene ointment. A corticosteroid lotion is used daily on the scalp; topical tar preparations are added when necessary. These therapies have produced a partial improvement response of approximately 80% plaque clearance, leaving less than 250 square centimeters of chronic plaques resistant to topical therapy. The patient continues to suffer from significant erythema, induration, pruritus, and desquamation of thick scales from these non responsive areas. The severity of the disease is documented and the decision is made to utilize laser treatment for recurrent psoriatic plaques. Activities of daily living and quality of life are negatively impacted by the presence of symptomatic lesions.

Description of Procedure (96920)

The affected area is draped and the lesion site(s) prepped with a clarifying agent such as mineral oil or other moisturizing agent. The physician assesses the redness of the lesions and any erythema. Pain or blistering from the previous therapy or treatment methodology is also assessed. The physician determines the laser dosage level from an assessment of the minimum erythema dosage of laser light on normal skin. The physician treats area of inflamed lesions or plaque with the laser. The physician monitors for pain as well as skin surface reaction throughout the process.

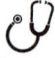

Clinical Example (96921)

The patient is a 35-year-old Caucasian male with a 10-year history of stable moderate plaque psoriasis, which worsens during the winter months. There is a family history of psoriasis. Physical findings include inflamed, scaly, somewhat tender lesions present on the extensor surfaces of elbows and knees, hips, sacrum, and scalp involving 10% of the body surface area, or about 1500 square centimeters.

Currently, the patient's therapy includes daily use of both moderate-potency topical corticosteroid ointment and calcipotriene ointment. A corticosteroid lotion is used daily on the scalp; topical tar preparations are added when necessary. These therapies have produced a partial improvement response of approximately 85% plaque clearance, leaving less than 250 square centimeters of chronic plaques resistant to topical therapy. The patient continues to suffer from significant erythema, induration, pruritus, and desquamation of thick scales from these non-responsive areas. The severity of the disease is documented and the decision is made to utilize laser treatment for recurrent psoriatic plaques. Activities of daily living and quality of life are negatively impacted by the presence of symptomatic lesions.

Description of Procedure (96921)

The patient is positioned, the affected area draped, and the lesion site(s) prepped with a clarifying agent such as mineral oil or other moisturizing agent. The physician assesses the redness of the lesions and any erythema. Pain or blistering from the previous therapy or treatment methodology is also assessed. The physician determines the laser dosage level from an assessment of the minimum erythema dosage of laser light on normal skin. The physician treats each lesion or plaque with the laser. The physician monitors for pain as well as skin surface reaction throughout the process.

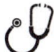

Clinical Example (96922)

The patient is a 35-year-old Caucasian male with a 10-year history of stable moderate plaque psoriasis, which worsens during the winter months. There is a family history of psoriasis. Physical findings include inflamed, scaly, somewhat tender lesions present on the extensor surfaces of elbows and knees, hips, sacrum, and scalp involving 10% of the body surface area, or about 1500 square centimeters.

Currently the patient's therapy includes daily use of both moderate-potency topical corticosteroid ointment and calcipotriene ointment. A corticosteroid lotion is used daily on the scalp; topical tar preparations are added when necessary. These therapies have produced a partial improvement response of approximately 65% plaque clearance, leaving over 500 square centimeters of chronic plaques resistant to topical therapy. The patient continues to suffer from significant erythema, induration, pruritus, and desquamation of thick scales from these non-responsive areas. The severity of the disease is documented and the decision is made to utilize laser treatment for recurrent psoriatic plaques. Activities of daily living and quality of life are negatively impacted by the presence of symptomatic lesions.

Description of Procedure (96922)

The patient is positioned, the affected area draped, and the lesion site(s) prepped with a clarifying agent such as mineral oil or other moisturizing agent. The physician assesses the redness of the lesions and any erythema. Pain or blistering from the previous therapy or treatment methodology is also assessed. The physician determines the laser dosage level from an assessment of the minimum erythema dosage of laser light on normal skin. The physician treats each lesion or plaque with the laser. The physician monitors for pain as well as skin surface reaction throughout the process.

Special Services, Procedures and Reports

Miscellaneous Services

●**99026**   Hospital mandated on-call service; in-hospital, each hour

●**99027**   out-of-hospital, each hour

▶(For physician standby services requiring prolonged physician attendance, use 99360, as appropriate. Time spent performing separately reportable procedure(s) or service(s) should not be included in the time reported as mandated on-call service)◀

 Rationale
Two new codes 99026 and 99027 are established in the Medicine subsection of the CPT book to report physician hospital mandated on-call services. In support of this action, a cross-reference was added following 99360 to instruct that hospital mandated on-call services are reported with codes 99026 and 99027.

Qualifying Circumstances for Anesthesia

99100   Anesthesia for patient of extreme age, under 1 year and over 70 (List separately in addition to code for primary anesthesia procedure)

▶(For procedure performed on infants less than one year of age at time of surgery, see 00833, 00834)◀

 Rationale
New code 00326 was added to reflect the increased work, method, and risk associated with providing anesthesia for procedures on the larynx and trachea for children less than 1 year of age. Two new codes, 00834 and 00836, were created to recognize the anesthetic complexity involved in hernia repairs for infants under 1 year of age.

In support of these actions, a correlating cross-reference following code 99100 was created.

Note: The parenthetic note that follows code 99100 will be changed for *CPT 2004*.

Home Health Procedures/Services

These codes are used by non-physician health care professionals. Physicians should utilize the home visit codes 99341-99350, and utilize CPT codes other than 99500▶-99600◀ for any additional procedure/service provided to a patient living in a residence.

The following codes are used to report services provided in a patient's residence (including assisted living apartments, group homes, non-traditional private homes, custodial care facilities, or schools).

Health care professionals who are authorized to use Evaluation and Management Home Visit codes (99341-99350) may report codes 99500▶-99600◀ in addition to codes 99341-99350 if both services are performed. Evaluation and Management services may be reported separately, using the modifier '-25', if the patient's condition requires a significant separately identifiable E/M service, above and beyond the home health service(s)/procedure(s) codes 99500▶-99600.◀

▶Codes 99551-99600 include a home visit by a health care professional in a single 24-hour period. All solutions, equipment, supplies and drugs are excluded and should be reported separately. If more than one therapy is given in a 24-hour period, the most complex therapy should be reported first and 99600 should be reported separately for each additional therapy given in that 24-hour period. These codes do not represent self-administration of medications by the patient.◀

99500   Home visit for prenatal monitoring and assessment to include fetal heart rate, non-stress test, uterine monitoring, and gestational diabetes monitoring

99501   Home visit for postnatal assessment and follow up care

99502   Home visit for newborn care and assessment

99503   Home visit for respiratory therapy care (eg, bronchodilator, oxygen therapy, respiratory assessment, apnea evaluation)

▲99504   Home visit for mechanical ventilation care

99505   Home visit for stoma care and maintenance including colostomy and cystostomy

99506   Home visit for intramuscular injections

99507   Home visit for care and maintenance of catheter(s) (eg, urinary, drainage, and enteral)

▶(99508 has been deleted. To report see 95806-95811)◀

99509   Home visit for assistance with activities of daily living

99510   Home visit for individual, family, or marriage counseling

99511   Home visit for fecal impaction management and enema administration

99512   Home visit for hemodialysis

(For home infusion of peritoneal dialysis, use 99559)

▶(99539 has been deleted. To report, use 99600)◀

Home Infusion Procedures▶/Services◀

▲99551   Home infusion for pain management (intravenous or subcutaneous), per visit

▲99552   Home infusion for pain management (epidural or intrathecal), per visit

▲99553   Home infusion for tocolytic therapy, per visit

▲99554   Home infusion for hematopoietic hormones (eg, erythropoietin, G-CSF, GM-CSF) or platelets, per visit

▲99555   Home infusion for chemotherapy, per visit

▲99556   Home infusion for antibiotics/antifungals/antivirals, per visit

▲99557   Home infusion of continuous anticoagulant therapy (eg, heparin), per visit

▲99558   Home infusion of immunotherapy, per visit

▲99559   Home infusion of peritoneal dialysis, per visit

(For home visit for hemodialysis, use 99512)

▲99560   Home infusion of enteral nutrition, per visit

▲99561   Home infusion of hydration therapy, per visit

▲99562   Home infusion of total parenteral nutrition, per visit

▲99563   Home administration of aerosolized pentamidine, per visit

▲99564   Home infusion for anti-hemophilic agents (eg, Factor VIII), per visit

▲99565   Home infusion of alpha-1-proteinase inhibitor (eg, Prolastin), per visit

▲99566   Home infusion for uninterrupted, long-term intravenous treatment (eg, epoprostenol), per visit

▲99567   Home infusion of sympathomimetic agents (eg, dobutamine), per visit

▲99568   Home infusion of miscellaneous drugs, per visit

+▲99569   Home infusion, each additional therapy given on same day (List separately in addition to code for primary visit), per visit

●99600   Unlisted home visit service or procedure

Rationale

For *CPT 2003*, the Home Infusion Procedure codes were combined under the same section as the Home/Health Procedures/Services with appropriate revisions to the Home Health Procedures/Services guidelines to reflect the revisions to the referenced code ranges. The descriptor in code 99504 was revised to provide consistency with the other Home Health code descriptors. In the introductory language, the phrase "and all necessary solutions, equipment, and supplies (except drugs) required to deliver a therapy" has been removed from the introductory language with the addition of instructions that all other solutions, equipment, supplies, drugs, etc, be reported separately. Previously, all necessary solutions, equipment, and supplies, except drugs, were included. Now these can be reported separately. Code 99539 was deleted for the purpose of relocation and renumbering, and code 99600 was added to accommodate the merging of the Home Infusion Procedure codes with the Home Health Procedures/Services and to allow expansion of this section. Code 99508 was deleted because CPT codes were previously available for reporting polysomnography and sleep study services. To remain consistent with other CPT code descriptors, the words "per diem" have been deleted and replaced with "per visit" in the nomenclature of each home infusion code.

Appendix—Modifiers

The revisions to this section consist of the addition of a new modifier for 2003 and the deletion of all language within the modifier descriptors referencing the use of five-digit modifier codes.

Appendix — Modifiers

This list includes all of the modifiers applicable to CPT 2003 codes.

-21 **Prolonged Evaluation and Management Service:** When the face-to-face or floor/unit service(s) provided is prolonged or otherwise greater than that usually required for the highest level of evaluation and management service within a given category, it may be identified by adding modifier '-21' to the evaluation and management code number. A report may also be appropriate.

-22 **Unusual Procedural Services:** When the service(s) provided is greater than that usually required for the listed procedure, it may be identified by adding modifier '-22' to the usual procedure number. A report may also be appropriate.

-23 **Unusual Anesthesia:** Occasionally, a procedure, which usually requires either no anesthesia or local anesthesia, because of unusual circumstances must be done under general anesthesia. This circumstance may be reported by adding the modifier '-23' to the procedure code of the basic service.

-24 **Unrelated Evaluation and Management Service by the Same Physician During a Postoperative Period:** The physician may need to indicate that an evaluation and management service was performed during a postoperative period for a reason(s) unrelated to the original procedure. This circumstance may be reported by adding the modifier '-24' to the appropriate level of E/M service.

-25 **Significant, Separately Identifiable Evaluation and Management Service by the Same Physician on the Same Day of the Procedure or Other Service:** The physician may need to indicate that on the day a procedure or service identified by a CPT code was performed, the patient's condition required a significant, separately identifiable E/M service above and beyond the other service provided or beyond the usual preoperative and postoperative care associated with the procedure that was performed. The E/M service may be prompted by the symptom or condition for which the procedure and/or service was provided. As such, different diagnoses are not required for reporting of the E/M services on the same date. This circumstance may be reported by adding the modifier '-25' to the appropriate level of E/M service. **Note**: This modifier is not used to report an E/M service that resulted in a decision to perform surgery. See modifier '-57.'

-26 **Professional Component:** Certain procedures are a combination of a physician component and a technical component. When the physician component is reported separately, the service may be identified by adding the modifier '-26' to the usual procedure number.

-32 **Mandated Services:** Services related to mandated consultation and/or related services (eg, PRO, third-party payer, governmental, legislative, or regulatory requirement) may be identified by adding the modifier '-32' to the basic procedure.

-47 **Anesthesia by Surgeon:** Regional or general anesthesia provided by the surgeon may be reported by adding the modifier '-47' to the basic service. (This does not include local anesthesia.) Note: Modifier '-47' would not be used as a modifier for the anesthesia procedures 00100-01999.

-50 **Bilateral Procedure:** Unless otherwise identified in the listings, bilateral procedures that are performed at the same operative session should be identified by adding the modifier '-50' to the appropriate five-digit code.

-51 **Multiple Procedures:** When multiple procedures, other than E/M Services, are performed at the same session by the same provider, the primary procedure or service may be reported as listed. The additional procedure(s) or service(s) may be identified by appending the modifier '-51' to the additional procedure or service code(s). **Note:** This modifier should not be appended to designated "add-on" codes (see Appendix E).

-52 **Reduced Services:** Under certain circumstances a service or procedure is partially reduced or eliminated at the physician's discretion. Under these circumstances the service provided can be identified by its usual procedure number and the addition of the modifier '-52,' signifying that the service is reduced. This provides a means of reporting reduced services without disturbing the identification of the basic service. **Note:** For hospital outpatient reporting of a previously scheduled procedure/service that is partially reduced or cancelled as a result of extenuating circumstances or those that threaten the well-being of the patient prior to or after administration of anesthesia, see modifiers '-73' and '-74' (see modifiers approved for ASC hospital outpatient use).

-53 **Discontinued Procedure:** Under certain circumstances, the physician may elect to terminate a surgical or diagnostic procedure. Due to extenuating circumstances or those that threaten the well-being of the patient, it may be necessary to indicate that a surgical or diagnostic procedure was started but discontinued. This circumstance may be reported by adding the modifier '-53' to the code reported by the physician for the discontinued procedure. **Note:** This modifier is not used to report the elective cancellation of a procedure prior to the patient's anesthesia induction and/or surgical preparation in the operating suite. For outpatient hospital/ambulatory surgery center (ASC) reporting of a previously scheduled procedure/service that is partially reduced or cancelled as a result of extenuating circumstances or those that threaten the well-being of the patient prior to or after administration of anesthesia, see modifiers '-73' and '-74' (see modifiers approved for ASC hospital outpatient use).

-54 **Surgical Care Only:** When one physician performs a surgical procedure and another provides preoperative and/or postoperative management, surgical services may be identified by adding the modifier '-54' to the usual procedure number.

-55 **Postoperative Management Only:** When one physician performed the postoperative management and another physician has performed the surgical procedure, the postoperative component may be identified by adding the modifier '-55' to the usual procedure number.

-56 **Preoperative Management Only:** When one physician performed the preoperative care and evaluation and another physician performed the surgical procedure, the preoperative component may be identified by adding the modifier '-56' to the usual procedure number.

-57 **Decision for Surgery:** An evaluation and management service that resulted in the initial decision to perform the surgery, may be identified by adding the modifier '-57' to the appropriate level of E/M service.

-58 **Staged or Related Procedure or Service by the Same Physician During the Postoperative Period:** The physician may need to indicate that the performance of a procedure or service during the postoperative period was: a) planned prospectively at the time of the original procedure (staged); b) more extensive than the original procedure; or c) for therapy following a diagnostic surgical procedure. This circumstance may be reported by adding the modifier '-58' to the staged or related procedure. Note: This modifier is not used to report the treatment of a problem that requires a return to the operating room. See modifier '-78.'

-59 **Distinct Procedural Service:** Under certain circumstances, the physician may need to indicate that a procedure or service was distinct or independent from other services performed on the same day. Modifier '-59' is used to identify procedures/services that are not normally reported together, but are appropriate under the circumstances. This may represent a different session or patient encounter, different procedure or surgery, different site or organ system, separate incision/excision, separate lesion, or separate injury (or area of injury in extensive injuries) not ordinarily encountered or performed on the same day by the same physician. However, when another already established modifier is appropriate it should be used rather than modifier '-59.' Only if no more descriptive modifier is available, and the use of modifier '-59' best explains the circumstances, should modifier '-59' be used.

-62 **Two Surgeons:** When two surgeons work together as primary surgeons performing distinct part(s) of a procedure, each surgeon should report his/her distinct operative work by adding the modifier '-62' to the procedure code and any associated add-on code(s) for that procedure as long as both surgeons continue to work together as primary surgeons. Each surgeon should report the co-surgery once using the same procedure code. If additional procedure(s) (including add-on procedure(s)), are performed during the same surgical session, separate code(s) may also be reported with the modifier '-62' added. **Note:** If a co-surgeon acts as an assistant in the performance of additional procedure(s) during the same surgical session, those services may be reported using separate procedure code(s) with the modifier '-80' or modifier '-82' added, as appropriate.

▶**-63** **Procedure Performed on Infants less than 4 kg:** Procedures performed on neonates and infants up to a present body weight of 4 kg may involve significantly increased complexity and physician work commonly associated with these patients. This circumstance may be reported by adding the modifier '-63' to the procedure number. Note: Unless otherwise designated, this modifier may only be appended to procedures/services listed in the 20000-69999 code series. Modifier '-63' should not be appended to any CPT codes listed in the Evaluation and Management Services, Anesthesia, Radiology, Pathology/ Laboratory, or Medicine sections.◀

-66 **Surgical Team:** Under some circumstances, highly complex procedures (requiring the concomitant services of several physicians, often of different specialties, plus other highly skilled, specially trained personnel, various types of complex equipment) are carried out under the "surgical team" concept. Such circumstances may be identified by each participating physician with the addition of the modifier '-66' to the basic procedure number used for reporting services.

-76 **Repeat Procedure by Same Physician:** The physician may need to indicate that a procedure or service was repeated subsequent to the original procedure or service. This circumstance may be reported by adding the modifier '-76' to the repeated procedure/service.

-77 **Repeat Procedure by Another Physician:** The physician may need to indicate that a basic procedure or service performed by another physician had to be repeated. This situation may be reported by adding modifier '-77' to the repeated procedure/service.

-78 **Return to the Operating Room for a Related Procedure During the Postoperative Period:** The physician may need to indicate that another procedure was performed during the postoperative period of the initial procedure. When this subsequent procedure is related to the first, and requires the use of the operating room, it may be reported by adding the modifier '-78' to the related procedure. (For repeat procedures on the same day, see '-76.')

-79 **Unrelated Procedure or Service by the Same Physician During the Postoperative Period:** The physician may need to indicate that the performance of a procedure or service during the postoperative period was unrelated to the original procedure. This circumstance may be reported by using the modifier '-79'. (For repeat procedure on the same day, see '-76'.)

-80 **Assistant Surgeon:** Surgical assistant services may be identified by adding the modifier '-80' to the usual procedure number(s).

-81 **Minimum Assistant Surgeon:** Minimum surgical assistant services are identified by adding the modifier '-81' to the usual procedure number.

-82 **Assistant Surgeon (when qualified resident surgeon not available):** The unavailability of a qualified resident surgeon is a prerequisite for use of modifier '-82' appended to the usual procedure code number(s).

-90 **Reference (Outside) Laboratory:** When laboratory procedures are performed by a party other than the treating or reporting physician, the procedure may be identified by adding the modifier '-90' to the usual procedure number.

-99 **Multiple Modifiers:** Under certain circumstances two or more modifiers may be necessary to completely delineate a service. In such situations modifier '-99' should be added to the basic procedure, and other applicable modifiers may be listed as part of the description of the service.

Modifiers Approved for Ambulatory Surgery Center (ASC) Hospital Outpatient Use

CPT Level I Modifiers

-25 **Significant, Separately Identifiable Evaluation and Management Service by the Same Physician on the Same Day of the Procedure or Other Service:** The physician may need to indicate that on the day a procedure or service identified by a CPT code was performed, the patient's condition required a significant, separately identifiable E/M service above and beyond the other service provided or beyond the usual preoperative and postoperative care associated with the procedure that was performed. The E/M service may be prompted by the symptom or condition for which the procedure and/or service was provided. As such, different diagnoses are not required for reporting of the E/M services on the same date. This circumstance may be reported by adding the modifier '-25' to the appropriate level of E/M service. **Note:** This modifier is not used to report an E/M service that resulted in a decision to perform surgery. See modifier '-57.'

-50 **Bilateral Procedure:** Unless otherwise identified in the listings, bilateral procedures that are performed at the same operative session should be identified by adding modifier '-50' to the appropriate five digit code.

-52 **Reduced Services:** Under certain circumstances a service or procedure is partially reduced or eliminated at the physician's discretion. Under these circumstances the service provided can be identified by its usual procedure number and the addition of the modifier '-52,' signifying that the service is reduced. This provides a means of reporting reduced services without disturbing the identification of the basic service. **Note:** For hospital outpatient reporting of a previously scheduled procedure/service that is partially reduced or cancelled as a result of extenuating circumstances or those that threaten the well-being of the patient prior to or after administration of anesthesia, see modifiers '-73' and '-74'.

-58 **Staged or Related Procedure or Service by the Same Physician During the Postoperative Period:** The physician may need to indicate that the performance of a procedure or service during the postoperative period was: a) planned prospectively at the time of the original procedure (staged); b) more extensive than the original procedure; or c) for therapy following a diagnostic surgical procedure. This circumstance may be reported by adding the modifier '-58' to the staged or related procedure. **Note:** This modifier is not used to report the treatment of a problem that requires a return to the operating room. See modifier '-78.'

-59 **Distinct Procedural Service:** Under certain circumstances, the physician may need to indicate that a procedure or service was distinct or independent from other services performed on the same day. Modifier '-59' is used to identify procedures/services that are not normally reported together, but are appropriate under the circumstances. This may represent a different session or patient encounter, different procedure or surgery, different site or organ system, separate incision/excision, separate lesion, or separate injury (or area of injury in extensive injuries) not ordinarily encountered or performed on the same day by the same physician. However, when another already established modifier is appropriate it should be used rather than modifier '-59'. Only if no more descriptive modifier is available, and the use of modifier '-59' best explains the circumstances, should modifier '-59' be used.

-73 **Discontinued Out-Patient Hospital/Ambulatory Surgery Center (ASC) Procedure Prior to the Administration of Anesthesia:** Due to extenuating circumstances or those that threaten the well-being of the patient, the physician may cancel a surgical or diagnostic procedure subsequent to the patient's surgical preparation (including sedation when provided, and being taken to the room where the procedure is to be performed) but prior to the administration of anesthesia (local, regional block(s) or general). Under these circumstances, the intended service that is prepared for but cancelled can be reported by its usual procedure number and the addition of the modifier '-73'. **Note:** The elective cancellation of a service prior to the administration of anesthesia and/or surgical preparation of the patient should not be reported. For physician reporting of a discontinued procedure, see modifier '-53.'

-74 **Discontinued Out-Patient Hospital/Ambulatory Surgery Center (ASC) Procedure After Administration of Anesthesia:** Due to extenuating circumstances or those that threaten the well being of the patient, the physician may terminate a surgical or diagnostic procedure after the administration of anesthesia (local, regional block(s), general) or after the procedure was started (incision made, intubation started, scope inserted, etc.) Under these circumstances, the procedure started but terminated can be reported by its usual procedure number and the addition of the modifier '-74'. **Note:** The elective cancellation of a service prior to the administration of anesthesia and/or surgical preparation of the patient should not be reported. For physician reporting of a discontinued procedure, see modifier '-53.'

-76 **Repeat Procedure by Same Physician:** The physician may need to indicate that a procedure or service was repeated subsequent to the original procedure or service. This circumstance may be reported by adding the modifier '-76' to the repeated procedure/service.

-77 **Repeat Procedure by Another Physician:** The physician may need to indicate that a basic procedure or service performed by another physician had to be repeated. This situation may be reported by adding modifier '-77' to the repeated procedure/service.

-78 **Return to the Operating Room for a Related Procedure During the Postoperative Period:** The physician may need to indicate that another procedure was performed during the postoperative period of the initial procedure. When this subsequent procedure is related to the first, and requires the use of the operating room, it may be reported by adding the modifier '-78' to the related procedure. (For repeat procedures on the same day, see '-76.')

-79   **Unrelated Procedure or Service by the Same Physician During the Postoperative Period:** The physician may need to indicate that the performance of a procedure or service during the postoperative period was unrelated to the original procedure. This circumstance may be reported by using the modifier '-79.' (For repeat procedure on the same day, see '-76.')

 ## Rationale for Modifier '-63'

The modifier '-63' was established to be appended only to invasive surgical procedures, and reported only for those for neonates/infants up to the 4-kg cut-off. In this population of patients there is a significant increase in work intensity, specifically related to temperature control, obtaining IV access (which may require upwards of 45 minutes), and the operation itself which is technically more difficult, especially with regard to maintenance of homeostasis.

The procedures with which modifier '-63' cannot be reported are generally procedures performed on infants for the correction of congenital abnormalities and are exempt from appending the modifier '-63.' It is not appropriate to report the modifier '-63' with these procedures because the additional work that the modifier '-63' is intended to represent has been previously identified as an inherent element within the procedures in this list. When appended to a procedure, the modifier '-63' indicates the additional difficulty of performing a procedure, which may involve significantly increased complexity and physician work commonly associated with neonates and infants up to a body weight of 4 kg.

Examples of procedures that the modifier '-63' might typically be appended to would include codes 44120, Enterectomy, resection of small intestine; 44140, Enterectomy, for necrotizing enterocolitis; 33820, Repair of patent ductus arteriosus; 43220, Esophagoscopy with balloon dilation (less than 30 mm diameter), post-tracheoesophageal fistula repair; 43246, percutaneous gastrostomy placement for feeding problems; 47000, Liver biopsy; or 44055, reduction of malrotation for diagnosis of midgut volvulus.

The instructional notes pertaining to reporting five-digit modifiers have been deleted from the CPT code set to coincide with the HCFA (CMS) 1500 claim form reporting instructions, as this was in conflict with the previous instructions included in the CPT code set regarding the use of a separate five-digit modifier. According to the Chair of the National Uniform Claim Committee (NUCC), the electronic claim format for the HCFA (CMS) 1500 claim form that is under development (10/02 implementation) in compliance with the regulations that apply to the Health Insurance Portability and Accountability Act (HIPAA) will not accommodate a five-digit modifier. The current field length of the electronic format that holds a modifier is limited to two characters.

Category III Codes

Eighteen new codes have been added to the Category III section for 2003. The most significant of these is the series of eight new codes for reporting procedures related to thoracic aortic aneurysm repair.

Category III Codes

● **0027T** Endoscopic lysis of epidural adhesions with direct visualization using mechanical means (eg, spinal endoscopic catheter system) or solution injection (eg, normal saline) including radiologic localization and epidurography

▶(For diagnostic epiduroscopy, use 64999)◀

 Rationale

This Category III code was added to describe endoscopic lysis of adhesions. In relation to the addition of code 0027T, "Epiduroscope" was stricken from the parenthetical phrase associated with code 62263 in order to distinguish this code from code 0027T. Finally, a cross-reference was added following code 0027T to clarify that code 0027T should not be reported for a diagnostic epiduroscopy. Instead, diagnostic epiduroscopy should continue to be reported by 64999 Unlisted procedure, nervous system.

● **0028T** Dual energy x-ray absorptiometry (DEXA) body composition study, one or more sites

 Rationale

Category III code 0028T has been added to provide a reporting mechanism to describe a procedure for assessing body fat composition using dual energy x-ray absorptiometry (DEXA). DEXA has been used extensively for assessing bone density (codes 76075 and 76076). A cross-reference following code 76076 has been added to direct users to this new code.

DEXA, performed to estimate body fat composition, requires a different procedure than when used for assessing bone density. The reasons for estimation of body fat composition include:

1. Children with growth disorders
2. Patients with eating disorders
3. Patients with rapid intentional or unintentional weight loss including malabsorptive disorders, secondary hyperparathyroidism, renal disease, AIDS
4. Athletes
5. Patients on long-term total parenteral nutrition
6. Adults with growth hormone deficiency

DEXA is widely used for the measurement of bone mineral and forms an integral part of the four-compartment model. In recent years, the software has been developed to divide the soft tissue into fat and fat free mass (bones, muscles, viscera). In its own right, DEXA therefore provides an example of a three-compartment model (bone, fat, and fat-free soft tissue). With the additional measurement of total body water, an alternative four-compartment mode can be derived (bone, water, fat, and dry fat-free soft tissue).

Soft tissue composition is measured in a whole-body scan, which takes between 5 and 20 minutes depending on the particular machine. The body is scanned in a rectilinear or fan-beam manner using two low-dose x-rays at different energies, typically 70 and 140 keV. The effective dose equivalent is similar to a day's background radiation and this low dose makes the procedure suitable for most groups of subjects, including babies and children, although it remains prudent not to scan pregnant women. It is also acceptable to make longitudinal measurements in individual subjects. DEXA is one of the very few techniques to bridge the gap between body composition analysis in the laboratory and the clinic.

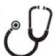

Clinical Example #1 (0028T)

A 36-year-old woman with a BMI of 40 kg/m^2 undergoes a gastric bypass procedure and loses about 50 pounds in a 3-month period. She also notes generalized weakness. A complete history and physical did not reveal any localizing findings. There was concern regarding possible malnutrition and degree of muscle versus fat loss.

The physician orders body composition assessment by DEXA. This is performed either in the ambulatory clinical diagnostic center or in a hospital's diagnostic center. The DEXA was obtained and revealed that her lean body mass was appropriate and that most of her weight loss was due to reduction in fat.

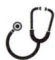

Clinical Example #2 (0028T)

A 21-year-old woman with anorexia enters an eating disorder clinic for assessment. There are no medical, gastrointestinal or hormonal causes for her weight loss. Baseline body composition data is obtained for subsequent comparison to objectively assess changes in body composition in response to therapy.

Description of Procedure (0028T)

The patient enters the examination suite and lays on the scanning table. The body is scanned in a rectilinear or fan-beam manner using two low-dose x-rays at different energies, typically at 70 and 140 keV. The effective dose of radiation is equal to one day's background radiation. A whole-body scan is performed and takes between 5 and 20 minutes depending on the machine used. The body can then be analyzed by region with respect to grams of fat and total body mass. A percentage of fat is then calculated for each region as well as for the total body.

The interpreting physician assesses the quality of images and data obtained prior to releasing the report to the patient and/or referring physician.

●0029T   Treatment(s) for incontinence, pulsed magnetic neuromodulation, per day

Rationale

A Category III code has been added for the treatment of urinary incontinence utilizing extracorporeal magnetic innervation. This technology involves the delivery of non-invasive magnetic pulses resulting in depolarization of neuron membranes, which cause the induction of nerve impulses in the pudendal and splanchnic nerves (and their branches) for the purpose of restoration of neuromuscular control in the treatment of urinary incontinence. A specially designed chair has been developed to ensure the pelvic floor and sphincter muscles are correctly positioned to receive the therapeutic pulsed magnetic field. The magnetic impulses induce a corresponding pattern of contractions in the muscles of the pelvic floor and urinary sphincters. Because urinary leakage is typically caused by weakness of pelvic muscles and the urethral sphincter (stress incontinence), or muscle spasms in the detrusor muscle (urge incontinence), this therapy may help patients by building strength and endurance in pelvic muscles, and assist patients by decoupling muscle fibers to restore urinary control.

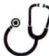

Clinical Example (0029T)

The patient is a 55-year-old woman who is complaining of involuntary loss of urine with activities such as coughing or lifting. The patient has had symptoms for at least 3 months and is having to use pads or other protection for daily activities. The initial evaluation has confirmed symptoms and signs of urinary incontinence and has excluded transient causes. Urinalysis fails to reveal evidence of hematuria or active urinary infection. Urinary retention is excluded by clinical examination, post-void catheterization or ultrasound scan. The patient has used Kegel exercises without success. The clinician ensures that there is no contra-indication to ExMI, such as pregnancy, major pelvic organ prolapse, or cardiac pacemaker.

Description of Procedure (0029T)

Based on the diagnosis, the physician determines dosage and modulation parameters. This prescription is encoded on a treatment card. The patient treatment involves patient instruction and positioning on the NeoControl system. The therapy head, which is positioned in the seat of the treatment chair, produces a rapidly changing pulsed magnetic field that will induce neuron depolarization resulting in contractions of the muscles of the pelvic floor. Patient tolerance is tested and output power adjusted as required. The treatment cycle includes 20 to 30 minutes of intermittent stimulation to improve sphincter function and bladder control. During the interval treatment, the patient follows a program of education using an interactive video screen technology. The patient learns about the causes of incontinence, the factors that may worsen or improve symptoms, and strategies to maintain bladder health during and after ExMI treatment. This procedure is repeated 16 to 20 times to complete a course of therapy. Patient progress is assessed after 8 treatments or sooner if changes in patient condition present. Treatment parameters may need to be adjusted.

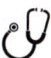

Clinical Example (0029T)

The patient is a 75-year-old woman who is complaining of involuntary loss of urine with activities such as standing up from sitting. The patient has had symptoms for at least 3 months and is having to use pads or other protection for daily activities. The initial evaluation has confirmed symptoms and signs of urinary incontinence and has excluded transient causes. Urinalysis fails to reveal evidence of hematuria or active urinary infection. Urinary retention is excluded by clinical examination, post-void catheterization, or ultrasound scan. The patient has used Kegel exercises without success. The therapist ensures that there is no contra-indication to ExMI such as major pelvic organ prolapse or cardiac pacemaker.

Description of Procedure (0029T)

Based on the diagnosis, the physician will determine dosage and modulation parameters. This prescription is encoded on a treatment card. The patient treatment involves patient instruction and positioning on the NeoControl system. The therapy head, which is positioned in the seat of the treatment chair, produces a rapidly changing pulsed magnetic field that will induce neuron depolarization resulting in contractions of the muscles of the pelvic floor. Patient tolerance is tested and output power adjusted as required. The treatment cycle includes 20 to 30 minutes of intermittent stimulation to improve sphincter function and bladder control. During the interval treatment, the patient follows a program of education using an interactive video screen technology. The patient learns about the causes of incontinence, the factors that may worsen or improve symptoms, and strategies to maintain bladder health during and after ExMI treatment. This procedure is repeated 16 to 20 times to complete a course of therapy. Patient progress is assessed after 8 treatments or sooner if changes in patient condition present. Treatment parameters may need to be adjusted.

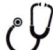

Clinical Example (0029T)

The patient is a 65-year-old woman who is complaining of urinary frequency, urgency, and involuntary loss of urine before she is able to make it to the bathroom. Leakage may be provoked by standing or by the sound of running water. The patient has had symptoms for at least 3 months and is having to use pads or other protection for daily activities. The initial evaluation has confirmed symptoms and signs of urinary incontinence and has excluded transient causes. Urinalysis has failed to reveal evidence of hematuria or active urinary infection. Urinary retention is excluded by clinical examination, post-void catheterization or ultrasound scan. The patient has used Kegel exercises without success. The therapist ensures that there is no contra-indication for ExMI such as major pelvic organ prolapse, severe estrogen deficiency, or cardiac pacemaker.

Description of Procedure (0029T)
See previous descriptive listing.

● **0030T**   Antiprothrombin (phospholipid cofactor) antibody, each Ig class

Rationale

Category III code 0030T has been added to describe antiprothrombin (phospholipid cofactor) antibody testing, which is currently being used as serologic markers for the antiphospholipid syndrome (APS) to assess those patients who may be at risk for recurrent arterial or venous thrombosis, thrombocytopenia, and/or fetal loss. Testing for antibodies to prothrombin provides valuable information as an aid in the diagnosis and thrombotic risk assessment in antiphospholipid syndrome.

The term "antiphospholipid antibodies" is used to describe a heterogeneous group of autoantibodies with specificity toward several negatively charged phospholipids and phospholipid/protein (cofactor) complexes. Elevated levels of antiphospholipid antibodies are recognized as serological markers for the antiphospholipid syndrome

(APS), characterized clinically by recurrent venous and/or arterial thrombosis, thrombocytopenia, and spontaneous abortion. Currently, CPT codes exist for two of these antibodies: anti-cardiolipin (aCL), 86147, and anti-phosphatidylserine (aPS), 86148. Protein targets, commonly referred to as antiphospholipid cofactors, are thought to play an important role in the pathogenesis of thrombosis in the antiphospholipid syndrome (APS).

Lupus anticoagulants (LA) are a heterogeneous sub-group of antiphospholipid antibodies that inhibit in vitro phospholipid-dependent coagulation assays. LA also require prothrombin or beta-2-glycoprotein I as cofactors for optimal immunologic binding. In vitro, anti-Prothrombin (aPT) antibodies induce lupus anticoagulant (LA) activity in a manner similar to anti-B2GPI antibodies, by competing with other coagulation factors for available phospholipid binding sites on exposed surfaces (prothrombinase complex).

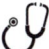
Clinical Example (0030T)
A middle-aged male presents with arthritis, fever, progressive weight loss, generalized lymphadenopathy, and erythematous skin rash. Lymph node biopsy shows atypical plasmacytosis. Serum protein electrophoresis shows hypergammaglobulinemia, serum IgM is elevated to 1030 mg/dL (normal, 60-263 mg/dL), and lupus anticoagulant (LA) test is performed with strongly positive results.

Description of Procedure (0030T)
The strongly positive LA results prompted an antiphospholipid antibody evaluation to determine the risk for thrombosis and consider anticoagulation therapy. Patient sera are tested for anti-cardiolipin (aCL), anti-phosphatidylserine (aPS), anti-beta 2 glycoprotein I (aB2GPI), and anti-prothrombin (aPT). Antibody levels are positive for aCL IgG and IgM, aPS IgG and IgM, and aPT IgM, but negative for aB2GPI. The strong lupus anticoagulant activity in this patient is most likely due to the elevated anti-Prothrombin antibody levels, since aB2GPI levels are negative. The patient later develops arterial thrombosis (stroke). Risk for thrombosis in this patient is due to elevated aPT levels. Without the aPT levels being tested, the risk of thrombosis would have been misinterpreted due to the normal aB2GPI levels.

●0031T   Speculoscopy;

●0032T   with directed sampling

Rationale
Two new Category III codes were created to describe a magnified chemiluminescent light examination of the cervix and specimen collection. This examination is performed to identify potentially abnormal lesions of the uterine ecto-cervix for detection of dysplasia (both low and high grade).

●0033T   Endovascular repair of descending thoracic aortic aneurysm, pseudoaneurysm or dissection; involving coverage of left subclavian artery origin, initial endoprosthesis

▶(For radiological supervision and interpretation, use 0038T)◀

●**0034T**   not involving coverage of left subclavian artery origin, initial endoprosthesis

    ▶(For radiological supervision and interpretation, use 0039T)◀

●**0035T**   Placement of proximal or distal extension prosthesis for endovascular repair of descending thoracic aortic aneurysm, pseudoaneurysm or dissection; initial extension

    ▶(For radiological supervision and interpretation, use 0040T)◀

    ▶(Do not report 0034T and 0035T, when placement of extension converts repair to cover left subclavian origin, use only 0033T)◀

+●**0036T**   each additional extension (List separately in addition to code for primary procedure)

    ▶(Use 0036T in conjunction with code 0035T)◀

    ▶(For radiological supervision and interpretation, use 0040T)◀

●**0037T**   Open subclavian to carotid artery transposition performed in conjunction with endovascular thoracic aneurysm repair, by neck incision, unilateral

    ▶(For bilateral procedure, use modifier '-50')◀

    ▶(Do not report 0037T in addition to 35694)◀

●**0038T**   Endovascular repair of descending thoracic aortic aneurysm, pseudoaneurysm or dissection involving coverage of left subclavian artery origin, initial endoprosthesis, radiological supervision and interpretation

    ▶(For implantation of endovascular graft, use 0033T)◀

●**0039T**   Endovascular repair of descending thoracic aortic aneurysm, pseudoaneurysm or dissection not involving coverage of left subclavian artery origin, initial endoprosthesis; radiological supervision and interpretation

    ▶(For implantation of endovascular graft, see 0034T)◀

●**0040T**   Placement of proximal or distal extension prosthesis for endovascular repair of descending thoracic aortic aneurysm, pseudoaneurysm or dissection, each extension, radiological supervision and interpretation

    ▶(For implantation of endovascular graft extensions, see 0035T, 0036T)◀

Rationale

Codes were added for services involving endovascular thoracic aortic aneurysm (TAA) repair. These codes identify a new method to repair aortic aneurysms. Other codes included in the CPT code set that identify endovascular aortic aneurysm repair (34800-34832) identify abdominal repairs and are, therefore, not specific to these procedures. TAA repair employs new and different devices and delivery systems and requires use of fluoroscopic guidance. Parenthetical notes have been added identifying the codes to use for guidance. It also demands different physician skills than those necessary for traditional, open surgical TAA repair.

Codes 0033T-0040T identify these endovascular thoracic aortic aneurysm repair services and are part of a number of additions to the CPT book regarding these types of procedures. These changes include the addition of two new headings, addition of new introductory notes, addition of cross-references specific to the establishment of new CPT codes describing endovascular repair of aneurysms, false aneurysms, and dissections of the descending thoracic aorta, and correlating CPT additions/revisions to cross-references in the Surgery and Radiology sections.

Codes 0033T and 0034T identify initial endovascular repair of TAAs through use of an endoprosthesis. They vary according to whether the left subclavian artery origin is covered (0033T) or not (0034T).

Codes 0035T and 0036T identify placement of extensions for the endovascular repair. This includes the initial extension placement (0035T) and subsequent extensions (0036T). In addition, code 0036T is intended to be used once for each additional extension device placed. Note that the parenthetical note that follows code 0035T indicates that this code should not be used when the endovascular device covers the left subclavian artery origin. If this vessel's origin is covered by the device placed, then code 0033T should be reported instead to identify the specific procedure performed.

Code 0037T identifies open arterial transposition of the subclavian artery to the carotid artery when performed in conjunction with endovascular TAA repair. When performing the endovascular repair, the proximity of the TAA to the left subclavian may require deployment of the endoprosthesis directly across the subclavian origin to achieve an adequately hemostatic "seal zone" during aneurysm repair. For this procedure, in order to maintain blood flow to the left arm, the subclavian artery is re-implanted onto the left common carotid artery through a separate neck incision. The transposition may be performed simultaneously with the endovascular repair, but if it is known in advance that transposition will be required, some surgeons prefer to do it a day or two prior to the endovascular TAA operation. The surgical work of this transposition is essentially the same as that in the 90-day global service 35694 (arterial transposition, subclavian to carotid artery). Therefore, the rationale and intended use for this code is to eliminate the risk of double-counting of post-service work.

Codes 0038T-0040T identify the supervision and interpretation procedures necessary to perform each of the aforementioned services. Cross-referenced parenthetical notes have been placed in this section to instruct on appropriate reporting of these codes, to identify the component S&I procedure codes and appropriate use of the interventional codes.

●**0041T** Urinalysis infectious agent detection, semi-quantitative analysis of volatile compounds

 Rationale

Category III code 0041T has been added to report a new technique/methodology for diagnosing urinary tract infections (UTIs). The new methodology employs the conducting polymer array sensing (CPAS) testing technique. A correlating cross-reference in the Pathology and Laboratory subsection has been added directing the user to this newly established code.

The CPAS technique is an automated in vitro diagnostic test that measures volatile compounds released into the headspace of a urine sample as a detector of bacterial infection using gas sensors and conducting polymer technology. Typically, CPAS requires specialized equipment consisting of an autosampler, sensor analyzer unit, carousel, incubator, and humidifier. Software algorithms define the presence of a urinary tract infection, and clinical interpretation is not required.

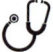

Clinical Example (0041T)

A symptomatic patient presents with a chief complaint of urinary frequency, burning, and urgency consistent with a UTI. There is no history of recurrent UTI. A clean-catch midstream urine specimen is slightly cloudy and straw colored. The specimen is sent to the laboratory in a vessel without preservatives for determination of the presence of bacteriuria using the CPAS method.

Description of Procedure (0041T)

The CPAS uses "electronic nose" technology for the detection of volatile metabolites released from microorganisms in human specimens. The principle is based on the release of volatile compounds from bacteria into the headspace (the volume above the liquid samples) of the clinical sample. The volatile compounds are detected by an array of gas sensors based on patented conducting polymer technology.

In the laboratory, the midstream urine specimen is pipetted into a glass vial containing reagents. The vial is put into the instrument carousel. The specimen identification number is input to the instrument's computer. Once the system's checks have been satisfied and input is completed, the instrument automatically starts to analyze the samples. A report showing the patient ID and the diagnostic result as positive or negative is automatically printed out within 5 hours of the start of the analysis. The results are communicated with the referring physician.

●0042T   Cerebral perfusion analysis using computed tomography with contrast administration, including post-processing of parametric maps with determination of cerebral blood flow, cerebral blood volume, and mean transit time

Rationale

To address the increasing number of cerebral perfusion studies using CT scanning technology, new Category III code 0042T has been added. Also, a correlating cross-reference has been added in the Radiology section to direct the user to the newly established code.

The addition of this code reflects the utility and increasing number of cerebral perfusion studies using CT scanning technology in patients with cerebral ischemia, brain tumors, or vasospasm. Measurements of cerebral perfusion, including cerebral blood flow (CBF), cerebral blood volume (CBV), and mean transit time (MTT), provide useful physiologic data regarding the status of the intracranial circulation. This data may be clinically valuable in the evaluation of such diverse diseases as acute stroke, carotid occlusive disease, and vasospasm following aneurysm rupture, as well as in brain tumor grading, stereotactic biopsy guidance, and treatment response monitoring.

CT is typically the first imaging test performed in cases of acute stroke, dissection, or transient ischemic attack, and is also commonly used in planning stereotactic brain tumor biopsy. Unlike MRI perfusion maps, CT perfusion maps can provide quantitative assessment of the CBF, CBV, and MTT blood flow parameters, so that precise thresholds of ischemia can be calculated.

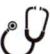

Clinical Example (0042T)

A 69-year-old male presents to a community hospital 1 hour after sudden onset of right hemiparesis and intermittent aphasia that occurred while playing golf. The patient has a regular pulse but is believed to have been in atrial fibrillation during symptom onset. An unenhanced CT scan is performed (coded separately), which shows no evidence of hemorrhage, but a subtle low density in the left insular cortex of undetermined age. The remainder of the scan is normal.

While the patient is still on the CT scanner table, a CT perfusion study is subsequently obtained (coded separately); CT perfusion analysis is performed by selecting the levels of major interest and scanning repeatedly before and during a 45-mL bolus of nonionic contrast administered at 5 mL/sec. CT perfusion is accomplished with the scanner in cine mode. Four contiguous 5- to 10-mm-thick axial images are obtained, which include visualization of the insula, lenticular nuclei, superior temporal lobes, inferior frontal lobes, inferior parietal lobes, and thalamus. After a 5-second prep delay, these levels are scanned at a rate of 1 image per second for 45 seconds. Within 5 to 10 minutes of scan completion, CT perfusion maps of cerebral blood flow (CBF), cerebral blood volume (CBV), and mean transit time (MTT) are constructed at a freestanding workstation using dedicated software by a radiologist in attendance. These images take approximately 15 to 20 minutes to generate. The images demonstrate a large region of delayed mean transit time in the distribution of the left middle cerebral artery, a portion of which demonstrates low cerebral blood volume. Because of the concern for a large-vessel distribution ischemic region, a CT angiogram may then be requested. In this case, a CTA demonstrated thrombus in the mid M1 division left MCA thrombus and the absence of a significant left internal carotid artery bifurcation stenosis. The patient is removed from the CT table in anticipation of IV thrombolytic treatment.

The CBV maps in this case show a small region of low blood volume, which corresponds to the untenanted CT findings. The cerebral blood flow and mean transit time maps, however, show a much larger surrounding area of diminished blood flow and increased blood transit time over the entire visualized MCA territory. Quantitative CBF values are at or below 20 mL/100 g/min at many locations; quantitative MTT values exceed 6 seconds at some locations. Because this data suggests an extensive area with poor collateral blood flow, unlikely to be irreversibly infarcted but potentially at risk for stroke in the absence of MCA recanalization (ischemic penumbra), and because recanalization is more likely to be successful in response to intra-arterial (IA) rather than IV thrombolysis, the decision is made to start IV thrombolysis and to immediately transport the patient to a nearby tertiary care center for definitive intra-arterial thrombolytic therapy. In this case, the CT perfusion demonstrated tissue at risk of infarction, leading to a CTA and more aggressive thrombolytic therapy.

●**0043T** Carbon monoxide, expired gas analysis (eg, ETCO$_c$/hemolysis breath test)

Rationale
Category III code 0043T has been added to allow a reporting mechanism for non-invasive testing for measurements of end-tidal carbon monoxide (ETCO$_c$) for the purpose of detecting the rate of hemolysis. A correlating cross-reference has been added to the Pathology and Laboratory subsection to direct the user to this new code.

The measurement of ETCO$_c$ corrected for background carbon monoxide (CO) in the breath represents a new technology that can detect the rate of hemolysis and/or assist in the tracking of hemolytic conditions. The technology can also measure end-tidal carbon dioxide (ETCO$_2$) and respiratory rate simultaneously. The test is non-invasive, it does not require the cooperation of the patient, and results are available immediately.

The catabolism of hemoglobin (Hgb) results in the equimolar formation of CO and bilirubin. ETCO$_c$ is an indicator of the rate of hemolysis and bilirubin production. Elevation of breath CO is indicative of pathological processes in newborn, pediatric, and adult populations. Currently available technologies to measure this parameter either are inaccurate, can be used only in the research arena, require the cooperation of patients, or are invasive and require laboratory analysis.

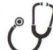
Clinical Example (0043T)
The patient is a male infant 39+ weeks of gestation, delivered by normal spontaneous vaginal delivery. There were no complications during pregnancy or delivery. Birth weight is 3100 g. Maternal blood type is O+; the baby's blood type is A+. At 24 hours of age, the ETCO$_c$ breath test for hemolysis is administered.

Description of Procedure (0043T)
Administration of the test involves placement of a catheter into a patient's nostril, secured to lip with adhesive; insertion of filter cartridge to analyzer port; and sampling of patient's breath with background air check for base levels.

Test results are documented in the patient's record. A normal ETCO$_c$ level could qualify the infant for early discharge. An elevated ETCO$_c$ indicates that the infant is at high risk for the development of hyperbilirubinemia. The cause of hemolysis should be identified, appropriate treatment should be initiated, and the patient should be monitored closely.

●**0044T** Whole body integumentary photography, at request of a physician, for monitoring of high-risk patients with dysplastic nevus syndrome or familial melanoma

Rationale
This code is specifically designed to accurately describe and report whole body imaging and comparative whole body imaging, and is intended for detection of atypical pigmented lesions and dysplastic nevi. The code includes more restrictive language within the code descriptor to reflect that the whole body photography is only for monitoring patients with atypical pigmented lesions or melanoma and not for monitoring patients with basal cell cancer or squamous cell cancer. Since

this code has been created as a Category III code, this code is intended to collect data on defined services, and to reflect actual medical practice. This descriptor language reduces distortion of the quality of the data collected. Finally, the intent of use of the language "atypical pigmented lesions" and "dysplastic nevi" are synonymous.

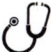

Clinical Example (0044T)

A 30-year-old woman has several moles, which vary in color, shape and size. She has noticed a slight change in size on one of the moles and doesn't know if there has been any changes in her other moles. She has fair skin and is concerned because she has had several sunburns in her youth. She is single and reports that it is virtually impossible for her to scan her body for changes and developments regarding moles and lesions. She is aware of skin cancer and how its occurrence is linked to sun exposure.

Description of Procedure (0044T)

A review of the woman's medical history is performed, as well as education regarding preventative programs designed to minimize skin cancer risk. Education can include the use of sunscreens, hats, UV sunglasses, long sleeves and pants, avoiding hottest part of the day, protection of children in the same manner, brochures and a web site containing information on the ABCs of skin cancer, monitoring suspect moles and lesions and the importance of scheduled screenings.

Two non-physician technicians perform a full body imaging procedure. Suspicious moles or lesions may be isolated and imaged on a micro basis and tagged with a millimeter measuring identification tag. The tag will specify the date, the patient's name and body section where the suspect mole or lesion is being micro imaged.

Once the images have been developed, a copy of the images will be forwarded to the referring physician for review. The physician will interpret the images and acknowledge any areas of concern and communicate his initial findings with his patient on the next office visit. A copy of the CD ROM disk will also be sent to the patient. This allows the patient to have a record of her skin, moles, and lesions and will help her to monitor her skin in between appointments with her doctor.

Tabular Review of the Changes

This table is provided to give you an "at-a-glance" review of the code changes included in *CPT 2003*. The table is divided into several columns as follows: "code" indicates the code involved in the change; "new" indicates that a new code was added; "revised" indicates that an existing code was changed; "deleted" indicates that a code was deleted; "Gr" indicates that a grammatical change was made to the code descriptor, but that this change did not change the intent of the code; and "cross" indicates that a cross-reference immediately preceding or following the code in the table was changed in some way.

Please note that headings in this table appear only if a code changed under that heading or subheading.

Tabular Review of the Changes

KEY: **Del** = Deleted
Rev = Revised
Gr = Grammar revision
Cross = Cross-reference

Section/Code	New	Del	Rev	Gr	Cross
Anesthesia					
Neck					
00320			x		
00326	x				x
Intrathoracic					
00528			x		x
00539	x				
00541	x				
Spine and Spinal Cord					
00640	x				
Lower Abdomen					
00832					x
00834	x				x
00836	x				x
00869		x			x
Perineum					
00921	x				
Knee and Popliteal Area					
01382			x		
01400			x		
Lower Leg (Below Knee, Includes Ankle and Foot)					
01464			x		

Section/Code	New	Del	Rev	Gr	Cross
Shoulder and Axilla					
01622			x		
01630			x		
Upper Arm and Elbow					
01732			x		
01740			x		
Forearm, Wrist, and Hand					
01829	x				
01830			x		
Obstetric					
01960			x		
01961			x		
01962			x		
01963			x		
01964			x		
01968			x		
01969			x		
Other Procedures					
01991	x				
01992	x				x
01996			x		x

Surgery

Section/Code	New	Del	Rev	Gr	Cross
General					
10022					x

Section/Code	New	Del	Rev	Gr	Cross
Integumentary System					
Skin, Subcutaneous and Accessory Structures					
Excision-Benign Lesions					
11400			X		
11401			X		
11402			X		
11403			X		
11404			X		
11406			X		
11420			X		
11421			X		
11422			X		
11423			X		
11424			X		
11426			X		
11440			X		
11441			X		
11442			X		
11443			X		
11444			X		
11446			X		
Excision-Malignant Lesions					
11600			X		
11601			X		
11602			X		
11603			X		
11604			X		
11606			X		
11620			X		
11621			X		

Section/Code	New	Del	Rev	Gr	Cross
11622			x		
11623			x		
11624			x		
11626			x		
11640			x		
11641			x		
11642			x		
11643			x		
11644			x		
11646			x		

Repair (Closure)

Other Flaps and Grafts

15756			x		

Destruction

Mohs Micrographic Surgery

17304			x		x
17310			x		x

Musculoskeletal System

General

Introduction or Removal

20550			x		
20552			x		
20553			x		
20600			x		
20605			x		
20612	x				x

Head

Excision

21030			x		
21034			x		

Section/Code	New	Del	Rev	Gr	Cross
21040			x		
21041		x			x
21046	x				
21047	x				
21048	x				
21049	x				

Neck (Soft Tissues) and Thorax

Repair, Revision, and/or Reconstruction

Section/Code	New	Del	Rev	Gr	Cross
21740			x		
21742	x				
21743	x				

Shoulder

Repair, Revision, and/or Reconstruction

Section/Code	New	Del	Rev	Gr	Cross
23410			x		
23412					x

Humerus (Upper Arm) and Elbow

Fracture and/or Dislocation

Section/Code	New	Del	Rev	Gr	Cross
24516			x		

Forearm and Wrist

Repair, Revision, and/or Reconstruction

Section/Code	New	Del	Rev	Gr	Cross
25320			x		

Hand and Fingers

Repair, Revision, and/or Reconstruction

Section/Code	New	Del	Rev	Gr	Cross
26440			x		

Pelvis and Hip Joint

Fracture and/or Dislocation

Section/Code	New	Del	Rev	Gr	Cross
27235			x		
27244			x		

Section/Code	New	Del	Rev	Gr	Cross
Femur (Thigh Region) and Knee Joint					
Repair, Revision, and/or Reconstruction					
27425			x		x
Leg (Tibia and Fibula) and Ankle Joint					
Repair, Revision, and/or Reconstruction					
27730			x		
Fracture and/or Dislocation					
27759			x		
Arthrodesis					
27870			x		x
Application of Casts and Strapping					
Lower Extremity					
Strapping-Any Age					
29540			x		
Endoscopy/Arthroscopy					
29808	x				
29827	x				x
29873	x				x
29899	x				x
Respiratory System					
Nose					
Repair					
30540					x
30545					x
Larynx					
Endoscopy					
31520					x
31578					x

Section/Code	New	Del	Rev	Gr	Cross
Trachea and Bronchi					
Endoscopy					
31625			x		
31628			x		x
31629			x		x
Cardiovascular System					
Heart and Pericardium					
Transmyocardial Revascularization					
33141					x
Pacemaker or Pacing Cardioverter-Defibrillator					
33215	x				
33216			x		
33224	x				
33225	x				x
33226	x				
Cardiac Valves					
Aortic Valve					
33401					x
33403					x
Pulmonary Valve					
33470					x
33472					x
Coronary Artery Anomalies					
33502					x
33503					x
33505					x
33506					x
Endoscopy					
33508	x				x

Section/Code	New	Del	Rev	Gr	Cross
Single Ventricle and Other Complex Cardiac Anomalies					
33610					x
33611					x
33619					x
Septal Defect					
33647					x
33670					x
33690					x
33694					x
Total Anomalous Pulmonary Venous Drainage					
33730					x
33732					x
Shunting Procedures					
33735					x
33736					x
33750					x
33755					x
33762					x
Transposition of the Great Vessels					
33778					x
Truncus Arteriosus					
33786					x
Pulmonary Artery					
33918					x
33919					x
33922					x
Cardiac Assist					
33961					x

Section/Code	New	Del	Rev	Gr	Cross
Arteries and Veins					
Endovascular Repair of Abdominal Aortic Aneurysm					
34812			x		
34825			x		
34826					x
34833	x				x
34834	x				x
Endovascular Repair of Iliac Aneurysm					
34900	x				x
Direct Repair of Aneurysm or Excision (Partial or Total) and Graft Insertion for Aneurysm, False Aneurysm, Ruptured Aneurysm, and Associated Occlusive Disease					
35001					x
Bypass Graft					
Vein					
35500					x
35572	x				x
Other Than Vein					
35606					x
35641					x
35646					x
Adjuvant Techniques					
Arterial Transposition					
35694					x
Venous					
36414	x				
36415			x		x
36416	x				x
36420					x
36450					x
36460					x
36510					x

Section/Code	New	Del	Rev	Gr	Cross
36511	x				
36512	x				
36513	x				
36514	x				
36515	x				
36516	x				
36520		x			x
36521		x			x
36533					x
36536	x				x
36537	x				x
36540			x		x
Arterial					
36660					x
Hemodialysis Access, Intravascular Cannulation for Extracorporeal Circulation, or Shunt Insertion					
36822					x
36830			x		
Portal Decompression Procedures					
37140			x		
37181					x
37182	x				x
37183	x				x
Endoscopy					
37300	x				x
37301	x				
Endoscopy					
37500	x				x
37501	x				

Section/Code	New	Del	Rev	Gr	Cross
Ligation and Other Procedures					
37606					x
37760			x		x

Hemic and Lymphatic Systems

General

38204	x				
38205	x				
38206	x				
38207	x				x
38208	x				x
38209	x				
38210	x				
38211	x				
38212	x				
38213	x				
38214	x				
38215	x				
Bone Marrow or Stem Cell Services/Procedures					
38220			x		
38221			x		
38231		x			x
38242	x				

Mediastinum and Diaphragm

Diaphragm

Repair

39503					x

Section/Code	New	Del	Rev	Gr	Cross
Digestive System					
Salivary Gland and Ducts					
Excision					
42400					x
Esophagus					
Endoscopy					
43201	x				x
43236	x				x
43245			x		x
Repair					
43313					x
43314					x
Stomach					
Incision					
43520					x
Other Procedures					
43831					x
Intestines (Except Rectum)					
Incision					
44055					x
Excision					
44126					x
44127					x
44128					x
44143					x
44145					x
44146					x
44150					x
44152					x
44153					x

Section/Code	New	Del	Rev	Gr	Cross
44155					X
Laparoscopy					
44206	X				X
44207	X				X
44208	X				X
44209		X			X
44210	X				X
44211	X				X
44212	X				X
44238	X				
44239	X				
Other Procedures					
44701	X				X
44799		X			X
Rectum					
Endoscopy					
45335	X				
45340	X				X
45343	X				
45344	X				X
45381	X				
45386	X				X
45388	X				
45389	X				X
Other Procedures					
45999					X
Anus					
Incision					
46070					X
Repair					

Section/Code	New	Del	Rev	Gr	Cross
46705					x
46706	x				
46715					x
46716					x
46735					x
46742					x
46744					x

Biliary Tract

Excision

47700					x
47701					x

Abdomen, Peritoneum, and Omentum

Excision, Destruction

49200			x		
49215					x

Introduction, Revision, and/or Removal

49419	x				x

Repair

Hernioplasty, Herniorrhaphy, Herniotomy

49491					x
49492					x
49495					x
49496					x
49600					x
49605					x
49606					x
49611					x

Suture

49904	x				x

Other Procedures

49905			x		x

Section/Code	New	Del	Rev	Gr	Cross
Urinary System					
Kidney					
Incision					
50010					X
Excision					
50200					X
50240					X
Laparoscopy					
50542	X				X
50543	X				X
Endoscopy					
50562	X				
Bladder					
Introduction					
51600					X
51701	X				
51702	X				
51703	X				
Urodynamics					
51798	X				
Endoscopy-Cystoscopy, Urethroscopy, Cystourethroscopy					
52001			X		
Ureter and Pelvis					
52354			X		
52355			X		
Urethra					
Incision					
53025					X
Repair					
53440			X		

Section/Code	New	Del	Rev	Gr	Cross
53442			x		
Manipulation					
53670		x			x
53675		x			x

Male Genital System

Penis

Section/Code	New	Del	Rev	Gr	Cross
Incision					
54000					x
Excision					
54150					x
54160					x

Prostate (For transurethral destruction of prostate, see 53850-53852)

Section/Code	New	Del	Rev	Gr	Cross
55845					x
Laparoscopy					
55866	x				x

Female Genital System

Vulva, Perineum and Introitus

Section/Code	New	Del	Rev	Gr	Cross
Endoscopy					
56820	x				
56821	x				x

Vagina

Section/Code	New	Del	Rev	Gr	Cross
Manipulation					
57420	x				
57421	x				x
Endoscopy					
57452			x		x
57454			x		
57455	x				
57456	x				
57460			x		

Section/Code	New	Del	Rev	Gr	Cross
57461	X				X

Cervix Uteri

Endoscopy

57500					X

Corpus Uteri

Excision

58140			X		
58146	X				X
58260			X		
58267				X	
58290	X				
58291	X				
58292	X				
58293	X				
58294	X				

Repair

58545	X				
58546	X				

Laparoscopy/Hysteroscopy

58550			X		
58551		X			X
58552	X				
58553	X				
58554	X				

Nervous System

Skull, Meninges, and Brain

Twist Drill, Burr Hole(s), or Trephine

61107					X
61210					X
61215					X

Section/Code	New	Del	Rev	Gr	Cross
61300	x				x
61301	x				x
61302	x				x
Craniectomy or Craniotomy					
61316	x				x
61322	x				x
61323	x				x
61340			x		x
61517	x				x
Endovascular Therapy					
61623	x				
61624			x		
Stereotaxis					
61751			x		
Neurostimulators (Intracranial)					
61862					x
Repair					
62148	x				x
Neuroendoscopy					
62160	x				x
62161	x				
62162	x				
62163	x				
62164	x				
62165	x				
Cerebrospinal Fluid (CSF) Shunt					
62201			x		x
62220					x
62223					x

Section/Code	New	Del	Rev	Gr	Cross
62225					x
62230					x

Spine and Spinal Cord

Injection, Drainage, or Aspiration

62263			x		x
62264	x				x
62269					x
62284			x		
62319					x

Catheter Implantation

62351					x

Reservoir/Pump Implantation

62368					x

Repair

63700					x
63702					x
63704					x
63706					x

Extracranial Nerves, Peripheral Nerves, and Autonomic Nervous System

Introduction/Injection of Anesthetic Agent (Nerve Block), Diagnostic or Therapeutic

Somatic Nerves

64415			x		
64416	x				x
64445			x		
64446	x				x
64447	x				x
64448	x				x

Section/Code	New	Del	Rev	Gr	Cross
Eye and Ocular Adnexa					
Anterior Segment					
Anterior Chamber					
Incision					
65820					x
Anterior Sclera					
Excision					
66031	x				x
Lens					
Removal Cataract					
66990	x				x
Posterior Segment					
Vitreous					
67040					x
Auditory System					
Middle Ear					
Incision					
69424			x		x

Radiology

Diagnostic Radiology (Diagnostic Imaging)

Section/Code	New	Del	Rev	Gr	Cross
Head and Neck					
70450			x		
70480			x		
70486			x		
70490			x		
Chest					
71250			x		
71275			x		

Section/Code	New	Del	Rev	Gr	Cross
Spine and Pelvis					
72125			X		
72128			X		
72131			X		
72192			X		
72275					X
Upper Extremities					
73200			X		
Lower Extremities					
73700			X		
Abdomen					
74022			X		
74150			X		
Veins and Lymphatics					
Transcatheter Procedures					
75901	X				X
75902	X				X
75953			X		
75954	X				X
Other Procedures					
76000					X
76005					X
76006			X		X
76070			X		
76071	X				
76076					X
76085			X		X
76091					X
76092					X
76355			X		

Section/Code	New	Del	Rev	Gr	Cross
76360			x		
76370			x		
76380			x		
76496	x				
76497	x				
76498	x				
76499			x		

Diagnostic Ultrasound

Spinal Canal

76801	x				
76802	x				x

Pelvis

Obstetrical

76805			x		
76810			x		x
76811	x				
76812	x				x
76815			x		x
76816			x		x
76817	x				x

Non-obstetrical

76830					x

Ultrasonic Guidance Procedures

Other Procedures

76999			x		

Radiation Oncology

Medical Radiation Physics, Dosimetry, Treatment Devices, and Special Services

77301					x
77326			x		

Section/Code	New	Del	Rev	Gr	Cross

Pathology and Laboratory

Organ or Disease Oriented Panels

80090		X			X

Urinalysis

81007					X

Chemistry

82205					X
83880	X				
83907	X				
84302	X				

Hematology and Coagulation

85004	X				
85007			X		
85008			X		
85009			X		
85013			X		X
85014			X		
85018			X		
85021		X			X
85022		X			X
85023		X			X
85024		X			X
85025			X		
85027			X		
85031		X			X
85032	X				
85041			X		X
85044			X		
85045			X		

Section/Code	New	Del	Rev	Gr	Cross
85048			x		x
85049	x				
85378			x		
85380	x				x
85576				x	
85585		x			x
85590		x			x
85595		x			x

Immunology

Section/Code	New	Del	Rev	Gr	Cross
86148					x
86348	x				

Transfusion Medicine

Section/Code	New	Del	Rev	Gr	Cross
86915		x			x
86930			x		
86931			x		
86932			x		

Microbiology

Section/Code	New	Del	Rev	Gr	Cross
87177					x
87207			x		x
87254			x		
87255	x				

Cytopathology

Section/Code	New	Del	Rev	Gr	Cross
88144		x			
88145		x			x
88170					x
88171					x
88174	x				
88175	x				x

Section/Code	New	Del	Rev	Gr	Cross
Cytogenetic Studies					
88240					X
88241					X
Other Procedures					
89310			X		
89360					X

Medicine

Section/Code	New	Del	Rev	Gr	Cross
Vaccines, Toxoids					
90709		X			X
Therapeutic, Prophylactic or Diagnostic Injections					
90788					X
Biofeedback					
90911					X
Special Otorhinolaryngologic Services					
92525		X			X
Audiologic Function Tests With Medical Diagnostic Evaluation					
92597					X
92598		X			X
Other Procedures					
92599		X			X
Evaluative and Therapeutic Services					
92601	X				X
92602	X				X
92603	X				
92604	X				X
92605	X				
92606	X				
92607	X				X

Section/Code	New	Del	Rev	Gr	Cross
92608	X				X
92609	X				X
92610	X				X
92611	X				X
92612	X				
92613	X				X
92614	X				
92615	X				X
92616	X				
92617	X				X

Other Procedures

92700	X				

Cardiovascular

Cardiography

93012			X		
93268			X		

Cardiac Catheterization

93506	X				X

Repair of Septal Defect

93580	X				X
93581	X				X

Intracardiac Electrophysiological Procedures/Studies

Definitions

93609					X
93613					X
93620			X		
93621			X		
93622			X		

Pulmonary

94640			X		X

Section/Code	New	Del	Rev	Gr	Cross
94650		x			
94651		x			
94652		x			x
94664			x		x
94665		x			x

Allergy and Clinical Immunology Allergy Testing

Allergy Testing

95015			x		
95024			x		
95027			x		
95028			x		

Neurology and Neuromuscular Procedures

Sleep Testing

95812			x		
95816			x		x
95819			x		x
95822			x		x
95827			x		x

Electromyography and Nerve Conduction Tests

95860				x	
95861				x	
95863				x	
95864				x	
95867			x		
95868				x	
95869			x		
95870					x
95875			x		

Intraoperative Neurophysiology

95920					x

Section/Code	New	Del	Rev	Gr	Cross
Evoked Potentials and Reflex Tests					
95927					x
Special EEG Tests					
95954					x
Neurostimulators, Analysis-Programming					
95990	x				x
Health and Behavior Assessment/Intervention					
96150					x
96155					x
Chemotherapy Administration					
96414					x
96425					x
96498	x				
96530			x		x
Special Dermatological Procedures					
96900					x
96920	x				
96921	x				
96922	x				
Special Services, Procedures and Reports					
Miscellaneous Services					
99026	x				
99027	x				x
Qualifying Circumstances for Anesthesia					
99100					x

Evaluation and Management

Pediatric Critical Care Patient Transport

99289			x		

Section/Code	New	Del	Rev	Gr	Cross
99290					X
Pediatric Critical Care					
99293	X				
99294	X				
Neonatal Critical Care					
99295			X		
99296			X		
99297		X			X
Intensive (Non-Critical) Low Birth Weight Services					
99298			X		
99299	X				
Prolonged Services					
Physician Standby Services					
99360					X
Home Health Procedures/Services					
99504			X		
99508		X			X
99539		X			X
Home Infusion Procedures/Services					
99551			X		
99552			X		
99553			X		
99554			X		
99555			X		
99556			X		
99557			X		
99558			X		
99559			X		
99560			X		

Section/Code	New	Del	Rev	Gr	Cross
99561			x		
99562			x		
99563			x		
99564			x		
99565			x		
99566			x		
99567			x		
99568			x		
99569			x		
99600	x				

Category III Codes

Section/Code	New	Del	Rev	Gr	Cross
0027T	x				x
0028T	x				
0029T	x				
0030T	x				
0031T	x				
0032T	x				
0033T	x				x
0034T	x				x
0035T	x				x
0036T	x				x
0037T	x				x
0038T	x				x
0039T	x				x
0040T	x				x
0041T	x				
0042T	x				
0043T	x				
0044T	x				

CPT 2003 Errata

The following are errors that were detected at the time *CPT 2003* was published. If additional errors are identified, please call CPT Editorial Research and Development at 312 464-4723.